ADVANCES IN STEM CELL RESEARCH

STEM CELL RESEARCH

NEW DEVELOPMENTS

ADVANCES IN STEM CELL RESEARCH

Additional books in this series can be found on Nova's website under the Series tab.

Additional E-books in this series can be found on Nova's website under the E-book tab.

STEM CELLS - LABORATORY AND CLINICAL RESEARCH

Additional books in this series can be found on Nova's website under the Series tab.

Additional E-books in this series can be found on Nova's website under the E-book tab.

ADVANCES IN STEM CELL RESEARCH

STEM CELL RESEARCH

NEW DEVELOPMENTS

HIROSHI TANAKA
AND
MICHAEL C. F. CHANG
EDITORS

Nova Science Publishers, Inc.
New York

For permission to use material from this book please contact us:
Telephone 631-231-7269; Fax 631-231-8175
Web Site: http://www.novapublishers.com

Additional color graphics may be available in the e-book version of this book.

LIBRARY OF CONGRESS CATALOGING-IN-PUBLICATION DATA

Stem cell research : new developments / editors, Hiroshi Tanaka and Michael C.F. Chang.
p. cm.
Includes index.
ISBN 978-1-61942-081-6 (hardcover)
1. Stem cells--Research. I. Tanaka, Hiroshi. II. Chang, Michael C. F.
QH588.S83S73998 2011
616.02'774--dc23
2011043206

Published by Nova Science Publishers, Inc. † New York

CONTENTS

PREFACE

Among the many applications of stem cell research are nervous system diseases, diabetes, heart disease, autoimmune diseases as well as Parkinson's disease, end-stage kidney disease, liver failure, cancer, spinal cord injury, multiple sclerosis, Parkinson's disease, and Alzheimer's disease. Stem cells are self-renewing, unspecialized cells that can give rise to multiple types all of specialized cells of the body. Stem cell research also involves complex ethical and legal considerations since they involve adult, fetal tissue and embryonic sources. This book brings together leading research from throughout the world in this frontier field.

Chapter 1 - Tissue is frequently damaged or lost in injury and disease. There has been an increasing interest in stem cell applications and tissue engineering approaches in surgical practice to deal with damaged or lost tissue. Tissue engineering is an exciting strategy being explored to deal with damaged or lost tissue. It is the science of generating tissue using molecular and cellular techniques, combined with material engineering principles, to replace tissue. This could be in the form of cells with or without matrices. There have been developments in almost all surgical disciplines, including plastic surgery. Unfortunately significant hurdles remain to be overcome in many areas before tissue engineering becomes more routinely used in clinical practice.

In this paper the tissue engineering approaches relevant to plastic surgery for tendons and skin are discussed.

Chapter 2 - Tissue is frequently damaged or lost in injury and disease. There has been an increasing interest in stem cell applications and tissue engineering approaches in surgical practice to deal with damaged or lost tissue. Tissue engineering is an exciting strategy being explored to deal with damaged or lost tissue. It is the science of generating tissue using molecular and cellular techniques, combined with material engineering principles, to replace tissue. This could be in the form of cells with or without matrices. There have been developments in almost all surgical disciplines including plastic surgery. Unfortunately significant hurdles remain to be overcome in many areas before tissue engineering becomes more routinely used in clinical practice. In this paper tissue engineering approaches relevant to neurovascular structures is discussed.

Chapter 3 - Tissue is frequently damaged or lost in injury and disease. There has been an increasing interest in stem cell applications and tissue engineering approaches in surgical practice to deal with damaged or lost tissue. Tissue engineering is an exciting strategy being explored to deal with damaged or lost tissue. It is the science of generating tissue using molecular and cellular techniques, combined with material engineering principles, to replace tissue. This could be in the form of cells with or without matrices. Although there have been developments in almost all surgical disciplines, the greatest advances are being made in orthopaedics, especially in bone repair. This is due to many factors including the familiarity with bone marrow derived mesenchymal stem cells and bone grafting. Unfortunately significant hurdles remain to be overcome in many areas before tissue engineering becomes more routinely used in clinical practice. In this paper the tissue engineering approaches relevant to bone repair are discussed. Significant hurdles however remain to be overcome before tissue engineering becomes more routinely used in surgical practice.

Chapter 4 - Allogeneic hematopoietic stem cell transplantation (allo-HSCT) in humans results in true biological chimeras. While circulating hematopoietic and immune cells and their tissue derivatives (e.g. Kupffer cells, Langerhans cells) become donor genotype after transplantation, other cells remain recipient in origin. This unphysiological formation of biological chimeras is not free of consequences. The first sequel which has been recognized in the development of chimerical organisms after allo-HSCT is the graft versus host reaction, in which the new developed immune cells from the graft recognize the host's epithelial cells as foreign and kill them. There is now accumulating evidence that there are also other consequences in the co-existence of two genetically distinct populations in the transplant recipient. First, epithelial cells with donor-derived genotype emerge. Second, epithelial tissues of the host acquire genomic alterations. The current chapter discusses existing data on these recently discovered phenomena and focuses on their pathogenesis, clinical significance and therapeutic implications.

Chapter 5 - Transforming growth factor-beta 1 (TGF-β1) is part of a large family of proteins which control a number of cellular responses in cells derived from a variety of tissues. TGF- β1 and its signalling pathways can inhibit proliferation in a number of cell types (e.g. non-transformed epithelial and endothelial cells) but causes proliferation in a number of transformed cells and immortalised fibroblasts. TGF-β1 binds to its heterodimeric receptors, of which there are a number and in some cell types such as endothelial derived cells it appears that the receptor can determine whether the cells undergo proliferation. Further, the signalling pathways involved in TGF-β appear to play a role in determining if cells proliferate. Aberrant TGF- β1 and its signalling is known to play a role in a number of diseases; this review will discuss the pathways involved in a number of cell types and discuss the effect of abnormal TGF-β1 and its signalling in a number of diseases.

Chapter 6 - Oral Squamous Cell Carcinoma (OSCC) is the sixth most common malignant tumor and its incidence is increasing worldwide. The overall five-year survival rate in patients with OSCC is still lower than 50%. The classification and prognostic assessment of oral cancer is currently based on clinical and histopathologic biomarkers. Availability of an increasing number of molecular biomarkers provides with the potential for redefining diagnostic and prognostic categories and utilizing pharmacogenomics for the treatment of patients. The aim of the present chapter is to provide a basis that will allow the reconstruction of future oral cancer research. The authors critically review the common medical databases (PubMed, EMBASE, Scopus and Cochrane CENTRAL) for studies reporting on molecular biomarkers for oral carcinoma. In this chapter the authors will try to focus on oral cancer biomarkers through a cell cycle perspective. For this, the hallmarks proposed by Hanahan and Weinberg offer a good basis for segregation of various biomarkers. The authors further discuss the genetic basis of oral cancer with regard to the possible stem cell origin of cancer cells and the role of alcohol and tobacco in carcinogenesis.

Substantial evidence points to genomic instability as a cause rather than as a consequence of malignant transformation. In cell cycle reality, molecular and genetic changes interplay to give birth to a population of cells with enhanced properties. Cancer may be considered a process of "natural selection." If these new cells acquired properties that give them advantage over the remainder of cells in a multicellular organism, they would proliferate. Once these cells reach a significant number (clinically manifesting as cancer) they could attempt a "mutiny" and subsequently destroy the host organism-cell community.

Oral cancer will eventually end being a "black box" for researchers. Cancer precursor cells -stem cells more likely- undergo several genome changes. These changes could be either mutations or epigenetic. These changes provide the stem cells with the ability to self-invoke growth signals, the ability to suppress anti-growth signals, to avoid apoptosis, to replicate without limit, to invade, proliferate and sustain blood supply. Stem cells are able to collect progressively these changes in their genome. Mutations, epigenetic changes, nemosis, neosis and meiomitosis all have roles in the machinery that moves precursor stem cells round the hallmarks of cancer. Contemporary use of biomarkers although limited, is a reality, with HPV tumor discrimination, EGFR targeted therapy and aneuploidy being the most well documented.

Chapter 7 - Colorectal cancer is the second leading cause of cancer-related death in the United States. Among many gene mutations associated with colorectal cancer, mutation of APC (adenomatous polyposis coli) or β-catenin, which activates Wnt signaling, represents the initiation step of colon tumorigenesis. Wnt signaling is known to play multiple roles in early development and formation of human cancers. In addition, Wnt signaling also regulates the self-renewal and differentiation of adult stem cells. Recently, cancer stem cells have emerged as an exciting new concept in cancer research. However, many challenging questions have also arisen. What is the definition of a cancer stem cell? Where do such cells originate and what are the markers for these cells? What's the genetic and epigenetic machinery that regulate the homeostasis of this cell population? What is the mechanism underlying the process of cancer stem cell-involved tumorigenesis? In this review, the authors will discuss the development and trends in the field of cancer stem cell research, with emphasis on colon cancer stem cells. Since Wnt signaling is involved in both intestinal stem cells and colon cancers, the authors will first discuss the mechanisms of the Wnt signal transduction pathway, and then discuss the roles of Wnt signaling in normal intestine and in colon cancer. Finally, the authors will discuss the challenges and opportunities in colon cancer stem cell research.

Chapter 8 - Of the many markers for cancer stem cells (CSCs) in lung cancer reported to date, the cell surface antigen CD133, nuclear β-catenin accumulation, the side population phenotype, and high aldehyde dehydrogenase (ALDH) activity seem to be most reliable. In this chapter, the authors review the results of studies on lung CSCs and discuss the significance of these markers from a biological, pathological, and clinical viewpoint. In addition, the authors present their own data, focusing primarily upon ALDH1A1. Twenty-seven lung cancer cell lines (nine small cell lung carcinoma (SCLC) cell lines and eighteen non-small cell lung carcinoma (NSCLC) cell lines) were examined for mRNA and protein expression and fractions of cells with activity. ALDH1A1 mRNA was strongly expressed in five cell lines, of which three were SCLC cell lines and two were NSCLC cell lines. Two of the SCLC cell lines consistently expressed the protein and had a large fraction of cells with ALDH activity, but the third did not. Both the NSCLC cell lines expressed the protein, but only one had a large fraction of cells with strong ALDH activity. In brief, the level of

ALDH1A1 mRNA did not always parallel that of the protein in SCLC cell lines, while the level of ALDH1A1 protein did not necessarily parallel that of ALDH activity in NSCLC cell lines. The ALDH1A1 protein level or ALDH activity level was well associated with the mRNA level of CD133, which is the most commonly used marker for CSCs, in SCLC cell lines, but not in NSCLC cell lines, suggesting an abundance of CSC populations in SCLC compared to in NSCLC. From the current findings, the mechanism and pathway that regulate the expression of ALDH1A1 mRNA and its protein, and its enzymatic activity as well differ greatly between SCLC and NSCLC cells. The authors speculate that ALDH (its expression and activity) is only one of the factors determining the stemness of CSCs in lung cancers. In conclusion, the CSCs in SCLC and NSCLC differ distinctly in terms not only of their abundance but also of the regulatory mechanism of ALDH1A1 expression and activity, as well as its role in the maintenance/activation of stemness. Exploring the mechanism of ALDH's activation and its role in the maintenance of the stemness not only of CSCs but also of normal stem cells would provide a novel paradigm for stem cell biology.

Chapter 9 - The biology of stem cells and their properties have already been recognized as integral to tumour pathogenesis in several types of cancer. A role for stem cells has been demonstrated, so far, for the hematopoietic system diseases, as well as for several solid tumours such as breast, brain and lung cancer. There is a rising interest in the field of oncology in order to understand if cancer stem cells can play a key role also in the pathogenesis of head and neck tumours. It is likely that cancer stem cells are a minor population of tumour cells that possess the stem cell property of self-renewal. The evidence that the development of a tumour comes from a small number of cells with stem-like characteristic, could bring to the identification of therapies against these cellular targets, fundamental for maintenance and progression of the lesion. This new model for cancer will have significant implications for the way the authors will study and treat tumours.

Head and neck cancer is still the sixth most common cancer type worldwide. Disappointingly, despite significant advances in surgical and other treatments that enhance quality of life, survival rates have only moderately improved during the last 20 years.

Aim of this chapter is to discuss among this new model of cancerogenesis.

Chapter 10 - Acute myeloid leukemia has emerged as a paradigm for the concept of the cancer stem cell. This hypothesis presumes that the disease is maintained by a rare population of leukemia-initiating stem cells which have acquired genetic or epigenetic changes. It is most likely that a single (epi)genetic event will not be sufficient to cause leukemia, but that a number of sequential events are required. Similar to normal hematopoietic stem cells, both intrinsic as well as extrinsic factors that arise from the bone marrow niche, provide essential cues that regulate cell fate decisions such as leukemic stem cell self-renewal and differentiation. In this chapter, the authors will review the genetic and epigenetic abnormalities that underlie the process of leukemic transformation, and will discuss which events potentially co-operate to induce leukemia.

Chapter 11 - Mesenchymal stem cells (MSCs) are adult stem cells that derive from the bone marrow. A major feature of these cells is their ability to differentiate into adipocytes, chondrocytes or osteocytes. They are also defined by the expression of certain markers, such as CD105, CD73 and CD90, and the lack of others (CD45, CD34, CD14, CD79a and HLA-DR). This expression profile makes them distinct from other bone-derived cells. Several functions have been attributed to MSCs. E.g., MSCs modulate immune responses by suppressing the activities of a number of immune cells. This function is thought to be important to prevent excessive inflammation in the wound healing process. MSCs are chemoattracted to wounds. Probably mistaking tumors for wounds, MSCs also enter solid tumors, where they modulate the activities of tumor cells by exposing them to a plethora of cyto- and chemokines. Recently, MSC-secreted CCL5 has been shown to trigger breast cancer cells to metastasize to lung. Moreover, MSCs are able to differentiate into carcinoma-associated fibroblasts (CAF) which are known to have tumor-promoting activity. This review will summarize the current knowledge on the functions of MSCs in tumor progression.

Chapter 12 - Recent insights regarding the function of cancer stem cells are particularly intriguing when considered in the context of the metastatic cascade. As evidence for the direct involvement of cancer stem cells in initiating the growth of metastatic lesions is scant, this chapter will focus on known events in malignant transformation that are likely to involve or affect cancer stem cells, which may give rise to primary tumors of varying degrees of malignancy and metastatic potentials. The role of cancer stem cells in the later steps of the metastasis cascade will also be discussed. Finally, this chapter will explore potential characteristics vulnerabilities of cancer stem cells involved in metastasis, and speculate on how these weaknesses may be exploited to generate novel therapeutic and diagnostic approaches.

Chapter 13 - To examine the factors involving human carcinogenesis in order to design new strategies for prevention and treatment, a new approach from the current reductionalistic molecular oncological view will have to be made. In addition, this view must take into account both biological and cultural evolutionary factors that interact with the biology of the pathogenesis of cancer. An integrated hypothesist that links many incomplete hypotheses, such as the stem cell or de-differentiation theories of cancer, the multi-stage, multi-mechanism or "initiation/promotion/progression" theory, the mutation and epigenetic theories of carcinogenesis, and the "cancer stem cells" hypothesis, has been outlined. The emergence of somatic and germ-line stem cells during the biological evolution of the multi-cellular organism created new functions to regulate, homeostatically, phenotypes, such as growth control, differentiation, apoptosis, senescence and adaptive functions of terminally differentiated cells. The evidence supporting the stem cells as target cells for the initiation process was reviewed. The biological consequence of the initiation of an adult stem cell appears to be the inhibition of asymmetric cell division, or the blockage of "mortalization" of a normal "immortal" stem cell, not the "immortalization" of a normal, "mortal" cell. Promotion, functionally, is the clonal expansion of initiated stem cells by both mitogenesis and the inhibition of apoptosis. These promoting conditions occur during wound healing, compensatory hyperplasia after cell death, chronic inflammation, growth factors and by many dietary and environmental, non-mutagenic chemicals. All of these promoting conditions inhibit cell-cell communication, either by disruption of gap junctions in progenitor cells or by interfering with secreted negative growth regulator-receptor signalling in cells not having functional gap junctions, thereby releasing initiated stem cells from mitotic inhibition. Tumor promoters are characterized by threshold levels, exposing the initiated cells for regular and long periods of time in the absence of anti-promoters and having species, gender, cell-type specificities. The normal stem cell appears to give rise to the initiated stem cell which ultimately can accrue all the phenotypes of an invasive, metastatic "cancer stem cell". As the tumor grows, some of these cancer stem cells can partially differentiate to become cancer "non-stem cells". Finally, to understand how cultural evolution affects the human cancer patterns, domestication of certain animals helped to change dietary habits which can influence the carcinogenic process. These dietary factors can influence the adult stem cells, in utero and postnatally, so as to either increase or decrease the risk to cancer by altering the stem cell pools and by increasing or decreasing the promotion of the initiated stem cells. This might provide a mechanistic basis for the "Barker hypothesis".

Versions of these chapters were also published in *Stem Cell Research Journal*, Volume 2, Numbers 1-3, edited by Frank Columbus, published by Nova Science Publishers, Inc. They were submitted for appropriate modifications in an effort to encourage wider dissemination of research.

In: Stem Cell Research: New Developments
Editors: Hiroshi Tanaka and Michael C. F. Chang
ISBN: 978-1-61942-081-6

Chapter 1

PRINCIPLES OF TISSUE ENGINEERING APPROACHES IN PLASTIC SURGERY: TENDONS AND SKIN

***Faizal Rayanmarakkar*[1], *Wasim S. Khan*[1,*], *Atif Malik*[1] *and Timothy E. Hardingham*[2]**

[1]University College London Institute of Orthopaedics and Musculoskeletal Sciences, Royal National Orthopaedic Hospital, Stanmore, London, UK

[2]United Kingdom Centre for Tissue Engineering and Wellcome Trust Centre for Cell Matrix Research, Faculty of Life Sciences, University of Manchester, Oxford Road, Manchester, UK

ABSTRACT

Tissue is frequently damaged or lost in injury and disease. There has been an increasing interest in stem cell applications and tissue engineering approaches in surgical practice to deal with damaged or lost tissue. Tissue engineering is an exciting strategy being explored to deal with damaged or lost tissue. It is the science of generating tissue using molecular and cellular techniques, combined with material engineering principles, to replace tissue. This could be in the form of cells with or without matrices. There have been developments in almost all surgical disciplines, including plastic surgery. Unfortunately significant hurdles remain to be overcome in many areas before tissue engineering becomes more routinely used in clinical practice.

In this paper the tissue engineering approaches relevant to plastic surgery for tendons and skin are discussed.

* Corresponding Author: Mr Wasim S Khan, Academic Clinical Fellow, University College London Institute of Orthopaedics and Musculoskeletal Science, Royal National Orthopaedic Hospital, Stanmore, London, HA7 4LP, UK. Telephone number: +44 (0) 7971 190720. Fax number: +44 (0) 20 8570 3864. E-mail address: wasimkhan@doctors.org.uk.

INTRODUCTION

Tissue engineering has been defined as the application of scientific principles to the design, construction, modification and growth of living tissue using biomaterials, cells and factors alone and in combination [33] (Langer and Vacanti, 1993). In essence three elements are central in tissue engineering; stem or precursor cells; an appropriate biological scaffold and growth factors. It generally involves the use of cells with a matrix or scaffold that guides the cells during tissue repair or regeneration. The use of more undifferentiated cell types, such as stem cells or early mesenchymal progenitors that retain multi-lineage and self renewal potential is preferable to the use of terminally differentiated cells. The scaffold could be natural or biosynthetic. Cells harvested from donor tissues, including adult stem cells, can be expanded in culture and associated with resorbable biomaterials forming the scaffold. The cells can be stimulated by specific bioactive molecules such as growth factors. The cells can also be genetically modified via genomic insertion of a new healthy copy of a gene before expansion and subsequent tissue reconstitution. To date the use of gene technology has not been applied to humans. The cells could be stimulated in-vitro to form tissue for future re-implantation in-vivo. Below applications of tissue engineering principles are discussed relevant to tendons and skin.

1. TENDONS

In the united states hand injuries account for 5–10% of annual emergency department visits nationwide and hand surgeons repair nearly one-third of a million digital flexor tendon injuries per year in the United States [48]. Outcome is often unsatisfactory and recovery after surgery takes longer time. Also the repaired tendon regains only half of its initial mechanical properties due to 1) the difficulty to anchorage the tendon in muscle, 2) the high mechanical constraint on the repair structure, 3) the unavailability of ideal tendon grafts, 4) adhesion formation is a major problem, not only in primary repair but also in tendon reconstruction using autografts as well as allografts. Tendon tissue engineering offers an alternative approach to the pitfalls faced in tendon surgery. The main aim is to restore the injured tendon with tissue engineered graft with good structural and functional properties.

Successful repair of ruptured flexor tendons, as measured by restoration of digital flexion function, is a great challenge to hand surgeons because of the lack of adequate donor tendon and flexor tendon adhesions. The first problem arises in loss of tendon substance. The material requirement exceeds availability in devastating injuries although autologous palmaris and plantaris longus tendon grafts are used. The second problem of flexor tendon adhesions is caused by factors like the site and type of injury, the surgical technique and the wound healing response which is most relevant in zone II flexor tendon injuries. The main issue is the 'no-man's land' or Zone II as they are associated with poor prognosis and were treated non-operatively. The biological cascade of events during healing often causes the tendon proper to adhere indiscriminately to its surrounding tissue [37 1]. Clinical and experimental observations suggest that formation of adhesions is precipitated by injury to the tendon sheath, surgical manipulation, and immobilization [18 55 2,3]. Extrasynovial tendons are dependent on peripheral neovascularisation, which causes adhesions, but there is a lack of accessible donor intrasynovial tendons for which tissue engineering of intrasynovial tendon grafts would provide a solution to this problem.

The transplantation of a tendon graft is an alternative to primary repair for the hand surgeon. The graft is positioned outside the confines of the flexor sheath in zone II and attached distally in Zone I and proximally in Zone III to the flexor digitorum profundus tendon. Cellular necrosis, inflammation and adhesion may result from routine surgical manipulation of flexor tendon grafts. To address this, devitalised structures such as freeze-dried tendon allografts or tissue-engineered biomaterial scaffolds can be used as alternatives to live autografts in reconstructing the digital flexor mechanism [5].

Tendons are bands of dense connective tissue that help normal joint movement and stability. They protect the muscle (fascia) and fix the length of the muscle belly. They also play a role of damper and shock absorber. They are composed of collagen fibers, and the function and behaviour of tendons depend on of their mechanical properties. They consist of fascicles, fibrils, subfibrils, microfibrils and tropocollagen. Tendon is covered by epitenon which is contiguous paratenon on its outer surface and endotenon on its inner surface. Peritenon with paratenon and epitenon surrounds the tendon and supports gliding. Flexor tendons of the hand are covered by a well defined sheath of synovial cells. Here they (paratenon) are mentioned as tenosynovium, but if there is no synovial lining, the paratenon is called tenovagium. At the musculo-tendinous junction, the perimysium is continuous with the endotenon. At the other extremity on the tendon–bone interface, the collagen fibers and the endotenon become continuous with the periosteum. The tendon insertion into bone is of two types. The first one described by Cooper and Misol shows a transition from the tendon to a layer of fibrocartilage with digitations in the periosteum [16]. Around 50-70% of the tendon is comprised of water and 60-85% of the tendon comprises of type I and type III collagen. Collagen type I is responsible for 70% of the dry weight of the tendon structure. Proteoglycans and leucine-rich protein also play a role in the organisation and mechanical properties of the tissue.

Tendon healing consists of three phases: inflammatory, proliferative and remodeling. During the initial phase of inflammation, fibroblasts and macrophages are recruited to the site of injury, and phagocytosis of the necrotic tissue ensues. During the proliferative phase there is proliferation of fibroblasts and formation of the scar (formed from immature and disorganized collagen matrix). In the final phase of remodelling the immature collagen fibers in the scar tissue become organised and align with the tendon fibers. Therefore the etiology of adhesion formation has been linked to the remodelling phase [37] (Lilly et al 2006).

There are mechanical and biochemical strategies to avoid adhesion formation. Mechanical interventions include post-operative passive motion and rehabilitation protocols post- operatively. Good surgical techniques to minimise the trauma of the tendon, graft, and the surrounding tissues, and the use of anti-adhesion surface coating of the graft as a physical barrier against adhesion formation [40 8 25 41] (Meislin et al. 1990; Boyer et al. 2005; Hatano et al 2000; Mentzel et al. 2000).

We have to yet define success in creating an ideal tendon substitute using current tissue engineering strategies e.g. synthetic biomaterial scaffolds, in order to improve healing. These engineered scaffolds can be impregnated with genes or growth factors for targeted and timed release at the site of implantation [5] (Basile et al 2008). The main problems are 1) their mechanical strength do not match with those of native tissue, so there is a delay in restoration of function, 2) they do not remodel in response to daily activity, 3) they break down producing by-products that induce inflammation and compromise the repair process [66 5]. Naturally derived materials processed from animal tissue or produced using recombination technology may be better tolerated when implanted [5]. The one that is derived from allogeneic tendon tissue is an ideal example for a naturally derived biomaterial scaffold for tendon tissue engineering. Whitlock et al. had described that a naturally derived biomaterial scaffold from tendon tissue are open to host cell-mediated remodelling and are devoid of cellular material to minimise inflammatory potential. They also possess biomechanical integrity. The tendon designs should allow cell to cell connectivity to allow intracellular communication. Biological and biochemical intervention strategies primarily rely upon growth factor delivery to accelerate the rate of tendon healing and remodelling. While a number of growth factors could potentially improve the repair of tendons, their effects on tendon adhesion have been left largely unexplored [61 19 58 1 29] (Towler DA and Gelberman RH 2006; Hsu C and Chang J 2004; Thomopoulos, 2005; Gelberman, 2007; Wang, 2005; Abrahamsson, 1996; Kashiwagi, 2004). A rational design for a growth-factor delivery therapy should be based on the natural history of gene expression of growth factors during the different phases of tendon repair, a thorough understanding of the molecular action of these factors, and a sustained delivery mechanism to maximise the therapeutic effects of these factors.

Tissue engineering techniques have developed biologic and synthetic scaffolds which can repair tendon defects and improve healing by regeneration of the tendon's natural biologic composition to restore its mechanical capacity. One of the most promising scaffold developments from biomechanical and biocompatible points of view would be based on biomimetic strategy. In this approach, the scaffold should include polymeric collagen as the fundamental fibrous phase and being cross linked to give the mechanical strength of the engineered tendon. The combination of scaffold, cell and stimulation, and their applications is the soul of tissue engineering [17] (DeFranco MJ, 2004). This branch also provides new biomaterials that mimic real tissues which induce in vivo regeneration and in vitro functional replacement tissue. The organised collagen structure surrounded by proteoglycans allows tendons to face a wide range of non-linear mechanical deformation which is the main issue in tissue engineering of tendons. Smaller defects are treated by in vivo techniques involving the in situ delivery of genetically modified cells on a scaffold providing immediate mechanical support and boosting the regeneration and healing process. Larger defects or tissue replacement are dealt by in vitro tissue engineering.

Incorporation of cells increases the healing potential of the tendons. Fibroblasts from tendon or skin are used commonly for this purpose. Stem cells are used because of the low mitotic activity of native mature tendon fibroblasts, has proved to be popular. Under mechanical stimulation, MSCs differentiated in fibroblasts, aligned themselves in collagen gel and helped in vivo tendon regeneration. The cells cause gel contraction that improves the biomechanical properties. The cells can be genetically modified to produce growth factors which can amplify healing. DNA synthesis of tendon fibroblasts can be stimulated by treatment with growth factors like PDGF and IGF-1 [4] (Banes et al, 1995). Cross linking (with di-catecholnordihydroguaiaretic acid) and hybridisation (with PLA) techniques have been introduced to augment mechanical properties [31]. Another method is acellular collagen scaffolds, which is in its infancy. Future work in tendon tissue engineering have to focus on biomimetism as defined by Koob (2002) where tendon is engineered by combining scaffold and gene therapy either with cells or with gene activated matrix [31].

2. SKIN

Skin, primarily is a protective barrier against the environment and has two layers. The skin is the largest organ of the body comprised of epidermis and dermis with a complex nerve and blood supply. The superficial epidermal layer provides a protection against infection and moisture loss. The deeper dermal layer provides elasticity and mechanical integrity of the skin, and contains the blood vessels that are responsible for the nutrition of the epidermal layer. They constitute the bulk of the skin and are composed of collagen with some elastin and glycosaminoglycans. Major cell type present in the dermis are the fibroblasts and are capable of producing remodelling enzymes such as proteases and collagenases, which play an important role in the wound healing process Appendages like hair follicles or sweat glands, breach the epidermal and dermal layers. Cutaneous sensory nerves pass through the dermal tissue into the epidermal tissue. Regeneration of the epidermis depends on remnants of epidermal cells that lie deep within dermal structures.

When the wound is more than a few cm across, in-growth from the edges of a wound will be insufficient. There is a dire need for skin grafts due to burns, diabetic ulcers and skin cancers. Each year in the United States there are 1.25 million cases of burns, more than 600,000 cases of diabetic ulcers, and another 600,000 cases of skin cancer requiring excision [13 43] (Brigham, 1996; Mooney, 1999). Majority of them would require skin grafting. Skin grafts were introduced by Reverdin in 1871 and since then various skin substitutes are in vogue. Due to the donor site morbidity associated with autografts and allografts, there is a great deal of demand for an alternative which led to significant advances in tissue engineering of skin e.g. cultured autologous and allogenic keratinocytes grafts, autologous or allogenic composites, acellular biological matrices, and cellular matrices including biological substances such as fibrin sealant. These substitutes ideally should have barrier function, even though none of them have shown better results than autologous split skin grafting. Moreover we have to tide over issues like the need for second procedure, infection, rejection, immune and allergic reaction. At the same time we have to replicate the anatomy, physiology, biologic stability, or aesthetic nature of uninjured skin. The disadvantages of autologous cells are lack of quicker access off-the-shelf for the treatment of burns and trauma. There are three locations from which cell types for skin substitutes can be derived: local, systemic, and progenitor cell populations.

Local cells that could be used for skin tissue engineering applications include fibroblasts, keratinocytes, melanocytes, adipocytes and hair follicle cells. The local quiescent fibroblasts migrate into the affected area, produce extra-cellular matrix proteins, and promote wound contraction. Wound fibroblasts produce extra-cellular matrix proteins including collagen types I and III, fibronectin and proteoglycans, and are responsible for tissue remodelling, scar formation and repair. Systemic cells resident in the blood or bone marrow play a key role in skin wound healing. Progenitor cells are present in hair follicles, bone marrow or could be cultured in vitro from embryonic stem cell line. Keratinocytes can be grown in relatively large numbers over a period of 3 to 4 weeks. They are expensive, are prone to infection and cosmetically poor due to the absence of basement membrane and dermis. Even if their colony forming efficiency is decreased by 50%, cultured epithelial autograft sheets have been stored as frozen suspensions to use them at their optimum. Self-renewing stem cells is a solution to recreate skin and these cells in a keratinocyte culture is all that required for generating epidermal grafts. The significance of dermis in skin healing has led to the development of different engineered skin substitutes e.g. cadaveric skin, collagen based dermal substitute, hyaluronic based membranes, synthetic polymers and composite of biologic and synthetic materials.

Apligraf is a composite derived by combining bovine collagen with fibroblasts with an epidermal layer of neonatal allogeneic keratinocytes. This composite is currently the most sophisticated commercially available tissue-engineered product, and also the most expensive. Its main role is in the treatment of chronic ulcers. Healing is speeded up in chronic wounds [26] (Jones 2002). Clinical applications of acellular human dermal substitute have shown good outcomes in hand and foot burns. It not only retains dermal elements and but also allows migration of keratinocytes [15] (Chong, 2006). Alloderm is processed human cadaveric skin from which the epidermis has been removed and the cellular components of the dermis have been extracted prior to cryopreservation in order to avoid a specific immune response. It is a good template for dermal regeneration. Take rates are good and it reduces scarring of full-thickness wounds and allows grafting of an ultra-thin split-skin graft as a one-stage procedure [26] (Jones 2002). Dermagraft, a cryopreserved living dermal structure, manufactured by cultivating neonatal allogeneic fibroblasts on a polymer scaffold (polyglycolic acid or polyglactin-910, marketed as Dexon or Vicryl, respectively) was developed in order to permanently implant to replace the patient's damaged dermis with a living human material. Dermagraft stimulates the ingrowth of fibrovascular tissue from the wound bed and cause re-epithelialisation from the wound edges.

Clinical failure due to delays in vascularisation is the main drawback of tissue-engineered skin products. Various techniques for increasing vascularisation and promoting wound healing have been developed. One of the methods consists of formation of a matrix comprising gel (denatured collagen) and a nitric oxide inhibitor (L-arginine analog such as N-nitro-L-arginine and D-arginine). The matrix also contains a nitric oxide scavenger, such as dextran, heparin, cysteine, or cystine. A better understanding of the factors influencing extra-cellular matrix formation in tissue-engineering scaffolds is essential to achieve further development in skin generation [70] (Priya et al).

References

[1] Abrahamsson, S. O., and Lohmander, S.: Differential effects of insulin-like growth factor-I on matrix and DNA synthesis in various regions and types of rabbit tendons. *J. Orthop. Res.,* 14(3): 370-6, 1996.

[2] Andriano, K. P.; Tabata, Y.; Ikada, Y.; and Heller, J.: In vitro and in vivo comparison of bulk and surface hydrolysis in absorbable polymer scaffolds for tissue engineering. *J. Biomed Mater Res,* 48(5): 602-12, 1999.

[3] Archibald, S. J.; Shefner, J.; Krarup, C.; and Madison, R. D.: Monkey median nerve repaired by nerve graft or collagen nerve guide tube. *J. Neurosci.,* 15(5 Pt 2): 4109-23, 1995.

[4] Banes, A. J.; Tsuzaki, M.; Hu, P.; Brigman, B.; Brown, T.; Almekinders, L.; Lawrence, W. T.; and Fischer, T.: PDGF-BB, IGF-I and mechanical load stimulate DNA synthesis in avian tendon fibroblasts in vitro. *J. Biomech.,* 28(12): 1505-13, 1995.

[5] Basile, P. et al.: Freeze-dried tendon allografts as tissue-engineering scaffolds for Gdf5 gene delivery. *Mol. Ther.,* 16(3): 466-73, 2008.

[6] Bianco, P.; Riminucci, M.; Gronthos, S.; and Robey, P. G.: Bone marrow stromal stem cells: nature, biology, and potential applications. *Stem Cells,* 19(3): 180-92, 2001.

[7] Boden, S. D.: Bioactive factors for bone tissue engineering. *Clin. Orthop Relat. Res,* (367 Suppl): S84-94, 1999.

[8] Boyer, M. I.; Goldfarb, C. A.; and Gelberman, R. H.: Recent progress in flexor tendon healing. The modulation of tendon healing with rehabilitation variables. *J. Hand Ther,* 18(2): 80-5; quiz 86, 2005.

[9] Braddock, M.; Houston, P.; Campbell, C.; and Ashcroft, P.: Born again bone: tissue engineering for bone repair. *News Physiol Sci,* 16: 208-13, 2001.

[10] Brandt, J.; Dahlin, L. B.; and Lundborg, G.: Autologous tendons used as grafts for bridging peripheral nerve defects. *J. Hand Surg [Br],* 24(3): 284-90, 1999.

[11] Breitbart, A. S.; Grande, D. A.; Mason, J. M.; Barcia, M.; James, T.; and Grant, R. T.: Gene-enhanced tissue engineering: applications for bone healing using cultured periosteal cells transduced retrovirally with the BMP-7 gene. *Ann. Plast Surg,* 42(5): 488-95, 1999.

[12] Brekke, J. H., and Toth, J. M.: Principles of tissue engineering applied to programmable osteogenesis. *J. Biomed. Mater Res.,* 43(4): 380-98, 1998.

[13] Brigham, P. A., and McLoughlin, E.: Burn incidence and medical care use in the United States: estimates, trends, and data sources. *J. Burn Care Rehabil,* 17(2): 95-107, 1996.

[14] Cancedda, R.; Bianchi, G.; Derubeis, A.; and Quarto, R.: Cell therapy for bone disease: a review of current status. *Stem Cells,* 21(5): 610-9, 2003.

[15] Chong, A. K., and Chang, J.: Tissue engineering for the hand surgeon: a clinical perspective. *J Hand Surg [Am],* 31(3): 349-58, 2006.

[16] Cooper, R. R., and Misol, S.: Tendon and ligament insertion. A light and electron microscopic study. *J. Bone Joint Surg Am,* 52(1): 1-20, 1970.

[17] DeFranco, M. J.; Derwin, K.; and Iannotti, J. P.: New therapies in tendon reconstruction. *J. Am. Acad Orthop Surg,* 12(5): 298-304, 2004.

[18] Gelberman, R. H., and Manske, P. R.: Factors influencing flexor tendon adhesions. *Hand Clin.,* 1(1): 35-42, 1985.

[19] Gelberman, R. H.; Thomopoulos, S.; Sakiyama-Elbert, S. E.; Das, R.; and Silva, M. J.: The early effects of sustained platelet-derived growth factor administration on the functional and structural properties of repaired intrasynovial flexor tendons: an in vivo biomechanic study at 3 weeks in canines. *J. Hand Surg. [Am],* 32(3): 373-9, 2007.

[20] Glasby, M. A.; Gschmeissner, S. E.; Huang, C. L.; and De Souza, B. A.: Degenerated muscle grafts used for peripheral nerve repair in primates. *J. Hand Surg. [Br],* 11(3): 347-51, 1986.

[21] Govender, S. et al.: Recombinant human bone morphogenetic protein-2 for treatment of open tibial fractures: a prospective, controlled, randomized study of four hundred and fifty patients. *J. Bone Joint Surg. Am.,* 84-A(12): 2123-34, 2002.

[22] Grigolo, B.; Roseti, L.; Fiorini, M.; Fini, M.; Giavaresi, G.; Aldini, N. N.; Giardino, R.; and Facchini, A.: Transplantation of chondrocytes seeded on a hyaluronan derivative (hyaff-11) into cartilage defects in rabbits. *Biomaterials,* 22(17): 2417-24, 2001.

[23] Guenard, V.; Kleitman, N.; Morrissey, T. K.; Bunge, R. P.; and Aebischer, P.: Syngeneic Schwann cells derived from adult nerves seeded in semipermeable guidance channels enhance peripheral nerve regeneration. *J. Neurosci,* 12(9): 3310-20, 1992.

[24] Gundle, R.; Joyner, C. J.; and Triffitt, J. T.: Human bone tissue formation in diffusion chamber culture in vivo by bone-derived cells and marrow stromal fibroblastic cells. *Bone,* 16(6): 597-601, 1995.

[25] Hatano, I.; Suga, T.; Diao, E.; Peimer, C. A.; and Howard, C.: Adhesions from flexor tendon surgery: an animal study comparing surgical techniques. *J. Hand Surg. [Am],* 25(2): 252-9, 2000.

[26] Jones, I.; Currie, L.; and Martin, R.: A guide to biological skin substitutes. *Br. J. Plast Surg,* 55(3): 185-93, 2002.

[27] Kadiyala, S.; Young, R. G.; Thiede, M. A.; and Bruder, S. P.: Culture expanded canine mesenchymal stem cells possess osteochondrogenic potential in vivo and in vitro. *Cell Transplant,* 6(2): 125-34, 1997.

[28] Kale, S.; Biermann, S.; Edwards, C.; Tarnowski, C.; Morris, M.; and Long, M. W.: Three-dimensional cellular development is essential for ex vivo formation of human bone. *Nat. Biotechnol.,* 18(9): 954-8, 2000.

[29] Kashiwagi, K.; Mochizuki, Y.; Yasunaga, Y.; Ishida, O.; Deie, M.; and Ochi, M.: Effects of transforming growth factor-beta 1 on the early stages of healing of the Achilles tendon in a rat model. *Scand. J. Plast Reconstr Surg Hand Surg,* 38(4): 193-7, 2004.

[30] Koeberle, P. D., and Bahr, M.: Growth and guidance cues for regenerating axons: where have they gone? *J Neurobiol,* 59(1): 162-80, 2004.

[31] Koob, T. J.: Biomimetic approaches to tendon repair. *Comp Biochem Physiol A Mol Integr Physiol,* 133(4): 1171-92, 2002.

[32] Kruyt, M. C.; van Gaalen, S. M.; Oner, F. C.; Verbout, A. J.; de Bruijn, J. D.; and Dhert, W. J.: Bone tissue engineering and spinal fusion: the potential of hybrid constructs by combining osteoprogenitor cells and scaffolds. *Biomaterials,* 25(9): 1463-73, 2004.

[33] Langer, R., and Vacanti, J. P.: Tissue engineering. *Science,* 260(5110): 920-6, 1993.

[34] Lee, C. H.; Singla, A.; and Lee, Y.: Biomedical applications of collagen. *Int. J. Pharm,* 221(1-2): 1-22, 2001.

[35] Lee, K. Y.; Peters, M. C.; Anderson, K. W.; and Mooney, D. J.: Controlled growth factor release from synthetic extracellular matrices. *Nature,* 408(6815): 998-1000, 2000.

[36] LeGeros, R. Z.: Properties of osteoconductive biomaterials: calcium phosphates. *Clin. Orthop Relat. Res.,* (395): 81-98, 2002.

[37] Lilly, S. I., and Messer, T. M.: Complications after treatment of flexor tendon injuries. *J. Am. Acad. Orthop Surg,* 14(7): 387-96, 2006.

[38] Lundborg, G.: A 25-year perspective of peripheral nerve surgery: evolving neuroscientific concepts and clinical significance. *J. Hand Surg. [Am],* 25(3): 391-414, 2000.

[39] Lundborg, G.; Dahlin, L.; Dohi, D.; Kanje, M.; and Terada, N.: A new type of "bioartificial" nerve graft for bridging extended defects in nerves. *J. Hand Surg [Br],* 22(3): 299-303, 1997.

[40] Meislin, R. J.; Wiseman, D. M.; Alexander, H.; Cunningham, T.; Linsky, C.; Carlstedt, C.; Pitman, M.; and Casar, R.: A biomechanical study of tendon adhesion reduction using a biodegradable barrier in a rabbit model. *J. Appl. Biomater,* 1(1): 13-9, 1990.

[41] Mentzel, M.; Hoss, H.; Keppler, P.; Ebinger, T.; Kinzl, L.; and Wachter, N. J.: The effectiveness of ADCON-T/N, a new anti-adhesion barrier gel, in fresh divisions of the flexor tendons in Zone II. *J. Hand Surg [Br],* 25(6): 590-2, 2000.

[42] Merzenich, M. M.; Kaas, J. H.; Wall, J.; Nelson, R. J.; Sur, M.; and Felleman, D.: Topographic reorganization of somatosensory cortical areas 3b and 1 in adult monkeys following restricted deafferentation. *Neuroscience,* 8(1): 33-55, 1983.

[43] Mooney, D. J., and Mikos, A. G.: Growing new organs. *Sci. Am.,* 280(4): 60-5, 1999.

[44] Muschler, G. F.; Nitto, H.; Matsukura, Y.; Boehm, C.; Valdevit, A.; Kambic, H.; Davros, W.; Powell, K.; and Easley, K.: Spine fusion using cell matrix composites enriched in bone marrow-derived cells. *Clin. Orthop. Relat Res,* (407): 102-18, 2003.

[45] Olmsted, E. A.; Blum, J. S.; Rill, D.; Yotnda, P.; Gugala, Z.; Lindsey, R. W.; and Davis, A. R.: Adenovirus-mediated BMP2 expression in human bone marrow stromal cells. *J. Cell Biochem.,* 82(1): 11-21, 2001.

[46] Oreffo, R. O., and Triffitt, J. T.: Future potentials for using osteogenic stem cells and biomaterials in orthopedics. *Bone,* 25(2 Suppl): 5S-9S, 1999.

[47] Partridge, K. A., and Oreffo, R. O.: Gene delivery in bone tissue engineering: progress and prospects using viral and nonviral strategies. *Tissue Eng,* 10(1-2): 295-307, 2004.

[48] Pennisi, E.: Tending tender tendons. *Science,* 295(5557): 1011, 2002.

[49] Perry, C. R.: Bone repair techniques, bone graft, and bone graft substitutes. *Clin. Orthop. Relat Res.,* (360): 71-86, 1999.

[50] Petite, H.; Viateau, V.; Bensaid, W.; Meunier, A.; de Pollak, C.; Bourguignon, M.; Oudina, K.; Sedel, L.; and Guillemin, G.: Tissue-engineered bone regeneration. *Nat. Biotechnol.,* 18(9): 959-63, 2000.

[51] Quirk, R. A.; Chan, W. C.; Davies, M. C.; Tendler, S. J.; and Shakesheff, K. M.: Poly(L-lysine)-GRGDS as a biomimetic surface modifier for poly(lactic acid). *Biomaterials,* 22(8): 865-72, 2001.

[52] Raivich, G., and Kreutzberg, G. W.: Peripheral nerve regeneration: role of growth factors and their receptors. *Int. J. Dev. Neurosci,* 11(3): 311-24, 1993.

[53] Sakkers, R. J.; Dalmeyer, R. A.; de Wijn, J. R.; and van Blitterswijk, C. A.: Use of bone-bonding hydrogel copolymers in bone: an in vitro and in vivo study of expanding PEO-PBT copolymers in goat femora. *J. Biomed. Mater Res.,* 49(3): 312-8, 2000.

[54] Shin, H.; Jo, S.; and Mikos, A. G.: Biomimetic materials for tissue engineering. *Biomaterials,* 24(24): 4353-64, 2003.

[55] Silva, M. J.; Boyer, M. I.; and Gelberman, R. H.: Recent progress in flexor tendon healing. *J. Orthop. Sci.,* 7(4): 508-14, 2002.

[56] Stewart, K.; Walsh, S.; Screen, J.; Jefferiss, C. M.; Chainey, J.; Jordan, G. R.; and Beresford, J. N.: Further characterization of cells expressing STRO-1 in cultures of adult human bone marrow stromal cells. *J. Bone Miner Res.,* 14(8): 1345-56, 1999.

[57] Tepper, O. M.; Capla, J. M.; Galiano, R. D.; Ceradini, D. J.; Callaghan, M. J.; Kleinman, M. E.; and Gurtner, G. C.: Adult vasculogenesis occurs through in situ recruitment, proliferation, and tubulization of circulating bone marrow-derived cells. *Blood,* 105(3): 1068-77, 2005.

[58] Thomopoulos, S.; Harwood, F. L.; Silva, M. J.; Amiel, D.; and Gelberman, R. H.: Effect of several growth factors on canine flexor tendon fibroblast proliferation and collagen synthesis in vitro. *J. Hand Surg [Am],* 30(3): 441-7, 2005.
[59] Tohill, M., and Terenghi, G.: Stem-cell plasticity and therapy for injuries of the peripheral nervous system. *Biotechnol. Appl. Biochem.,* 40(Pt 1): 17-24, 2004.
[60] Tong, X. J.; Hirai, K.; Shimada, H.; Mizutani, Y.; Izumi, T.; Toda, N.; and Yu, P.: Sciatic nerve regeneration navigated by laminin-fibronectin double coated biodegradable collagen grafts in rats. *Brain Res.,* 663(1): 155-62, 1994.
[61] Towler, D. A., and Gelberman, R. H.: The alchemy of tendon repair: a primer for the (S)mad scientist. *J. Clin. Invest,* 116(4): 863-6, 2006.
[62] Urist, M. R.: Bone: formation by autoinduction. *Science,* 150(698): 893-9, 1965.
[63] Walton, R. L.; Brown, R. E.; Matory, W. E., Jr.; Borah, G. L.; and Dolph, J. L.: Autogenous vein graft repair of digital nerve defects in the finger: a retrospective clinical study. *Plast Reconstr Surg,* 84(6): 944-9; discussion 950-2, 1989.
[64] Weber, R. A.; Breidenbach, W. C.; Brown, R. E.; Jabaley, M. E.; and Mass, D. P.: A randomized prospective study of polyglycolic acid conduits for digital nerve reconstruction in humans. *Plast Reconstr Surg,* 106(5): 1036-45; discussion 1046-8, 2000.
[65] Whitaker, M. J.; Quirk, R. A.; Howdle, S. M.; and Shakesheff, K. M.: Growth factor release from tissue engineering scaffolds. *J. Pharm. Pharmacol,* 53(11): 1427-37, 2001.
[66] Whitlock, P. W.; Smith, T. L.; Poehling, G. G.; Shilt, J. S.; and Van Dyke, M.: A naturally derived, cytocompatible, and architecturally optimized scaffold for tendon and ligament regeneration. *Biomaterials,* 28(29): 4321-9, 2007.
[67] Whitworth, I. H.; Brown, R. A.; Dore, C. J.; Anand, P.; Green, C. J.; and Terenghi, G.: Nerve growth factor enhances nerve regeneration through fibronectin grafts. *J. Hand Surg [Br],* 21(4): 514-22, 1996.
[68] Wu, D.; Razzano, P.; and Grande, D. A.: Gene therapy and tissue engineering in repair of the musculoskeletal system. *J. Cell Biochem.,* 88(3): 467-81, 2003.
[69] Yow, K. H.; Ingram, J.; Korossis, S. A.; Ingham, E.; and Homer-Vanniasinkam, S.: Tissue engineering of vascular conduits. *Br. J. Surg,* 93(6): 652-61, 2006.
[70] Zhang, W. J.; Liu, W.; Cui, L.; and Cao, Y.: Tissue engineering of blood vessel. *J. Cell Mol. Med.,* 11(5): 945-57, 2007.

Reviewed by Mr Manish Agarwal, FRCS (Orth), Department of Trauma and Orthopaedics, Pennine Acute Hospitals NHS Trust, North Manchester General Hospital, Manchester, M8 5RB, UK

In: Stem Cell Research: New Developments
Editors: Hiroshi Tanaka and Michael C. F. Chang

ISBN: 978-1-61942-081-6

Chapter 2

Advances in Tissue Engineering Approaches for Neurovascular Structures

***Faizal Rayanmarakkar*[1], *Wasim S. Khan**[*1] *and T. E. Hardingham*[2]**

[1]University College London Institute of Orthopaedics and Musculoskeletal Sciences, Royal National Orthopaedic Hospital, Stanmore, London, UK

[2]United Kingdom Centre for Tissue Engineering and Wellcome Trust Centre for Cell Matrix Research, Faculty of Life Sciences, University of Manchester, Oxford Road, Manchester, UK

Abstract

Tissue is frequently damaged or lost in injury and disease. There has been an increasing interest in stem cell applications and tissue engineering approaches in surgical practice to deal with damaged or lost tissue. Tissue engineering is an exciting strategy being explored to deal with damaged or lost tissue. It is the science of generating tissue using molecular and cellular techniques, combined with material engineering principles, to replace tissue. This could be in the form of cells with or without matrices. There have been developments in almost all surgical disciplines including plastic surgery. Unfortunately significant hurdles remain to be overcome in many areas before tissue engineering becomes more routinely used in clinical practice. In this paper tissue engineering approaches relevant to neurovascular structures is discussed.

Introduction

Tissue engineering has been defined as the application of scientific principles to the design, construction, modification and growth of living tissue using biomaterials, cells and factors alone and in combination [33] (Langer and Vacanti, 1993). In essence three elements

* Corresponding Author: Mr Wasim S Khan, Academic Clinical Fellow, University College London Institute of Orthopaedics and Musculoskeletal Science, Royal National Orthopaedic Hospital, Stanmore, London, HA7 4LP, UK. Telephone number: +44 (0) 7971 190720. Fax number: +44 (0) 20 8570 3864. E-mail address: wasimkhan@doctors.org.uk.

are central in tissue engineering; stem or precursor cells; an appropriate biological scaffold and growth factors. It generally involves the use of cells with a matrix or scaffold that guides the cells during tissue repair or regeneration. The use of more undifferentiated cell types, such as stem cells or early mesenchymal progenitors that retain multi-lineage and self renewal potential is preferable to the use of terminally differentiated cells. The scaffold could be natural or biosynthetic. Cells harvested from donor tissues, including adult stem cells, can be expanded in culture and associated with resorbable biomaterials forming the scaffold. The cells can be stimulated by specific bioactive molecules such as growth factors. The cells can also be genetically modified via genomic insertion of a new healthy copy of a gene before expansion and subsequent tissue reconstitution. To date the use of gene technology has not been applied to humans. The cells could be stimulated in-vitro to form tissue for future re-implantation in-vivo. Below applications of tissue engineering principles are discussed relevant neurovascular structures.

1. Nerve

Nerve regeneration is a complex biological phenomenon and their repair poses a great task as the effects of nerve injury are not localised to the site of injury. Nerves can regenerate on their own if injuries are small in the peripheral nervous system. Surgical treatment is imperative for larger injuries. There is not only functional loss, caused by lack of innervations, but also changes occur along the entire path of the nerve from the target end organ to the central nervous system, with great effect on eventual outcomes [38 42] (Lundborg G. 2000 Merzenich MM, 1983). Advances in neuroscience, cell culture, genetic techniques, and biomaterials have provided optimism for new treatments for nerve injuries. For peripheral nerves, we can use direct end-to end surgical reconnection of the nerve ends or use an autologous graft for a larger nerve defect. Loss of function at the donor site and the need for multiple surgeries are the main drawbacks. There are devices that are now FDA approved for short nerve defects including Integra Neuro sciences Type I collagen tube (NeuraGen Nerve Guide) and SaluMedica's SaluBridge Nerve Cuff [39 3] (Archibald SJ, 1995. Lundborg G, 1997).

Various treatment options are:

(I) Autologous tissue grafts e.g. nerve grafts, vein grafts, muscle grafts, epineurial sheaths and tendon grafts.

(II) Nonautologous/acellular grafts e.g. immunosuppression with allografts, acellular allografts and xenografts, thermal decellularisation, radiation treatment, chemical decellularisation, small intestinal submucosa.

(III) Natural-based materials e.g. extra-cellular matrix protein-based material, fibronectin, laminin, collagen and hyaluronic acid-based materials, fibrin/fibrinogen, alginate, agarose.

(IV) Synthetic materials. There are various types:

1. Biodegradable synthetic materials e.g. Polylactic acid (PLA), Polylactic-co-glycolic acid (PLGA), Polycaprolactone, Polyurethane, Polyorganophosphazene, Poly 3-hydroxybutyrate, Polyethylene glycol, Biodegradable glass.

2. Electrically active materials e.g. Piezoelectric Electrically conducting material.
3. Nonbiodegradable synthetic materials e.g. Silicone Gore-Tex or ePTFE.

The biologic substitutes e.g. vessels, muscle and tendon are biocompatible and will not induce a notable immune response and provide a support structure to promote cell adhesion and migration. On the downfall there are potential difficulties with isolation and controlled scale-up, they induce changes in the structural properties of the conduit and cause more scar formation and fibrosis [10,20,63] (Walton RL, 1989; Glasby MA, 1986; Brandt J, 1999).

Nonautologous tissue and extracellular matrix (ECM)-based materials has generated a lot of interest. Allogenic and xenogeneic tissues (donor tissue from cadavers and animals respectively) have the advantages that supplies can be large and their use does not require harvest from the patient. However, these tissues possess some risk of disease transmission and must either be used in conjunction with immunosuppressants or must be processed to remove immunogenic components. Many efforts are being made to process intact nonautologous tissue, rendering it less immunogenic for clinical use. These methods focus on removal or destruction of the immunogenic cells and the preservation of the ECM components that are essentially conserved between species. Many different methods have been explored, including thermal techniques, radiation, and chemical processes. Whereas the biodegradable synthetics grafts minimises the risk of late foreign-body response e.g. polyglycolic acid bioabsorbable conduit (Neurotube; Neuroregen LLC, Bel Air, MD) for digital nerve reconstruction showed superior sensory recovery compared with autografts for gaps less than 3 cm [64] (Weber RA, 2000). Schwann cells surround axons and are key players during the process of nerve regeneration. Scaffolds seeded with cultured Schwann cells seem to have improved nerve regeneration processes in experimental models [23,59] (Tohill M, 2004; Guenard V, 1992). The use of cultured Schwann cells has been limited by difficulty in culturing and expanding these cells *in vitro*. Both foetal and adult progenitor neuronal cells have been tried as alternative sources of cells, but these cells also have problems with harvest and expansion. More recently there has been interest in the use of bone-marrow stem cells to populate nerve conduits. At first glance this might seem counterintuitive because Schwann cells are of ectodermal origin and bone-marrow cells are of mesodermal origin, however there is evidence that stem cells can transdifferentiate across other lineages. These cells are promising because they potentially can be harvested in large amounts from bone-marrow aspiration or possibly even venipuncture. Apart from synthetic biodegradable acellular conduits that currently are available for clinical use, other advances in nerve tissue engineering remain experimental. Convincing outcomes data beyond histologic evidence of nerve regeneration needs to be shown in cell-based conduits before they can be translated from bench to bedside. Newer conduits also likely will incorporate elements of the extracellular matrix such as collagen, laminin, and fibronectin which provide cues to guide axonal regeneration and prevent fibrosis [60 67] (Tong XJ, 1994;Whitworth IH, 1996).

Growth factors such as nerve growth factor, brain-derived neurotrophic factor, acidic and basic fibroblast growth factors, neurotrophin-3, insulin-like growth factor, platelet-derived growth factor, ciliary neurotrophic factor, interleukin-1, and transforming growth factor also may be supplemented to improve the regeneration process [52] (Raivich G, 1993). New advances are likely to come from the field of developmental neurobiology. Unlike adults, in whom neuronal misdirection and incomplete regeneration are features of nerve regeneration, the development process is marked by accurate path-finding of the developing neuron from the central nervous system to its end organs [30] (Koeberle PD, 2004). As knowledge of these guidance cues increases, strategies based on this understanding will enable the development of improved conduits.

2. Blood Vessels

Blood vessels comprise of three layers, from outside to inside the tunica intima, the tunica media and the tunica adventitia. The vascular wall is mainly composed by three types of cells: the endothelial cells that line the tunica intima, the smooth muscle cells that are predominantly located in the tunica media and the adventitial fibroblasts in the tunica adventitia. The integrity of the vessel and mechanical properties are maintained by the endothelial cells and the smooth muscle cells. The endothelial layer not only provides a continuous selective permeable, thrombo-resistant barrier that facilitates laminar blood flow through the blood vessel but also controls vessel tone, platelet activation, adhesion and aggregation, leukocyte adhesion and smooth muscle cell migration and proliferation. Whereas smooth muscle cells play a major role in maintaining elasticity and radial compliance of the vessels by secreting elastic fibres, elastic lamellae and proteoglycans.

The deficiency of graft material due to varicose veins, trauma, prior surgery and the escalating number of reoperations due to the chronic nature of these diseases has led to a high demand of engineered vascular grafts. The incidence of peripheral arterial disease and end-stage renal failure requiring graft is increasing. Also intermediate and long term patency rates in smaller vessels with a calibre of less than 6 mm are poor.

The off-the-shelf availability, harvesting issues, propagation of autologous cells, long cultivation times, the limited conduit length generated in the bioreactors and the need for additional surgical interventions for sourcing autologous cells are the greatest obstacles to the widespread acceptance of tissue engineering technology in clinical practice.

The aim of vascular tissue engineering is to reproduce biocompatible scaffolds. They use autologous cells like endothelial cells, vascular smooth muscle cells (SMCs) and fibroblasts to preclude the complications like thrombogenicity and immunogenicity. Endothelium has antithrombotic, anticoagulant functions and resists intimal hyperplasia. They contribute to construct properties by extracellular matrix production, structural organisation, and contractilability. Genetic manipulation is being tested to improve the proliferation rate of autologous endothelial cells without losing their other properties. Immune rejection is still a major hurdle for allogeneic endothelial and smooth muscle cells. There are two types of stem cells based on their origin, the embryonic and adult stem cells used as cell sources. Embryonic stem cells are still not introduced in clinical application. The main problems are the ethical issues, immunogenic and tumourgenic problems which have to be dealt with before transplantation. Adult stem cells avoid all these issues [70] (Zhang 2007). Fibroblasts too have been used as a cell source in vascular tissue engineering

For the tissue regeneration process the three dimentional structure of scaffold provides an ideal template for cell growth, migration, differentiation, secretion of extracellular matrix proteins and for directing new tissue formation [70] (Zhang 2007). Scaffolds can be either natural proteins, synthetic or biologic polymers. The main aim is to provide vascular cell remodelling and the structural support. Collagen, elastin and fibronectin are the major components of extra-cellular matrix in the body. The first tissue engineered vascular graft by Weinberg and Bell was created using collagen gel. The methods used to strengthen the collagen gel construct are the use of glycation, wrapping the constructs with Dacron mesh or polyurethane film, the use of non-degradable or degradable meshes as sleeves, and the application of dynamic mechanical stimulation.

Synthetic polymers include polyglycolic acid (PGA), poly-L-lactic acid and polyurethanes. Degradation products, degradation time, compliance, tensile strength, conduit size and configuration can be accurately modified at the point of manufacture to adjust their biocompatibility, degradation rate and elasticity. They are cheap and can be reproduced easily. But synthetic scaffolds do not grow, they lack cell attachment factors and their degradation products may cause intimal hyperplasia. To overcome these setbacks, biologic scaffolds were developed. There are three types of biological scaffold: decellularised allogeneic and xenogeneic blood vessel, decellularised non-vascular conduits and prefabricated extracellular matrices. Decellularisation is achieved chemically by treating with a combination of detergents, enzyme inhibitors and buffers. Decellularisation can be done mechanically by eversion and surface abrasion. They preserve the extra-cellular matrix components like elastin, collagen and glycasminoglycans which are vital for retention of tensile strength, elasticity, endothelial cell adhesion, proliferation, inhibition of smooth muscle cell proliferation (prevents intimal hyperplasia), migration and antithrombotic properties. The main risk of using xenogeneic scaffolds is transmission of animal pathogens [69] (Yow et al, 2006). The mechanical and haemodynamic properties of vascular grafts are crucial for their long-term survival. Bioreactors have been used to produce functional graft in culture with the desired biomechanical properties. Mechanical property of the engineered graft could be controlled by chemical reagents and growth factors e.g. transforming growth factor 1 (TGF-1), insulin, aprotinin, hyaluronan and retinoic acid. Another most exciting option is the rising potential of EPCs which are mobilised into the circulation in response to vessel injury, are significant source of endothelial cells in the face of vascular injury, forming new blood vessels via vasculogenesis (Tepper et al, 2005). They do not have the capacity of self renewal, but they can differentiate into endothelial cells. They can be augmented by statins or erythropoietin to mobilise EPCs to areas of denuded vessels [57](Tepper et al, 2005).

REFERENCES

[1] Abrahamsson, S. O., and Lohmander, S.: Differential effects of insulin-like growth factor-I on matrix and DNA synthesis in various regions and types of rabbit tendons. *J. Orthop. Res.,* 14(3): 370-6, 1996.

[2] Andriano, K. P.; Tabata, Y.; Ikada, Y.; and Heller, J.: In vitro and in vivo comparison of bulk and surface hydrolysis in absorbable polymer scaffolds for tissue engineering. *J. Biomed. Mater. Res.,* 48(5): 602-12, 1999.

[3] Archibald, S. J.; Shefner, J.; Krarup, C.; and Madison, R. D.: Monkey median nerve repaired by nerve graft or collagen nerve guide tube. *J. Neurosci.,* 15(5 Pt 2): 4109-23, 1995.

[4] Banes, A. J.; Tsuzaki, M.; Hu, P.; Brigman, B.; Brown, T.; Almekinders, L.; Lawrence, W. T.; and Fischer, T.: PDGF-BB, IGF-I and mechanical load stimulate DNA synthesis in avian tendon fibroblasts in vitro. *J. Biomech.,* 28(12): 1505-13, 1995.

[5] Basile, P. et al.: Freeze-dried tendon allografts as tissue-engineering scaffolds for Gdf5 gene delivery. *Mol. Ther.,* 16(3): 466-73, 2008.

[6] Bianco, P.; Riminucci, M.; Gronthos, S.; and Robey, P. G.: Bone marrow stromal stem cells: nature, biology, and potential applications. *Stem Cells,* 19(3): 180-92, 2001.

[7] Boden, S. D.: Bioactive factors for bone tissue engineering. *Clin. Orthop. Relat Res,* (367 Suppl): S84-94, 1999.

[8] Boyer, M. I.; Goldfarb, C. A.; and Gelberman, R. H.: Recent progress in flexor tendon healing. The modulation of tendon healing with rehabilitation variables. *J. Hand Ther.,* 18(2): 80-5; quiz 86, 2005.

[9] Braddock, M.; Houston, P.; Campbell, C.; and Ashcroft, P.: Born again bone: tissue engineering for bone repair. *News Physiol. Sci.,* 16: 208-13, 2001.

[10] Brandt, J.; Dahlin, L. B.; and Lundborg, G.: Autologous tendons used as grafts for bridging peripheral nerve defects. *J. Hand Surg. [Br],* 24(3): 284-90, 1999.

[11] Breitbart, A. S.; Grande, D. A.; Mason, J. M.; Barcia, M.; James, T.; and Grant, R. T.: Gene-enhanced tissue engineering: applications for bone healing using cultured periosteal cells transduced retrovirally with the BMP-7 gene. *Ann. Plast. Surg,* 42(5): 488-95, 1999.

[12] Brekke, J. H., and Toth, J. M.: Principles of tissue engineering applied to programmable osteogenesis. *J. Biomed. Mater. Res.,* 43(4): 380-98, 1998.

[13] Brigham, P. A., and McLoughlin, E.: Burn incidence and medical care use in the United States: estimates, trends, and data sources. *J. Burn Care Rehabil.,* 17(2): 95-107, 1996.

[14] Cancedda, R.; Bianchi, G.; Derubeis, A.; and Quarto, R.: Cell therapy for bone disease: a review of current status. *Stem Cells,* 21(5): 610-9, 2003.

[15] Chong, A. K., and Chang, J.: Tissue engineering for the hand surgeon: a clinical perspective. *J. Hand Surg. [Am],* 31(3): 349-58, 2006.

[16] Cooper, R. R., and Misol, S.: Tendon and ligament insertion. A light and electron microscopic study. *J. Bone Joint Surg Am.,* 52(1): 1-20, 1970.

[17] DeFranco, M. J.; Derwin, K.; and Iannotti, J. P.: New therapies in tendon reconstruction. *J. Am. Acad. Orthop Surg.,* 12(5): 298-304, 2004.

[18] Gelberman, R. H., and Manske, P. R.: Factors influencing flexor tendon adhesions. *Hand Clin.,* 1(1): 35-42, 1985.

[19] Gelberman, R. H.; Thomopoulos, S.; Sakiyama-Elbert, S. E.; Das, R.; and Silva, M. J.: The early effects of sustained platelet-derived growth factor administration on the functional and structural properties of repaired intrasynovial flexor tendons: an in vivo biomechanic study at 3 weeks in canines. *J. Hand Surg [Am],* 32(3): 373-9, 2007.

[20] Glasby, M. A.; Gschmeissner, S. E.; Huang, C. L.; and De Souza, B. A.: Degenerated muscle grafts used for peripheral nerve repair in primates. *J. Hand Surg [Br],* 11(3): 347-51, 1986.

[21] Govender, S. et al.: Recombinant human bone morphogenetic protein-2 for treatment of open tibial fractures: a prospective, controlled, randomized study of four hundred and fifty patients. *J. Bone Joint Surg Am.,* 84-A(12): 2123-34, 2002.

[22] Grigolo, B.; Roseti, L.; Fiorini, M.; Fini, M.; Giavaresi, G.; Aldini, N. N.; Giardino, R.; and Facchini, A.: Transplantation of chondrocytes seeded on a hyaluronan derivative (hyaff-11) into cartilage defects in rabbits. *Biomaterials,* 22(17): 2417-24, 2001.

[23] Guenard, V.; Kleitman, N.; Morrissey, T. K.; Bunge, R. P.; and Aebischer, P.: Syngeneic Schwann cells derived from adult nerves seeded in semipermeable guidance channels enhance peripheral nerve regeneration. *J. Neurosci.,* 12(9): 3310-20, 1992.

[24] Gundle, R.; Joyner, C. J.; and Triffitt, J. T.: Human bone tissue formation in diffusion chamber culture in vivo by bone-derived cells and marrow stromal fibroblastic cells. *Bone,* 16(6): 597-601, 1995.

[25] Hatano, I.; Suga, T.; Diao, E.; Peimer, C. A.; and Howard, C.: Adhesions from flexor tendon surgery: an animal study comparing surgical techniques. *J. Hand Surg [Am],* 25(2): 252-9, 2000.

[26] Jones, I.; Currie, L.; and Martin, R.: A guide to biological skin substitutes. *Br. J. Plast Surg,* 55(3): 185-93, 2002.

[27] Kadiyala, S.; Young, R. G.; Thiede, M. A.; and Bruder, S. P.: Culture expanded canine mesenchymal stem cells possess osteochondrogenic potential in vivo and in vitro. *Cell Transplant,* 6(2): 125-34, 1997.

[28] Kale, S.; Biermann, S.; Edwards, C.; Tarnowski, C.; Morris, M.; and Long, M. W.: Three-dimensional cellular development is essential for ex vivo formation of human bone. *Nat. Biotechnol,* 18(9): 954-8, 2000.

[29] Kashiwagi, K.; Mochizuki, Y.; Yasunaga, Y.; Ishida, O.; Deie, M.; and Ochi, M.: Effects of transforming growth factor-beta 1 on the early stages of healing of the Achilles tendon in a rat model. *Scand J. Plast Reconstr Surg Hand Surg,* 38(4): 193-7, 2004.

[30] Koeberle, P. D., and Bahr, M.: Growth and guidance cues for regenerating axons: where have they gone? *J. Neurobiol.,* 59(1): 162-80, 2004.

[31] Koob, T. J.: Biomimetic approaches to tendon repair. *Comp. Biochem. Physiol. A Mol. Integr. Physiol.,* 133(4): 1171-92, 2002.

[32] Kruyt, M. C.; van Gaalen, S. M.; Oner, F. C.; Verbout, A. J.; de Bruijn, J. D.; and Dhert, W. J.: Bone tissue engineering and spinal fusion: the potential of hybrid constructs by combining osteoprogenitor cells and scaffolds. *Biomaterials,* 25(9): 1463-73, 2004.

[33] Langer, R., and Vacanti, J. P.: Tissue engineering. *Science,* 260(5110): 920-6, 1993.

[34] Lee, C. H.; Singla, A.; and Lee, Y.: Biomedical applications of collagen. *Int J Pharm,* 221(1-2): 1-22, 2001.

[35] Lee, K. Y.; Peters, M. C.; Anderson, K. W.; and Mooney, D. J.: Controlled growth factor release from synthetic extracellular matrices. *Nature,* 408(6815): 998-1000, 2000.

[36] LeGeros, R. Z.: Properties of osteoconductive biomaterials: calcium phosphates. *Clin. Orthop. Relat Res.,* (395): 81-98, 2002.

[37] Lilly, S. I., and Messer, T. M.: Complications after treatment of flexor tendon injuries. *J. Am. Acad. Orthop. Surg.,* 14(7): 387-96, 2006.

[38] Lundborg, G.: A 25-year perspective of peripheral nerve surgery: evolving neuroscientific concepts and clinical significance. *J. Hand Surg. [Am],* 25(3): 391-414, 2000.

[39] Lundborg, G.; Dahlin, L.; Dohi, D.; Kanje, M.; and Terada, N.: A new type of "bioartificial" nerve graft for bridging extended defects in nerves. *J. Hand Surg. [Br],* 22(3): 299-303, 1997.

[40] Meislin, R. J.; Wiseman, D. M.; Alexander, H.; Cunningham, T.; Linsky, C.; Carlstedt, C.; Pitman, M.; and Casar, R.: A biomechanical study of tendon adhesion reduction using a biodegradable barrier in a rabbit model. *J. Appl. Biomater.,* 1(1): 13-9, 1990.

[41] Mentzel, M.; Hoss, H.; Keppler, P.; Ebinger, T.; Kinzl, L.; and Wachter, N. J.: The effectiveness of ADCON-T/N, a new anti-adhesion barrier gel, in fresh divisions of the flexor tendons in Zone II. *J. Hand Surg. [Br],* 25(6): 590-2, 2000.

[42] Merzenich, M. M.; Kaas, J. H.; Wall, J.; Nelson, R. J.; Sur, M.; and Felleman, D.: Topographic reorganization of somatosensory cortical areas 3b and 1 in adult monkeys following restricted deafferentation. *Neuroscience,* 8(1): 33-55, 1983.

[43] Mooney, D. J., and Mikos, A. G.: Growing new organs. *Sci. Am.,* 280(4): 60-5, 1999.

[44] Muschler, G. F.; Nitto, H.; Matsukura, Y.; Boehm, C.; Valdevit, A.; Kambic, H.; Davros, W.; Powell, K.; and Easley, K.: Spine fusion using cell matrix composites enriched in bone marrow-derived cells. *Clin. Orthop. Relat. Res.,* (407): 102-18, 2003.

[45] Olmsted, E. A.; Blum, J. S.; Rill, D.; Yotnda, P.; Gugala, Z.; Lindsey, R. W.; and Davis, A. R.: Adenovirus-mediated BMP2 expression in human bone marrow stromal cells. *J. Cell Biochem.,* 82(1): 11-21, 2001.

[46] Oreffo, R. O., and Triffitt, J. T.: Future potentials for using osteogenic stem cells and biomaterials in orthopedics. *Bone,* 25(2 Suppl): 5S-9S, 1999.

[47] Partridge, K. A., and Oreffo, R. O.: Gene delivery in bone tissue engineering: progress and prospects using viral and nonviral strategies. *Tissue Eng,* 10(1-2): 295-307, 2004.

[48] Pennisi, E.: Tending tender tendons. *Science,* 295(5557): 1011, 2002.

[49] Perry, C. R.: Bone repair techniques, bone graft, and bone graft substitutes. *Clin. Orthop. Relat Res.,* (360): 71-86, 1999.

[50] Petite, H.; Viateau, V.; Bensaid, W.; Meunier, A.; de Pollak, C.; Bourguignon, M.; Oudina, K.; Sedel, L.; and Guillemin, G.: Tissue-engineered bone regeneration. *Nat. Biotechnol.,* 18(9): 959-63, 2000.

[51] Quirk, R. A.; Chan, W. C.; Davies, M. C.; Tendler, S. J.; and Shakesheff, K. M.: Poly(L-lysine)-GRGDS as a biomimetic surface modifier for poly(lactic acid). *Biomaterials,* 22(8): 865-72, 2001.

[52] Raivich, G., and Kreutzberg, G. W.: Peripheral nerve regeneration: role of growth factors and their receptors. *Int. J. Dev. Neurosci.,* 11(3): 311-24, 1993.

[53] Sakkers, R. J.; Dalmeyer, R. A.; de Wijn, J. R.; and van Blitterswijk, C. A.: Use of bone-bonding hydrogel copolymers in bone: an in vitro and in vivo study of expanding PEO-PBT copolymers in goat femora. *J. Biomed. Mater. Res.,* 49(3): 312-8, 2000.

[54] Shin, H.; Jo, S.; and Mikos, A. G.: Biomimetic materials for tissue engineering. *Biomaterials,* 24(24): 4353-64, 2003.

[55] Silva, M. J.; Boyer, M. I.; and Gelberman, R. H.: Recent progress in flexor tendon healing. *J. Orthop. Sci.,* 7(4): 508-14, 2002.

[56] Stewart, K.; Walsh, S.; Screen, J.; Jefferiss, C. M.; Chainey, J.; Jordan, G. R.; and Beresford, J. N.: Further characterization of cells expressing STRO-1 in cultures of adult human bone marrow stromal cells. *J. Bone Miner Res.,* 14(8): 1345-56, 1999.

[57] Tepper, O. M.; Capla, J. M.; Galiano, R. D.; Ceradini, D. J.; Callaghan, M. J.; Kleinman, M. E.; and Gurtner, G. C.: Adult vasculogenesis occurs through in situ

recruitment, proliferation, and tubulization of circulating bone marrow-derived cells. *Blood,* 105(3): 1068-77, 2005.

[58] Thomopoulos, S.; Harwood, F. L.; Silva, M. J.; Amiel, D.; and Gelberman, R. H.: Effect of several growth factors on canine flexor tendon fibroblast proliferation and collagen synthesis in vitro. *J. Hand Surg [Am],* 30(3): 441-7, 2005.

[59] Tohill, M., and Terenghi, G.: Stem-cell plasticity and therapy for injuries of the peripheral nervous system. *Biotechnol. Appl. Biochem.,* 40(Pt 1): 17-24, 2004.

[60] Tong, X. J.; Hirai, K.; Shimada, H.; Mizutani, Y.; Izumi, T.; Toda, N.; and Yu, P.: Sciatic nerve regeneration navigated by laminin-fibronectin double coated biodegradable collagen grafts in rats. *Brain Res,* 663(1): 155-62, 1994.

[61] Towler, D. A., and Gelberman, R. H.: The alchemy of tendon repair: a primer for the (S)mad scientist. *J. Clin. Invest,* 116(4): 863-6, 2006.

[62] Urist, M. R.: Bone: formation by autoinduction. *Science,* 150(698): 893-9, 1965.

[63] Walton, R. L.; Brown, R. E.; Matory, W. E., Jr.; Borah, G. L.; and Dolph, J. L.: Autogenous vein graft repair of digital nerve defects in the finger: a retrospective clinical study. *Plast Reconstr Surg,* 84(6): 944-9; discussion 950-2, 1989.

[64] Weber, R. A.; Breidenbach, W. C.; Brown, R. E.; Jabaley, M. E.; and Mass, D. P.: A randomized prospective study of polyglycolic acid conduits for digital nerve reconstruction in humans. *Plast Reconstr Surg,* 106(5): 1036-45; discussion 1046-8, 2000.

[65] Whitaker, M. J.; Quirk, R. A.; Howdle, S. M.; and Shakesheff, K. M.: Growth factor release from tissue engineering scaffolds. *J. Pharm. Pharmacol.,* 53(11): 1427-37, 2001.

[66] Whitlock, P. W.; Smith, T. L.; Poehling, G. G.; Shilt, J. S.; and Van Dyke, M.: A naturally derived, cytocompatible, and architecturally optimized scaffold for tendon and ligament regeneration. *Biomaterials,* 28(29): 4321-9, 2007.

[67] Whitworth, I. H.; Brown, R. A.; Dore, C. J.; Anand, P.; Green, C. J.; and Terenghi, G.: Nerve growth factor enhances nerve regeneration through fibronectin grafts. *J. Hand Surg. [Br],* 21(4): 514-22, 1996.

[68] Wu, D.; Razzano, P.; and Grande, D. A.: Gene therapy and tissue engineering in repair of the musculoskeletal system. *J. Cell Biochem.,* 88(3): 467-81, 2003.

[69] Yow, K. H.; Ingram, J.; Korossis, S. A.; Ingham, E.; and Homer-Vanniasinkam, S.: Tissue engineering of vascular conduits. *Br. J. Surg.,* 93(6): 652-61, 2006.

[70] Zhang, W. J.; Liu, W.; Cui, L.; and Cao, Y.: Tissue engineering of blood vessel. *J. Cell Mol. Med.,* 11(5): 945-57, 2007.

Reviewed by Mr Manish Agarwal, FRCS (Orth), Department of Trauma and Orthopaedics, Pennine Acute Hospitals NHS Trust, North Manchester General Hospital, Manchester, M8 5RB, UK

In: Stem Cell Research: New Developments
Editors: Hiroshi Tanaka and Michael C. F. Chang
ISBN: 978-1-61942-081-6

Chapter 3

Tissue Engineering Approaches for Bone Repair: Cells, Scaffolds, Growth Factors and Gene Therapy

Wasim S. Khan* and David Marsh
University College London Institute of Orthopaedics and Musculoskeletal Sciences, Royal National Orthopaedic Hospital, Stanmore, London, UK

Abstract

Tissue is frequently damaged or lost in injury and disease. There has been an increasing interest in stem cell applications and tissue engineering approaches in surgical practice to deal with damaged or lost tissue. Tissue engineering is an exciting strategy being explored to deal with damaged or lost tissue. It is the science of generating tissue using molecular and cellular techniques, combined with material engineering principles, to replace tissue. This could be in the form of cells with or without matrices. Although there have been developments in almost all surgical disciplines, the greatest advances are being made in orthopaedics, especially in bone repair. This is due to many factors including the familiarity with bone marrow derived mesenchymal stem cells and bone grafting. Unfortunately significant hurdles remain to be overcome in many areas before tissue engineering becomes more routinely used in clinical practice. In this paper the tissue engineering approaches relevant to bone repair are discussed. Significant hurdles however remain to be overcome before tissue engineering becomes more routinely used in surgical practice.

* Corresponding Author: Mr Wasim S Khan, Academic Clinical Fellow, University College London Institute of Orthopaedics and Musculoskeletal Science, Royal National Orthopaedic Hospital, Stanmore, London, HA7 4LP, UK. Telephone number: +44 (0) 7971 190720. Fax number: +44 (0) 20 8570 3864. E-mail address: wasimkhan@doctors.org.uk.

INTRODUCTION

Regeneration involves replacement of old tissue with new tissue. It occurs readily in the embryo but is slow in most adult tissue. This may be because of the relatively large number of undifferentiated progenitor cells in the embryo (1 in 10,000) compared with adults (1 in 2,000,000) as shown by Haynesworth et al in 1994. Repair mechanisms in post-embryonic tissue, other than bone, result in scar formation instead of tissue regeneration. Repair is more rapid and designed for survival. It involves the inflammatory cell cascade followed by matrix deposition and the remodeling process which attempts to regenerate damaged tissue.

Bone is continually remodeled as a result of the balance between the activities of the osteoclasts and the osteoblasts. Because of the potential of bone to spontaneously regenerate, most bone lesions, such as fractures, heal well with conventional therapy or surgery. The osteogenic process that commences after the inflammatory phase, under the influence of bone-derived bioactive factors, is initiated by precursor cells from the periosteum adjacent to the fracture site. This generates hard callus by intramemembranous bone formation. A bone graft or substitute is often required to assist in orthopaedic surgery healing of a large traumatic or post-surgical defect and of osseous congenital deformities. The majority of bone formation however is by enchondral ossification of the soft callus that appears after infiltrated mesenchymal cells are induced to chondrogenesis. This improved understanding of repair and regeneration has helped with the development of orthopaedic tissue engineering [32] (Kruyt et al, 2004).

CURRENT TREATMENT

Current surgical treatment of large bone defects falls into two groups; Illizarov method or bone transport and bone graft transplant (auto-, allo-, xeno-grafts, different biomaterial implants). The lllizarov technique entails an osteotomy followed by bone distraction allowing regeneration of bone. The disadvantages include long recovery period and a high complication rate. The clinical gold standard for bone repair is an autologous graft that is effective, but is limited by the availability of sufficient donor tissue and donor site morbidity. As for graft transplants, vascularised autografts are presently mostly used e.g. autografting cancellous bone applying vascularised grafts of the fibula and iliac crest [49] (Perry, 1999). The disadvantages include problems related to anatomical limitations, graft integration, donor site morbidity including infection and haematoma and limitation of size of reconstruction.

TISSUE ENGINEERING

Tissue engineering has been defined as the application of scientific principles to the design, construction, modification and growth of living tissue using biomaterials, cells and factors alone and in combination [33] (Langer and Vacanti, 1993). In essence three elements are central in tissue engineering; stem or precursor cells; an appropriate biological scaffold and growth factors. All three are discussed in detail below. It generally involves the use of cells with a matrix or scaffold that guides the cells during tissue repair or regeneration. The use of more undifferentiated cell types, such as stem cells or early mesenchymal progenitors that retain multi-lineage and self renewal potential is preferable to the use of terminally differentiated cells. The scaffold could be natural or biosynthetic. Cells harvested from donor tissues, including adult stem cells, can be expanded in culture and associated with resorbable biomaterials forming the scaffold. The cells can be stimulated by specific bioactive molecules such as growth factors. The cells can also be genetically modified via genomic insertion of a new healthy copy of a gene before expansion and subsequent tissue reconstitution. To date the use of gene technology has not been applied to humans. The cells could be stimulated in-vitro to form tissue for future re-implantation in-vivo.

A tissue engineering approach to treat skeletal defects involves the use of osteoconductive biomaterial scaffolds with osteogenic cell populations and osteoinductive bioactive factors. A possible tissue engineering approach for bone repair is to use autologous bone marrow stem cells (BMSC) loaded on a scaffold [14] (Cancedda et al, 2003). The three constituents are discussed below.

1. Identification of Appropriate Cell Type

Differentiated cells released from adult tissue exhibit a limited proliferation capacity. This has limitations for their expansion in culture and in vitro reconstruction of tissue. Culturing undifferentiated cells (stem cells or progenitor cells) that have a higher proliferative capacity is more promising. Differentiation of these cells can be obtained in vitro by changing the culture conditions after their expansion or by providing a new physiological micro-environment in the transplant area in vivo.

A stem cell is a cell from the embryo, fetus or adult that, under certain conditions, can reproduce for long periods. It can also give rise to specialised cells of body tissues and organs. The use of stem cells from the embryo or fetus has many ethical considerations whereas the use of adult stem cells is generally well accepted by society. An adult stem cell is an undifferentiated or unspecialized cell present in differentiated tissue, which renews itself; and becomes specialized to yield all of the cell types of the tissue from which it was originated. Their progeny includes both new stem cells and committed progenitors with a more restricted differentiation potential. These progenitor cells in turn give rise to more differentiated cell types. The advantages of using stem cells rather than differentiated cells are a higher proliferative capacity, a higher regenerative potential over time and the ability to allow revascularization of the avascular scaffold. Cells with osteoprogenitor features have been isolated from several tissues including periosteum, bone marrow, adipose tissue and retina. The choice of source depends on accessibility, frequency of cells and information of a particular cell system.

Research suggests that stem cells derived from bone marrow (BMSC) can be expanded for a significant number of cell doublings without cell senescence. In vitro multi-differentiation potentials are gradually lost on expansion [14] (Cancedda et al , 2003). The harvest of bone marrow samples is an easy and relatively safe procedure. The bone marrow is a reservoir of multipotent stem cells for mesenchymal tissues. These multipotential stromal stem cells can differentiate into fibroblastic, osteogenic, adipogenic and reticular cells [6] (Bianco et al, 2001). A large number of BMSCs can be obtained in culture. Culture conditions remain essentially the same as the ones originally described by Friedenstein in 1966;

however, to increase the yield of osteoprogenitor cells, the effects of several growth factors on proliferation and differentiation of BMSC have been investigated. In addition, human bone marrow osteoprogenitor cells can be isolated and enriched using monoclonal antibodies as selective markers, such as STRO-1 from a CD34+ fraction, SB-10 (reacting with ALCAM), SH-2 (reacting with CD105) and HOP-26 (reacting with CD63) [46 47 56] (Oreffo and Triffitt, 1999; Stewart et al, 1999; Partridge and Oreffo, 2004). FGF-2 supplementation to the culture medium promotes cell proliferation and maintains their multi-lineage potential during expansion [14] (Cancedda et al, 2003).

Intraoperative adult stem cells technologies are being developed to enhance bone repair in delayed or non-union fractures as shown by Muschler et al in 2003 [44]. One in 23,000 adult bone marrow cells is an osteogenic precursor cell. These cells can potentially be separated by selective cell absorption in the operating theatre making viable implants for immediate surgical use. These cells can be combined with a suitable scaffold and used as an alternative to conventional bone autograft. The transplanted osteogenic stem cells can immediately begin to proliferate and lay down new bone matrix without removing the old matrix present in the autograft. The development of these cell based technologies may result in decreased use of conventional bone banks use dead bone to induce new bone formation.

2. Identification of Appropriate Scaffolds

Mesenchymal stem cells alone are unlikely to be sufficient for bone regeneration. Although marrow injections are simple and provide a reduced risk of morbidity, for large skeletal defects, a scaffold of appropriate shape, size and mechanical competence is required for fracture repair. The use of the scaffold or matrix is not only in controlling growth factor and cell delivery but also to provide a structural template to fill the tissue lesion. These could be naturally occurring or synthetic polymers or bioceramics. Biodegradable scaffolds provide t e initial structure and stability for tissue formation but degrade as tissue forms, providing room for matrix deposition and tissue growth. They can be used alone or in combination with growth factors or osteoconductive materials.

The scaffold aims to mimic the extracellular matrix in a regenerating bone viromnent. It has to be informative to the cells as well as provide mechanical support. A biomaterial should easily integrate with the adjacent bone and favour new tissue ingrowth (osteo-conduction). It should allow colonization by the host blood vessels, be biocompatible and resorbable.

Polymers include collagen that can be prepared in solution or shaped into membrane films, threads, sponges and acidic hydrogels. It is derived from xenogenic sources and purifcationtechniques are used to eliminate the immunogenic telopeptides. The primary obstacle to their use is the possibility of xenozoonoses [34] (Lee et al, 2001). Heparin-coating fibrin hydrogels can be used to slowly and regularly deliver growth factors with heparin binding affinity such as FGF-2. Alginates extracted from brown algae form a brown lattice hydrogel. It has large average mesh size allowing easy diffusion of macromolecules. Hyaluronic acid binds specifically to proteins. Its stability is increased by partial esterification making it particularly suitable for peptide release or protein delivery [22] (Grigolo et al, 2001).

Synthetic polymers include poly lactic acid (PLA), polyglycolic acid (PGA) and their co-polymer polylactic-co-glycolic acid (PLGA). They allow a better control of physicocliemical properties and delivery kinetics. They also reduce the risk of potential biohazardous complications. The disadvantages are the induction of some immune or inflammatory response after implantation. These polymers are currently used for a number of orthopaedic devices including suture anchors and interference screws) Other biodegradable materials for bone tissue engineering include Degrapol-foam and Polyactive that support bone cell adhesion and proliferation [53] (Sakkers et al, 2000). Surface eroding polymers, such as polyortho-esters may have advantages in load bearing bone applications as only the surface of these materials degrades leaving the bulk the mechanical strength [2] (Andriano et al, 1999).

Bioceramics act as a pre-existing bone surface on which bone cells deposit new bone matrix. Best results so far have been with porous bioceramics and BMSC. Bioceramics made from hydroxyapatite and tricalcium phosp ate are used for bone repair. They have osteoconductive properties and ability to integrate with bone tissue. They are not themselves osteoinductive and are resorbed relatively slow. Their resorbability can be increased by increasing the concentration of tricalcium phosphate. The production of porous scaffolds makes the interna architecture similar to that of cancellous bone. Advantages include large surface available for tissue regeneration and cell delivery and a favorable micro-environmental effect due to the presence of a mineralized matrix [36] (LeGeros, 2002). Problems include biodegradability and inflammatory and immunological reactions 46 (Oreffo and Triffitt, 1999).

Alternative scaffolds are derived from cadavers or animal skeletons and natural scaffolds for example the coral cytoskeleton. Mesenchymal stem cells mixed with coral implants have been shown to stimulate bone regeneration and achieve bone regeneration and achieve bone clinical union in an animal model of bone defect [50] (Petite et al, 2000). Biomimetic material chemistry attempts to reproduce the complex structures that occur in nature, such as coral, nacre and calcite shells and sea urchin spines, in synthetic systems and generate accurate and specific biomaterials. They potentially mimic many roles of the extracellular matrix by providing biological cues for cell-matrix interactions promoting tissue growth. They are modified with bioactive molecules and can be used as tissue engineering scaffolds that potentially serve as an artificial extracellular matrix providing biological cues to guide new tissue formation. More information on immunoreactivity and biocompatibility will be needed before clinical evaluation [54] (Shin et al, 2003).

Smart materials, for example, Arg-Gly-Asp (RGD) sequence peptides involved in integrin mediated cell adhesion can be incorporated onto the scaffold surface to enhance cell adhesion and spreading [51] (Quirk et al, 2001). Drug delivery techniques such as entrapment within a hydrogel matrix allowing growth factor to be released in a controlled fashion from the scaffold to aid the regenerating tissue have been applied [65] (Whitaker et al, 2001). This strategy has been applied in bone tissue engineering where growth factors such as recombinant human bone morphogenetic protein-2, basic fibroblast growth factor and vascular endothelial growth factor have all been successfully incorporated into a hydrogel prior to in vivo implantation [35] (Lee et al, 2000). A future goal will be the introduction of calcium based scaffolds that can gradually degrade at the same rate at which new bone is formed.

3. Growth Factors and Gene Therapy

Growth factors are cytokines that are secreted by many cell types and function as signaling molecules. Members of the TGF beta family, notably bone morphogenetic proteins (BMPs), are particularly relevant to skeletal tissue engineering. Other agents known to induce bone formation include FGF, PDGF and IGF-1, Indian sonic hedgehog and parathyroid hormone. One function of BMP is to induce the differentiation of undifferentiated mesenchymal cells into chondrogenic and osteogenic cells and to promote their proliferation (Saito and Takaota, 2003). BMPs have a role in bone development and thus their incorporation into tissue engineered scaffolds and delivery systems [7] (Boden, 1999).

The isolation of growth factors such as TGF beta 3 and its analogues such as BMPs e.g. BMP 2 and 7 has led to their use to enhance and accelerate bone repair and to replace the bone. Bone induction to assist and enhance bone deposition and repair was first introduced by Marshall Urist in 1965, and led to the isolation of BMPs, which could stimulate osteogenic precursor mesenchymal stem cells (MSCs) to form bone [62]. Human cDNA BMP 7 was cloned in 1990 and recombinant human form followed. It was shown to induce bone formation in animals by stimulating precursor MSCs. Recombinant human BMPs (rhBMPs) have been commercially available for over a decade but their bioavailability, bioactivity and costs have limited their clinical uptake. There are three methods by which BMPs can be used in bone tissue engineering and these include (a) cell therapy (b) gene therapy (c) cytokine therapy (Saito and Takaota, 2003).

Earlier examples include the use of porous PLGA scaffolds with high molecular weight hyaluronic acid for rhBMP-2 delivery [12] (Brekke and Toth, 1998). hnplantation of such constructs into long bone defects promoted cortical bone formation in vivo in rabbits (Mori et al, 2000). Another approach is to use collagens, the favoured carrier for BMPs, to generate composites with hydroxyapatite or PLA for use with rhBMP-2 for tissue engineering. This has shown to be successful in vivo by Winn et al in 1999: TGF beta 1 has been shown to stimulate the three-dimentional cellular development of human bone ex vivo [28] (Kale et al, 2000).

In 2002, injecting the rhBMP-7 into a bone non-union site resulted in healing of the site after 30 months as shown by Giltaij et al. The protein acts by recruiting adult osteogenic precursor MSCs. In a study by Giltaij et al 163 patients with non-union 23 months after injury received the recombinant protein implant and achieved clinical union in 70% andradiological union in 65% by 19 months. No significant adverse reactions were attributed to the implant. There was also a decreased incidence of osteomyelitis at the surgical site and decreased use of post-operative analgesia. A prospective randomized controlled trial of 450 patients concluded that the clinical use of rhBMP-2 as an adjunct to standard management of long bone fractures was safe, well tolerated and showed earlier functional recovery [21] (Govender et al, 2002).

Gene therapy is the science of the transfer of genetic material into individuals for therapeutic purposes by altering cellular function or structure at the molecular level. The ability to transfer genes into multipotent mesenchymal stem cells has many applications. Developments in gene technology offer the possibility of genetic modification of isolated and expanded cells to produce populations of progenitor cells over-expressing selected signaling molecules. The various techniques and methods currently available to enable gene transfer into a target population include viral methods (transduction) and nonviral methods (transfection). Viral delivery systems used for bone engineering include the retroviral and adenoviral systems. The advantages of viral expression of genes are a high efficiency of transduction (50-100%). The disadvantages include the potential for mutagenesis, carcinogenesis and the immune response to viral infection or proteins. Nonviral gene delivery makes use of lipopolyfection reagents such as liposomes, cationic lipids or cationic polymers complexed with a foreign DNA for transfection. Alternatively they can use physical methods such as microinjection, gene gun delivery or the use of uncomplexed plasmid DNA. The nonviral methods are safer but less efficient and some can cause immunological reactions [47] (Partridge and Oreffo, 2004). Another approach is to use matrices for gene or protein delivery. These provide a stable and sustained release include allogenic cortical bone and synthetic substances [9] (Braddok et al, 2001; Saito and Takaota, 2003).

Gene delivery can be direct in vivo or indirect ex vivo. The direct method involves transferring the genetic material into the target somatic cell in vivo. This is technically simpler to perform in a clinical setting. The indirect technique involves removal of cells from the patient, genetic modifications of the cells ex vivo and return of the cells to the patient. This is technically more complex but is relatively safer and allows for selection of cells for gene expression [68] (Wu et al, 2003). Lieberman et al have shown regional cell and gene therapy using BMP-2 producing bone marrow cells on the repair of segmental bone defects in rats. Brietbant et al have cultured periosteal cells retrovirally transduced with BMP-7 in a polyglycolic acid (PGA) scaffold in a critical sized calvarial defect model in rabbits [11]. Olmsted et al have indicated the potential to generate human bone marrow stromal cells expressing BMP-2 by adenoviral infection [45].

BONE REPAIR

The aim has been to provide the reconstructed segment with appropriate initial mechanical properties while encouraging new bone formation in the region. Bone formation by BMSC transplanted into small animals was first demonstrated by Friedenstein in 1966. Implanting BMSC combined with 3D mineralized bioceramic scaffolds subcutaneously into immunodeficient mice can be used to assess bone formation. Autologous BMSC and bioceramic composites have been used to repair experimentally induced bone defects (full thickness gaps in tibial diaphysis) in sheep. Gross morphology, radiographs and histology show complete integration of ceramic with bone and good functional recovery. Culture expanded bone marrow cells can heal a segmental bone defect following reimplantation (Kadiyala et al, 1997) and can give rise to osteogenic tissue within diffusion chambers in a variety of animal species (Gundle et al, 1995) [24, 27]. Similar results with carol scaffold and hydroxyapatite and beta tri-calcium phosphate scaffold have been described. The osteoprogenitor cells were harvested from the iliac crest and expanded in culture.

Based on the above pre-clinical trials, in 2001, autologous osteoprogenitor cells isolated from the bone marrow of patients and expanded in vitro were delivered in vivo with a microporous hydroxyapatite scaffold. This was for patients with 4-7 cm bone detects for whom a traditional therapeutic alternative was difficult or had previously failed. External fixation was provided initially for stability. By the second month, abundant callus formation along the implant and good integration at the interface with the bone were observed. No major complication was observed. All patients recovered limb function in 6-12 months. In cases where bone defects occur in positions requiring dynamic strength, such as long bones of the legs, an alternative to using an external fixator is BMP and polymer composites combined with solid materials with good affinity for bone. For instance a titanium implant with a porous surface on which the BMP and polymer composites are placed. This can be implanted into the bone defect and bone will form on the composite (Saito and Takaota, 2003).

REFERENCES

[1] Abrahamsson, S. O., and Lohmander, S.: Differential effects of insulin-like growth factor-I on matrix and DNA synthesis in various regions and types of rabbit tendons. *J. Orthop. Res.,* 14(3): 370-6, 1996.

[2] Andriano, K. P.; Tabata, Y.; Ikada, Y.; and Heller, J.: In vitro and in vivo comparison of bulk and surface hydrolysis in absorbable polymer scaffolds for tissue engineering. *J. Biomed. Mater Res.,* 48(5): 602-12, 1999.

[3] Archibald, S. J.; Shefner, J.; Krarup, C.; and Madison, R. D.: Monkey median nerve repaired by nerve graft or collagen nerve guide tube. *J. Neurosci.,* 15(5 Pt 2): 4109-23, 1995.

[4] Banes, A. J.; Tsuzaki, M.; Hu, P.; Brigman, B.; Brown, T.; Almekinders, L.; Lawrence, W. T.; and Fischer, T.: PDGF-BB, IGF-I and mechanical load stimulate DNA synthesis in avian tendon fibroblasts in vitro. *J. Biomech.,* 28(12): 1505-13, 1995.

[5] Basile, P. et al.: Freeze-dried tendon allografts as tissue-engineering scaffolds for Gdf5 gene delivery. *Mol. Ther,* 16(3): 466-73, 2008.

[6] Bianco, P.; Riminucci, M.; Gronthos, S.; and Robey, P. G.: Bone marrow stromal stem cells: nature, biology, and potential applications. *Stem Cells,* 19(3): 180-92, 2001.

[7] Boden, S. D.: Bioactive factors for bone tissue engineering. *Clin. Orthop. Relat Res.,* (367 Suppl): S84-94, 1999.

[8] Boyer, M. I.; Goldfarb, C. A.; and Gelberman, R. H.: Recent progress in flexor tendon healing. The modulation of tendon healing with rehabilitation variables. *J. Hand Ther,* 18(2): 80-5; quiz 86, 2005.

[9] Braddock, M.; Houston, P.; Campbell, C.; and Ashcroft, P.: Born again bone: tissue engineering for bone repair. *News Physiol Sci,* 16: 208-13, 2001.

[10] Brandt, J.; Dahlin, L. B.; and Lundborg, G.: Autologous tendons used as grafts for bridging peripheral nerve defects. *J. Hand Surg. [Br],* 24(3): 284-90, 1999.

[11] Breitbart, A. S.; Grande, D. A.; Mason, J. M.; Barcia, M.; James, T.; and Grant, R. T.: Gene-enhanced tissue engineering: applications for bone healing using cultured periosteal cells transduced retrovirally with the BMP-7 gene. *Ann. Plast. Surg,* 42(5): 488-95, 1999.

[12] Brekke, J. H., and Toth, J. M.: Principles of tissue engineering applied to programmable osteogenesis. *J. Biomed. Mater Res.,* 43(4): 380-98, 1998.

[13] Brigham, P. A., and McLoughlin, E.: Burn incidence and medical care use in the United States: estimates, trends, and data sources. *J. Burn Care Rehabil,* 17(2): 95-107, 1996.

[14] Cancedda, R.; Bianchi, G.; Derubeis, A.; and Quarto, R.: Cell therapy for bone disease: a review of current status. *Stem Cells,* 21(5): 610-9, 2003.

[15] Chong, A. K., and Chang, J.: Tissue engineering for the hand surgeon: a clinical perspective. *J. Hand Surg [Am],* 31(3): 349-58, 2006.

[16] Cooper, R. R., and Misol, S.: Tendon and ligament insertion. A light and electron microscopic study. *J. Bone Joint Surg Am,* 52(1): 1-20, 1970.

[17] DeFranco, M. J.; Derwin, K.; and Iannotti, J. P.: New therapies in tendon reconstruction. *J. Am. Acad. Orthop Surg,* 12(5): 298-304, 2004.

[18] Gelberman, R. H., and Manske, P. R.: Factors influencing flexor tendon adhesions. *Hand Clin.,* 1(1): 35-42, 1985.

[19] Gelberman, R. H.; Thomopoulos, S.; Sakiyama-Elbert, S. E.; Das, R.; and Silva, M. J.: The early effects of sustained platelet-derived growth factor administration on the functional and structural properties of repaired intrasynovial flexor tendons: an in vivo biomechanic study at 3 weeks in canines. *J. Hand Surg [Am],* 32(3): 373-9, 2007.

[20] Glasby, M. A.; Gschmeissner, S. E.; Huang, C. L.; and De Souza, B. A.: Degenerated muscle grafts used for peripheral nerve repair in primates. *J. Hand Surg. [Br],* 11(3): 347-51, 1986.

[21] Govender, S. et al.: Recombinant human bone morphogenetic protein-2 for treatment of open tibial fractures: a prospective, controlled, randomized study of four hundred and fifty patients. *J. Bone Joint Surg Am.,* 84-A(12): 2123-34, 2002.

[22] Grigolo, B.; Roseti, L.; Fiorini, M.; Fini, M.; Giavaresi, G.; Aldini, N. N.; Giardino, R.; and Facchini, A.: Transplantation of chondrocytes seeded on a hyaluronan derivative (hyaff-11) into cartilage defects in rabbits. *Biomaterials,* 22(17): 2417-24, 2001.

[23] Guenard, V.; Kleitman, N.; Morrissey, T. K.; Bunge, R. P.; and Aebischer, P.: Syngeneic Schwann cells derived from adult nerves seeded in semipermeable guidance channels enhance peripheral nerve regeneration. *J. Neurosci.,* 12(9): 3310-20, 1992.

[24] Gundle, R.; Joyner, C. J.; and Triffitt, J. T.: Human bone tissue formation in diffusion chamber culture in vivo by bone-derived cells and marrow stromal fibroblastic cells. *Bone,* 16(6): 597-601, 1995.

[25] Hatano, I.; Suga, T.; Diao, E.; Peimer, C. A.; and Howard, C.: Adhesions from flexor tendon surgery: an animal study comparing surgical techniques. *J. Hand Surg [Am],* 25(2): 252-9, 2000.

[26] Jones, I.; Currie, L.; and Martin, R.: A guide to biological skin substitutes. *Br. J. Plast Surg,* 55(3): 185-93, 2002.

[27] Kadiyala, S.; Young, R. G.; Thiede, M. A.; and Bruder, S. P.: Culture expanded canine mesenchymal stem cells possess osteochondrogenic potential in vivo and in vitro. *Cell Transplant,* 6(2): 125-34, 1997.

[28] Kale, S.; Biermann, S.; Edwards, C.; Tarnowski, C.; Morris, M.; and Long, M. W.: Three-dimensional cellular development is essential for ex vivo formation of human bone. *Nat. Biotechnol.,* 18(9): 954-8, 2000.

[29] Kashiwagi, K.; Mochizuki, Y.; Yasunaga, Y.; Ishida, O.; Deie, M.; and Ochi, M.: Effects of transforming growth factor-beta 1 on the early stages of healing of the Achilles tendon in a rat model. *Scand J. Plast Reconstr Surg Hand Surg,* 38(4): 193-7, 2004.

[30] Koeberle, P. D., and Bahr, M.: Growth and guidance cues for regenerating axons: where have they gone? *J. Neurobiol,* 59(1): 162-80, 2004.

[31] Koob, T. J.: Biomimetic approaches to tendon repair. *Comp. Biochem. Physiol. A Mol. Integr Physiol.,* 133(4): 1171-92, 2002.

[32] Kruyt, M. C.; van Gaalen, S. M.; Oner, F. C.; Verbout, A. J.; de Bruijn, J. D.; and Dhert, W. J.: Bone tissue engineering and spinal fusion: the potential of hybrid constructs by combining osteoprogenitor cells and scaffolds. *Biomaterials,* 25(9): 1463-73, 2004.
[33] Langer, R., and Vacanti, J. P.: Tissue engineering. *Science,* 260(5110): 920-6, 1993.
[34] Lee, C. H.; Singla, A.; and Lee, Y.: Biomedical applications of collagen. *Int. J. Pharm.,* 221(1-2): 1-22, 2001.
[35] Lee, K. Y.; Peters, M. C.; Anderson, K. W.; and Mooney, D. J.: Controlled growth factor release from synthetic extracellular matrices. *Nature,* 408(6815): 998-1000, 2000.
[36] LeGeros, R. Z.: Properties of osteoconductive biomaterials: calcium phosphates. *Clin. Orthop. Relat. Res.,* (395): 81-98, 2002.
[37] Lilly, S. I., and Messer, T. M.: Complications after treatment of flexor tendon injuries. *J. Am. Acad. Orthop. Surg.,* 14(7): 387-96, 2006.
[38] Lundborg, G.: A 25-year perspective of peripheral nerve surgery: evolving neuroscientific concepts and clinical significance. *J. Hand Surg [Am],* 25(3): 391-414, 2000.
[39] Lundborg, G.; Dahlin, L.; Dohi, D.; Kanje, M.; and Terada, N.: A new type of "bioartificial" nerve graft for bridging extended defects in nerves. *J. Hand Surg [Br],* 22(3): 299-303, 1997.
[40] Meislin, R. J.; Wiseman, D. M.; Alexander, H.; Cunningham, T.; Linsky, C.; Carlstedt, C.; Pitman, M.; and Casar, R.: A biomechanical study of tendon adhesion reduction using a biodegradable barrier in a rabbit model. *J. Appl. Biomater,* 1(1): 13-9, 1990.
[41] Mentzel, M.; Hoss, H.; Keppler, P.; Ebinger, T.; Kinzl, L.; and Wachter, N. J.: The effectiveness of ADCON-T/N, a new anti-adhesion barrier gel, in fresh divisions of the flexor tendons in Zone II. *J. Hand Surg [Br],* 25(6): 590-2, 2000.
[42] Merzenich, M. M.; Kaas, J. H.; Wall, J.; Nelson, R. J.; Sur, M.; and Felleman, D.: Topographic reorganization of somatosensory cortical areas 3b and 1 in adult monkeys following restricted deafferentation. *Neuroscience,* 8(1): 33-55, 1983.
[43] Mooney, D. J., and Mikos, A. G.: Growing new organs. *Sci Am,* 280(4): 60-5, 1999.
[44] Muschler, G. F.; Nitto, H.; Matsukura, Y.; Boehm, C.; Valdevit, A.; Kambic, H.; Davros, W.; Powell, K.; and Easley, K.: Spine fusion using cell matrix composites enriched in bone marrow-derived cells. *Clin. Orthop. Relat Res,* (407): 102-18, 2003.
[45] Olmsted, E. A.; Blum, J. S.; Rill, D.; Yotnda, P.; Gugala, Z.; Lindsey, R. W.; and Davis, A. R.: Adenovirus-mediated BMP2 expression in human bone marrow stromal cells. *J. Cell Biochem.,* 82(1): 11-21, 2001.
[46] Oreffo, R. O., and Triffitt, J. T.: Future potentials for using osteogenic stem cells and biomaterials in orthopedics. *Bone,* 25(2 Suppl): 5S-9S, 1999.
[47] Partridge, K. A., and Oreffo, R. O.: Gene delivery in bone tissue engineering: progress and prospects using viral and nonviral strategies. *Tissue Eng,* 10(1-2): 295-307, 2004.
[48] Pennisi, E.: Tending tender tendons. *Science,* 295(5557): 1011, 2002.
[49] Perry, C. R.: Bone repair techniques, bone graft, and bone graft substitutes. *Clin Orthop Relat Res,* (360): 71-86, 1999.
[50] Petite, H.; Viateau, V.; Bensaid, W.; Meunier, A.; de Pollak, C.; Bourguignon, M.; Oudina, K.; Sedel, L.; and Guillemin, G.: Tissue-engineered bone regeneration. *Nat. Biotechnol.,* 18(9): 959-63, 2000.

[51] Quirk, R. A.; Chan, W. C.; Davies, M. C.; Tendler, S. J.; and Shakesheff, K. M.: Poly(L-lysine)-GRGDS as a biomimetic surface modifier for poly(lactic acid). *Biomaterials,* 22(8): 865-72, 2001.

[52] Raivich, G., and Kreutzberg, G. W.: Peripheral nerve regeneration: role of growth factors and their receptors. *Int.J. Dev. Neurosci.,* 11(3): 311-24, 1993.

[53] Sakkers, R. J.; Dalmeyer, R. A.; de Wijn, J. R.; and van Blitterswijk, C. A.: Use of bone-bonding hydrogel copolymers in bone: an in vitro and in vivo study of expanding PEO-PBT copolymers in goat femora. *J. Biomed. Mater Res.,* 49(3): 312-8, 2000.

[54] Shin, H.; Jo, S.; and Mikos, A. G.: Biomimetic materials for tissue engineering. *Biomaterials,* 24(24): 4353-64, 2003.

[55] Silva, M. J.; Boyer, M. I.; and Gelberman, R. H.: Recent progress in flexor tendon healing. *J. Orthop. Sci.,* 7(4): 508-14, 2002.

[56] Stewart, K.; Walsh, S.; Screen, J.; Jefferiss, C. M.; Chainey, J.; Jordan, G. R.; and Beresford, J. N.: Further characterization of cells expressing STRO-1 in cultures of adult human bone marrow stromal cells. *J. Bone Miner Res.,* 14(8): 1345-56, 1999.

[57] Tepper, O. M.; Capla, J. M.; Galiano, R. D.; Ceradini, D. J.; Callaghan, M. J.; Kleinman, M. E.; and Gurtner, G. C.: Adult vasculogenesis occurs through in situ recruitment, proliferation, and tubulization of circulating bone marrow-derived cells. *Blood,* 105(3): 1068-77, 2005.

[58] Thomopoulos, S.; Harwood, F. L.; Silva, M. J.; Amiel, D.; and Gelberman, R. H.: Effect of several growth factors on canine flexor tendon fibroblast proliferation and collagen synthesis in vitro. *J. Hand Surg. [Am],* 30(3): 441-7, 2005.

[59] Tohill, M., and Terenghi, G.: Stem-cell plasticity and therapy for injuries of the peripheral nervous system. *Biotechnol. Appl. Biochem.,* 40(Pt 1): 17-24, 2004.

[60] Tong, X. J.; Hirai, K.; Shimada, H.; Mizutani, Y.; Izumi, T.; Toda, N.; and Yu, P.: Sciatic nerve regeneration navigated by laminin-fibronectin double coated biodegradable collagen grafts in rats. *Brain Res.,* 663(1): 155-62, 1994.

[61] Towler, D. A., and Gelberman, R. H.: The alchemy of tendon repair: a primer for the (S)mad scientist. *J. Clin. Invest,* 116(4): 863-6, 2006.

[62] Urist, M. R.: Bone: formation by autoinduction. *Science,* 150(698): 893-9, 1965.

[63] Walton, R. L.; Brown, R. E.; Matory, W. E., Jr.; Borah, G. L.; and Dolph, J. L.: Autogenous vein graft repair of digital nerve defects in the finger: a retrospective clinical study. *Plast Reconstr. Surg,* 84(6): 944-9; discussion 950-2, 1989.

[64] Weber, R. A.; Breidenbach, W. C.; Brown, R. E.; Jabaley, M. E.; and Mass, D. P.: A randomized prospective study of polyglycolic acid conduits for digital nerve reconstruction in humans. *Plast Reconstr. Surg,* 106(5): 1036-45; discussion 1046-8, 2000.

[65] Whitaker, M. J.; Quirk, R. A.; Howdle, S. M.; and Shakesheff, K. M.: Growth factor release from tissue engineering scaffolds. *J. Pharm. Pharmacol,* 53(11): 1427-37, 2001.

[66] Whitlock, P. W.; Smith, T. L.; Poehling, G. G.; Shilt, J. S.; and Van Dyke, M.: A naturally derived, cytocompatible, and architecturally optimized scaffold for tendon and ligament regeneration. *Biomaterials,* 28(29): 4321-9, 2007.

[67] Whitworth, I. H.; Brown, R. A.; Dore, C. J.; Anand, P.; Green, C. J.; and Terenghi, G.: Nerve growth factor enhances nerve regeneration through fibronectin grafts. *J. Hand Surg. [Br],* 21(4): 514-22, 1996.

[68] Wu, D.; Razzano, P.; and Grande, D. A.: Gene therapy and tissue engineering in repair of the musculoskeletal system. *J. Cell Biochem.,* 88(3): 467-81, 2003.
[69] Yow, K. H.; Ingram, J.; Korossis, S. A.; Ingham, E.; and Homer-Vanniasinkam, S.: Tissue engineering of vascular conduits. *Br. J. Surg,* 93(6): 652-61, 2006.
[70] Zhang, W. J.; Liu, W.; Cui, L.; and Cao, Y.: Tissue engineering of blood vessel. *J. Cell Mol. Med.,* 11(5): 945-57, 2007.

Manuscript reviewed by Mr Manish Agarwal, FRCS (Orth), Department of Trauma and Orthopaedics, Pennine Acute Hospitals NHS Trust, North Manchester General Hospital, Manchester, M8 5RB, UK

In: Stem Cell Research: New Developments
Editors: Hiroshi Tanaka and Michael C. F. Chang
ISBN: 978-1-61942-081-6

Chapter 4

NEW INSIGHTS IN THE DEVELOPMENT OF BIOLOGICAL CHIMERAS: GENOMIC INSTABILITY AND EPITHELIAL CHIMERISM AFTER HEMATOPOIETIC STEM CELL TRANSPLANTATION

Alexandros Spyridonidis[1,*], Yannis Metaxas[2], Maria Themeli[1], Hartmut Bertz[2], Nicholas Zoumbos[1] and Juergen Finke[2]
[1]Division of Hematology, University of Patras Medical Center, Patras, Greece
[2]Department of Hematology and Oncology,
Albert-Ludwigs University Medical Center, Freiburg, Germany

ABSTRACT

Allogeneic hematopoietic stem cell transplantation (allo-HSCT) in humans results in true biological chimeras. While circulating hematopoietic and immune cells and their tissue derivatives (e.g. Kupffer cells, Langerhans cells) become donor genotype after transplantation, other cells remain recipient in origin. This unphysiological formation of biological chimeras is not free of consequences. The first sequel which has been recognized in the development of chimerical organisms after allo-HSCT is the graft versus host reaction, in which the new developed immune cells from the graft recognize the host's epithelial cells as foreign and kill them. There is now accumulating evidence that there are also other consequences in the co-existence of two genetically distinct populations in the transplant recipient. First, epithelial cells with donor-derived genotype emerge. Second, epithelial tissues of the host acquire genomic alterations. The current chapter discusses existing data on these recently discovered phenomena and focuses on their pathogenesis, clinical significance and therapeutic implications.

* Correspondence: A. Spyridonidis, M.D. Division of Hematology, University of Patras Medical Center, 26500 Rio/Patras, Greece. Tel: +30-2610-999247. Fax: +30-2610-993950; E-mail: spyridonidis@med.upatras.gr.
Supported by Landesstiftung Baden Württemberg.

INTRODUCTION

Bone marrow (BM) consists one of the largest organs of our body. BM in adults has a weight of about 2.6 kg as compared to the 1.6 kg of the liver. The function of BM as the hematopoietic organ was first recognized in 1868 by Neumann in Germany and Bizzazero in Italy [1, 2]. Nearly 70 years later, Lorenz and colleagues showed that the hematopoietic activity of BM is transplantable by demonstrating that mice receiving an intravenous infusion of BM could be protected from the lethal effects of ionizing irradiation on hematopoiesis [3]. The first attempts to translate this exciting discovery into the clinic were disappointing [4]. Further research in bigger animals led to the first successful clinical BM transplantations (BMT) in the late ′60s, especially from the group of E. Donall Thomas who was therefore acknowledged with the Nobel Prize in 1990 [4]. The last 30 years BMT has become a standard treatment for many hematological malignancies and is now increasingly used also as immunotherapy for the treatment of solid tumours [4, 5]. Continuous experimental and clinical research led to further characterization and identification of the hematopoietic stem cells (HSC) within the BM leading to the refinement of this procedure which is now called Hematopoietic Stem Cell Transplantation (HSCT) or Hematopoietic Cell Transplantation (HCT).

As it is known, during allogeneic HCT (allo-HCT) the patient-recipient receives a preparative conditioning regimen (e.g. chemotherapy, radiotherapy) to destroy his hematopoiesis and immune system. This practice is followed by the administration of HSC harvested from the donor. The donor's HSC engraft, proliferate and finally reconstitute hematopoiesis in the recipient. The result is the creation of a biological chimera, a term used to describe the presence of tissues of different genetic origin in the same organism. The hematopoietic cells derive from the donor whilst the other tissues (e.g. epithelium) are genetically derived from the patient-recipient. This unphysiological formation of biological chimeras is not free of consequences. The first sequel which has been recognized in the development of chimeric organisms after allo-HCT is the graft versus host reaction (GvHR) in which the new developed immune cells from the graft recognize the host's epithelial cells as foreign and kill them [6]. There is now accumulating evidence that there are also other consequences in the co-existence of two genetically distinct populations in the transplant recipient. First, epithelial cells with donor-derived genotype emerge, a phenomenon which was initially misinterpreted and falsely described as "stem cell plasticity". Second, epithelial tissues of the host acquire genomic alterations. In the following we discuss existing data on these recently discovered phenomena occurring after allogeneic HCT and focus on their pathogenesis, clinical significance and their clinical and therapeutic implications.

A. EPITHELIAL CHIMERISM AFTER ALLOGENEIC HCT

Since the first experiments in mice performed by Lorenz et al. [3] researchers continued to perform murine and other animal bone marrow transplantations in order to understand this procedure in detail. The research was mainly focused on the hematopoiesis and immune-reconstitution in the transplanted animals and little attention has been paid to the effects of the Hematopoietic Cell Transplantation (HCT) on the non-hematopoietic tissues such as epithelium. A surprising result in 1998 revolutionized the bone marrow transplantation field and stem cell research. Ferrari et al. [7] presumed that fibroblasts, cells which normally make connective tissue, could also transdifferentiate to muscle cells. Therefore, the researchers injected purified fibroblasts in chemically-damaged muscles of mice and as controls they injected BM cells devoid of fibroblasts. To their surprise, new muscle cells were generated only in the mice that got the BM without the fibroblasts. This finding led to the speculation that BM is the source of tissue-specific stem cells. Indeed, a series of experimental hematopoietic cell transplantations performed in animals soon after the report by Ferrari et al. showed that the infusion of unfractionated bone marrow cells or bone-marrow cell subsets with high hematopoietic activity into irradiated mice, gave rise to hepatocytes, skin cells, pneumocytes, intestinal epithelium, pancreas cells, skeletal muscle, myocardium, neurons, and endothelium of donor origin[8-12]. Typically, in those experiments donor cells expressed either green fluorescent protein (GFP) or β-galactosidase (β-gal) and tissue-specific donor-derived cells after the transplantation were detected by expression of these markers in the tissue(s) of interest. These experimental animal results led to the exploration of similar events in humans. In humans, scientists mostly studied sex-mismatched allogeneic transplanted women and searched for Y+/tissue-specific cells. Indeed, many studies suggested the generation of donor-derived hepatocytes, cholangiocytes and colonic cells, among other epithelial cells [13-15]. Moreover, some of them claimed that up to 17% of the epithelial cells found were of donor origin. These initial reports proposing the robust generation of epithelial cells after murine or human HCT were published in reputable journals, and revealed probable new aspects of ontogenesis while also engendered expectations for novel therapies both in the scientific and the popular press. However, at the same time a significant number of studies failed to detect donor-derived epithelial cells after allo-HCT in similar experimental systems [16-18]. The debate on the developmental potential of adult hematopoietic stem cells became even more confusing since terms implicating mechanisms, such as "plasticity" and "transdifferentiation", were used in order to describe the above mentioned observations. To minimize confusion scientists started to use more precise terms in order to describe their findings. Epithelial chimerism or tissue-specific chimerism, like "myocardial chimerism", is used when cells obtained from hematopoietic tissues of a donor are transplanted into a host, and then marked donor cells are identified as epithelial cells in the host. On the other hand, the term "plasticity" is a functional characterization and is used only if stringent criteria are fulfilled, such as robust detection of epithelial chimerism, documentation of functionality of the chimerical epithelial cells and clonal analysis of the chimerical cells to verify their origin from a hematopoietic stem cell [19].

These new findings in HCT opened a new and very exciting era for intensive research for both stem cell biologists and clinicians. Moreover, it raised a significant number of questions to be answered. Does epithelial chimerism after HSC represent a real phenomenon? If epithelial chimerism really exists, is it an incidental by-product of transplantation without ancillary biological significance or does it have any clinical consequences? How does epithelial chimerism after HCT occur and which patterns does it follow? Are the chimerical epithelial cells functional and may HCT contribute to non-hematopoietic tissue repair? Adult hematopoietic stem cells do really transdifferentiate into non-hematopoietic lineages?

Epithelial Chimerism after Allogeneic HCT Is Real

Initial studies claiming to detect epithelial chimerism (or even more plasticity) after HCT were treated with doubt, because of methodological limitations. Alternative explanations were given for some of the suspected chimeric events found within histological sections. In animal models, the unanticipated endogenous β-gal signal might lead to false positive results when ROSA mice are used as donors for HCT [20, 21]. Lymphocytes entering epithelial tissues via the circulation, might act as "contaminants" and be easily mistaken as donor-derived epithelial cells, if the expression of hematopoietic markers is not examined. Tissue macrophages can down-regulate the expression of hematopoietic specific markers (CD45+) and therefore escape their detection as hematopoietic cells, if appropriate macrophage specific markers are not used [22]. Furthermore, in recent years it became clear that microscopic examinations of tissues may be tricky. Tissue is a compact, three-dimensional structure and this has to be taken in mind when interpretating the results of microscopic examinations. Indeed, overlapping cells in histological sections may produce artefacts showing marker co-localisation apparently within the same cell, although the markers are actually expressed in different cells [23]. Furthermore, the detection of tissue chimerism in female patients by the Y-chromosome is complicated by the fact that Y-chromosome material has been also found in maternal tissues from women which had a male fetus or had received blood transfusions from male donors [24]. These studies clearly show that detection of epithelial chimerism after HCT is not straightforward and requires unequivocal detection systems, like the use of combined stains within a single section and the use of laser scanning confocal and deconvolution microscopic methods for three dimensional analysis.

Despite the above methodological limitations, several carefully designed studies in recent years demonstrated that epithelial chimerism after HCT may in fact occur. In an elegant study Spyridonidis et al [23] applied a three-dimensional analysis on single colon sections from transplanted women after triple stain with donor specific, epithelial-specific and hematopoietic-specific markers, and could clearly show that epithelial chimerism after human HCT is a real phenomenon. This study was in accordance to other studies which strongly implied similar events in a human setting [15, 23, 25-27]. Because, as mentioned before, cells can wrap one another making tissue analysis very difficult, scientists further analysed isolated single epithelial cells for their origin after transplantation. Tran et al [28] and Metaxas et al [29] found that isolated buccal epithelial cells obtained by oral scraping from allo-transplanted women, contained the Y-chromosome within their nucleus, as detected by FISH, suggesting that HCT results in generation of individual epithelial cells with donor-derived genotype.

Are the Chimeric Epithelial Cells Functional?

The finding that transplanted cells derived from adult hematopoietic tissues are directly involved in the generation of epithelial cells raises the question of whether the generated cells are functional and whether HCT could functionally contribute to tissue repair by replacing damaged epithelia. In some animal HCT models, liver cells, pneumocytes and kidney tubular epithelial cells bearing donor specific DNA were found to express mRNA-albumin, mRNA-surfactant B and a specific cytochrome P450 enzyme (CYP1A2) respectively, indicating an appropriate cellular function [14]. However, since these cells appeared as isolated single cells it seems unlikely that they play an important role in the homeostasis, regeneration and function of epithelial tissue, at least in the setting of clinical HCT. In 2000, Lagasse et al [30] went a step further by demonstrating a robust and functional epithelial chimerism in a mice model of fatal hereditary tyrosinemia type I. The researchers performed transplantations of purified hematopoietic stem cells from ROSA wild-type mice to transgenic mice homozygous deficient for fumarylacetoacetate hydrolase (FAH–/-). These mice show progressive liver failure and renal tubular damage unless treated with 2-(2-nitro-4-trifluoro-methylbenzyol)-1,3-cyclohexanedione (NTBC). Three weeks after transplantation, they discontinued NTBC to allow selection of liver repopulating cells. They found that in contrast to control mice the transplanted mice survived the NTBC withdrawal and seemed clinically healthy. The liver of the survived mice revealed a high amount of donor-derived cells, presented as ß-gal+ nodes within damaged liver and making about 30–50% of the liver mass. Taken together, the results indicated that the donor-derived chimeric cells were responsible for the survival of the mice. The restoration of liver function through HCT in mice suffering from a lethal liver disease is a ground-breaking experiment, which has been reproduced in several laboratories [31, 32], and proves that murine HC-derived cells are directly involved in the generation of functional hepatocytes. In a similar experimental model, Hess et al [33] could restore damaged pancreatic function of streptozocin treated mice by transplantation of *c-kit*+ BM stem cells. Many studies since then were performed in order to find out the mechanism by which HCT may restore liver and pancreas function and rescue the mice. In the FAH-/- model hematopoietic cells were involved in the generation of functional hepatocyte-like cells through fusion. In the streptozocin treated mice the authors suggested that the HCT initiated the proliferation of endogenous pancreatic cells. A "paracrine effect" of BM-derived cells through release of cytokines within the damaged organ, or induction of neovascularization from BM-derived endothelial cells [34] are two possible mechanisms which may explain how the transplantation induced the endogenous tissue repair processes.

Aiming to find out whether besides murine HSC also human HSC has the potential to restore damaged organ function, Wang et al. [35] examined liver repopulation by human HSC in xenograft models. The authors treated NOD/SCID and NOD/SCID/β_2 microglobulin-null mice with carbon tetrachloride (CCl_4) in order to induce liver damage and then transplanted them with highly purified human hematopoietic stem cells. One month after transplantation the researchers detected human albumin in the serum of the mice, indicating that human derived albumin-secreting cells emerged. When they analyzed tissue sections of the liver, they detected human albumin along with human DNA sequences on hepatocyte-like liver cells. Almeida-Porada et al [36] performed similar studies in a mammalian non-injury model as they analyzed liver sections of sheep having undergone *in utero* HCT from human cells. As in the study of Wang, the researchers detected human hepatocyte-like cells and human albumin in the transplanted sheep.

Such reports suggesting that HCT may functionally contribute to non-hematopoietic tissue regeneration and restoration of damaged organ, stimulated investigators to seek rapid clinical translation. Human clinical trials investigating regenerative properties of HC-derived adult cells have already been started, especially in patients with heart diseases [37, 38]. However, for the clinical application of hematopoietic cells for regenerative purposes much remains to be determined. Whether observations made in selected experimental models also happen in humans is unclear. More importantly, the exact mechanism into how transplanted cells may actually improve organ function has not been elucidated. On the other side, such procedures may in fact cause opposite effects than tissue regeneration. In a very elegant study in mice, Houghton et al. [39] showed that transplanted bone marrow cells may transform into cancer cells under conditions of chronic inflammatory signals. The researchers used a Helicobacter felis (H. felis) C57BL/6 mouse strain which develops severe chronic gastritis and intestinal metaplasia after infection with H. felis [40]. These mice underwent bone marrow transplantation from ROSA26 transgenic mice expressing a non-mammalian β-galactosidase enzyme, so that bone marrow cells could be tracked by X-galactosidase (Xgal) staining. After hematopoietic reconstitution, the C57BL/6 mice were infected with H. felis, resulting in chronic inflammation of their gastric mucosa. The researchers observed that over time the dysplasia of the epithelium increased in severity, finally ending in the development of gastric cancer. When they examined sections of the gastric carcinoma they noticed that the majority of the glands stained blue with X-gal indicating their donor origin. A very recent study by Cogle et al [41] supported these results, even in a human setting, although the mechanisms suggested for the occurrence of the phenomenon differed between the two studies. Houghton et al based on their observations of the numerous donor-derived cancer cells proposed the bone marrow as a source for epithelial cancer, whereas Cogle et al for the exact opposite reason thought that bone-marrow cells rather adopt a cancerous phenotype via developmental mimicry.

Factors Contributing to the Development of Epithelial Chimerism after Allogeneic HCT

Epithelial chimerism after HCT is a rare and focal event with less than 1%, and probably less than 0.1%, of the overall tissue epithelial cells to contain donor genetic material. The reported higher incidence of epithelial chimerism found in some human studies (up to 17%) is most likely a methodological artefact resulting from counting the intraepithelial lymphocytes within the tissue as donor-derived epithelial cells. Although epithelial chimerism has been found in most of the epithelial tissues tested irrespective of the presence or absence of tissue damage, it seems that injury and high cell turnover play a role both in the occurrence and extent of chimeric events [8, 30, 42]. Most studies suggest that the more the degree of the tissue damage the greater the percentage of the detected chimeric cells [29, 42-44]. For example the percentage of the buccal chimeric cells in the allo-transplanted patients has been found to significantly correlate with the degree of oral mucositis in the early post transplantation period [29]. A recent study aimed to determine the degree of tissue damage required to produce chimeric events [45]. They used a mouse model having undergone allogeneic HCT and estimated the chimeric lung epithelial cells after various doses of irradiation. They concluded that only doses causing apparent tissue damage led to emergence of chimeric lung cells. A possible scenario explaining these results is that bone-marrow derived cells support tissue homeostasis when the extent of damage overwhelms the endogenous capacity of tissue regeneration.

Another critical factor for the development of chimerism in non-hematopoietic tissues is the type of tissue itself. It is suggested that the presence as well as the extent of this phenomenon is taking place in a tissue-dependent manner [46], with some tissues favouring the development of chimerical cells and others not.

To further support this notion, a recent study addressed the presence of donor-derived epithelial cells in multiple organs after HCT in murine embryos. They concluded that the different types of analyzed tissues showed variable degrees of chimerical events, although hematopoietic engraftment was always the same [47]. This could be attributed to micro-environmental cues provided by the tissue, which could induce a cell fate change in bone-marrow derived cells [48, 49]. Finally, there could be other factors affecting the emergence of epithelial chimerism, such as time elapsed after HCT. Herzog et al. [45] in mice and Metaxas et al. [29] in humans showed that time after HCT correlated positively with the degree of chimeric epithelial cells detected. Whatever the factors contributing to epithelial chimerism might be, they shed no light on the exact mechanisms responsible for this phenomenon.

Plasticity of Bone-Marrow Derived Cells?

Krause et al [50] demonstrated that a single cell capable of long-term reconstitution of hematopoiesis in lethally irradiated mice was also capable of differentiating into epithelial cells of the liver, lung, gastrointestinal tract and skin. The researchers used a membrane bound dye (PKH26) along with the stem cell markers CD34 and SCA-1 to track hematopoietic stem cells in sex-mismatched serial transplantations. After transplanting a first series of female mice with such cells isolated from male donors and establishing long-term hematopoiesis in them, they subsequently transplanted single hematopoietic stem cells from their bone marrow to a second series of female mice.

They sacrificed those secondary recipients after having established long-term repopulation of the hematopoietic system and evaluated different epithelial tissues for the presence of donor-derived non-hematopoietic cells. They detected such cells in different percentages, with the higher numbers being present in the alveoli of the lungs. These results suggested that in the adult bone marrow resides a cell(s) capable of both reconstituting the hematopoietic lineage and differentiating to non-hematopoietic cells, making the study of Krause et al. the best example of possible plasticity potential of hematopoietic stem cells. However, even this elegant study had some limitations and could not fulfil the previously mentioned criteria for demonstration of plasticity.

First, there was no 3D analysis of the examined tissues and there was no analysis of single chimeric cells; therefore overlapping events and hematopoietic "contaminants" residing within the examined tissue could not be unequivocally excluded. Second, there was no detection of robust epithelial chimerism. Third, although the researchers searched for tissue-specific genes, there was no clear evidence regarding the function of the chimeric cells. Fourth, there was no clonal analysis of the chimeric cells. And finally, the conclusion that "transdifferentiation" occurred, which was based on the detection of donor-derived epithelial cells after transplantation of a single hematopoietic cell, is not beyond question, since contaminants in the purified cell population cannot be entirely excluded. Taken together, the study of Krause et al lies very close, but the unambiguous proof of epithelial chimerism after HCT due to developmental plasticity and transdifferentiation of hematopoietic cells has not been clearly given.

Transdifferentiation is observed in lower vertebrates [51] and in some in vitro experiments with adult mammalian cells, but has been never clearly and unequivocally demonstrated that such an event could also occur naturally *in vivo*. Recently, Takahashi et al

[52] went a step further to this direction by demonstrating that differentiated fibroblasts can re-differentiate *in vitro* to embryonic-like stem cells, which are subsequent able to give rise *in vivo* to whole mice when injected to blastocysts.

Now other studies emerge in accordance to this new concept [53, 54], and it remains to be seen, if this phenomenon could take place in a large scale setting in *in vivo* experiments.

Possible Mechanisms Underlying Epithelial Chimerism

Other mechanisms have been suggested in order to explain how epithelial chimerism after HCT occurs. Avital et al [55] and Ratajczak et al [56] found cells in the BM and peripheral blood that express various early markers for hepatocytes (albumin, HNF-4, C/Eba, CYP3A2, CK19, fetoprotein) myocytes (Myf-5, MyoD), and neurons (GFAP, nestin), suggesting that tissue specific progenitors may exist in the BM and may also circulate in the blood. Others speculated that a universal type of stem cell, akin to an embryonic stem cell, exists in adult BM. Jiang et al. isolated "multipotent adult progenitor cells" (MAPCs) in the murine and human bone marrow capable to differentiate both in vitro and in vivo to various cell types such as muscle, cartilage, bone, liver, and different types of neurons and brain cells [57]. However, this work has not been replicated from other groups in its entirety [58] and Jiang et al. recently published some corrections of their initial work regarding mainly the detectable surface proteins of the presumed differentiated progenies of MAPCs [59]. Recently, the group of Ratajczak described another rare population of pluripotent stem cells in adult mice bone marrow [60] and in human cord blood [61] naming them Very Small Embryonic Like cells (VSELs) and having the phenotype CD45-/Lin-/CXCR4+/Oct-4+/Nanog+/SSEA- 1+. [62]. The authors showed that these cells have morphology and a phenotype similar to embryonic stem cells and possess the capacity to differentiate into all three germ lines in cultures *in vitro*. There is evidence that MAPCs and VSELs may be the same cell, as sharing many of their markers [63]. However, it is not unambiguously shown whether this capacity exist in a significant percentage *in vivo* or is induced mainly through *in vitro* manipulation [64].

Another proposed mechanism aiming to explain epithelial chimerism after allogeneic HCT is the fusion of bone-marrow derived stem cells with tissue-specific differentiated cells. However, different studies exploring this probability have yielded contradictory results. Vassilopoulos et al [65] showed that in FAH–/– mice fusion was the principal mechanism for the generation of chimeric liver cells, and Wang et al [66] agreed. However, in uninjured tissues fusion events are shown in a far smaller percentage [11]. Perhaps the liver regeneration in the FAH–/– liver favours the formation of heterokaryons through fusion, which could not be the case in other tissues. Furthermore, other studies in animal models using Cre/lox technology implied that fusion events may generally not occur during the generation of epithelial chimerism [12]. The results of our own group, where we detected only one X-chromosome in chimeric Y-chromosome positive buccal cells after male to female transplantation, were consisted with non-fusion mechanism for the generation of epithelial chimerism in humans [67] However, both studies have serious limitations since the Cre-recombinase enzyme is not expressed in all cells and X-chromosomes could be lost after cell fusion [35, 68].

Recent findings suggest a novel mechanism explaining epithelial chimerism after allogeneic HCT. Jang et al [8] found that when murine hematopoietic stem cells, enriched through phenotypical and functional assays (Fr25lin- PKH+ 2-d homed HSC), were co-cultured with injured liver separated by a barrier they may convert into liver-like cells. In a similar experimental system, Quesenberry et al [69] found that injured lung tissue induced *in vitro* bone marrow cells to express lung proteins. When these *in vitro* converted bone marrow cells were transplanted into lethally irradiated mice they were found again as type II pneumocytes. The group of Quesenberry went a step further and tried to find out which factors from the injured lung tissue induce the ectopic expression of lung proteins on bone marrow derived cells. Ultracentrifugation of the lung-conditioned medium revealed that the fraction able to induce lung-protein expression was the one which contained microvesicles carrying lung-specific mRNA. These microvesicles showed the ability to enter into subpopulations of the marrow cells thus mediating the marrow cell phenotype conversion. The authors suggest that the cell cycle status of the stem cells might relate to the ease of microvesicle cell entry into them. Thus, a possible scenario after HCT is that hematopoietic stem cells engraft in the tissues, incorporate microvesicles containing tissue-specific mRNA released from the tissue in case of injury and alter this way their phenotype leading to the observed epithelial chimerism.

Another mechanism explaining epithelial chimerism after allogeneic HCT which needs further exploration is horizontal gene transfer [70]. In this case, genetic material released from the hematopoietic-derived donor cells will be transferred, incorporated into the nucleus and eventually expressed by the recipient epithelial cell, ultimately leading to the emergence of epithelial cells with donor-derived genome. Horizontal gene transfer is well described in prokaryotic organisms as a mechanism for functional and phenotypic change in order to adapt to different enviromental conditions [71]. Horizontal gene transfer has also been shown in eukaryotic organisms both *in vitro* and *in vivo* [70, 72]. Large fragments of plasmid DNA fed to mice passed into the bloodstream and integrated into the nucleus of white blood cells, spleen and liver cells [73].

Table 1. Studies showing either epithelial chimerism or functionality of chimeric cells or plasticity potential of hematopoietic stem cells in animal and human setting

Epithelial Chimerism		Functional Epithelial Chimerism		Plasticity potential	
animal	human	animal	human	animal	human
Jang et al Ianus et al Mezey et al Harris et al	Alison et al Theise et al Körbling et al Tran et al Metaxas et al Spyridonidis et al	Lagasse et al Wang et al Houghton et al	never shown	Krause et al	never shown

Table 2. Proposed mechanisms for the development of epithelial chimerism

Possible Mechanism	Reference
tissue-specific progenitors in the bone marrow	Avital et al
multipotent adult progenitor cells, very small embryonic like cells	Jiang et al, Ratajczak et al
fusion	Vassilopoulos et al, Wang et al
transdifferentiation of terminally differentiated cells	Brockes et al, Takahashi et al
Horizontal transfer of tissue-specific microvesicles	Quesenberry et al

B. Genomic Instability in Epithelium after Allogeneic HCT

DNA is a reactive molecule and constantly attacked and modified by external and internal agents. A mammalian DNA molecule can undergo about 100.000 modifications per day and replicates with an error rate of one error per 10^{10} nucleotides [76]. Genome integrity is a basic element of the cellular homeostasis. To maintain genome integrity and ensure its stable inheritance during their replication, cells are equipped with several mechanisms, including DNA repair mechanisms, cell-cycle checkpoints and programmed cell death [77]. The term genomic instability (GI) describes the failure to transmit an accurate copy of the entire genome from one cell to its two daughter cells. The existence of genomic instability is a sign of the above mechanisms' failure, and has been correlated with cancer and cancerous transformation [78].

Microsatellites (MS) are short tandem repeat sequences (repeat units range from 1-6 bp in length) dispersed throughout the genome. There are more than 1 million MS loci in the human genome which comprises approximately 3% of the genome. MS are among the most variable types of DNA sequence in the genome. Their polymorphism derives mainly from variability in length rather than in primary sequence. Though highly polymorphic, as their length varies in a population, they are inherited stably and are unique to each individual, which means that the length of a MS is the same in all the cells of the same person [79]. For this reason the detection of different MS polymorphisms with PCR-based assays can be used for linkage mapping, paternity test, forensic purposes as well as for chimerism quantification after allo-HCT [79, 80]. The term MS instability (MSI) describes alterations in the length of a MS locus detected by PCR amplification of an individual's DNA [77]. The detection of MSI is considered to be indicative of a general genomic instability -which means the accumulation of mutations in the cells- and has been related to carcinogenesis [79, 81]. MSI was first detected and described in individuals with a type of hereditary colon cancer (HNPCC, hereditary non-polyposis colorectal carcinoma) which is caused by mutation of DNA-mismatch-repair gene MSH2 [81]. Besides HNPCC, MSI has also been reported in several sporadic cancers (colorectal, bladder, skin, lung, ovarian) [81-84]. Recently, MSI has also been observed in chronic inflammatory diseases such as ulcerative colitis and rheumatoid arthritis [85, 86]. The exact mechanisms through which chronic inflammation may lead to these genomic alterations are the subject of continuing debate. The biologic significance of genomic instability in chronic inflammation settings is yet unknown. Whilst in ulcerative colitis MSI has been associated with increased cancer risk [87], there is no such indication in rheumatoid arthritis [86]. After allogeneic HCT, epithelial tissues become injured through the preparative regimen and are then potentially attacked by alloreactive T cells. Graft-versus-host (GvH) reactions are complex processes developing after allo-HCT involving recruitment of alloreactive T-lymphocytes, release of cytokines (TNF-α, IL-1), production of free radicals and cellular cytotoxicity, among others [6, 88]. The net effect of these alloantigeneic reactions is tissue stress and apoptosis which we recognize clinically as GvH-disease (GvHD). Transplant survivors, especially those who suffer from chronic GvHD, are at risk for the development of secondary epithelial cancers [89]. The pathogenesis of solid tumours post-transplant is unknown.

Faber et al. [90] hypothesized that chronic tissue stress due to interaction of donor-derived lymphocytes with host epithelium in the biological chimeras developed after HCT may cause genomic alterations and therefore analysed epithelial tissues from allo-transplanted patients at molecular level. The authors found frequent genomic alterations measured as MSI in non-neoplastic epithelial tissues of patients who underwent allogeneic HCT. These genomic alterations were found only in allo-transplanted patients but not after autologous HCT or intensive chemotherapy, and therefore they suggested that allogeneic reactions after allo-HCT, e.g. GvH reactions, are substantially involved in the mutation process. In subsequent analyses performed in additional 70 patients who underwent allo-HCT, the authors confirmed their previous results by demonstrating GI in non-neoplastic tissues of nearly 50% of the allo-transplanted patients, especially in old recipients and those who suffered from chronic GvHD (unpublished results). The observation that biological chimeras after allo-HCT acquire genomic alterations initiates scientific questions and opens a new investigation field. What does the GI found in non-neoplastic tissues after transplantation point out? Replication errors during DNA synthesis occur with a certain probability in all cells and may result in a change of the length of MS loci, which are sequences particularly prone to DNA polymerase slippage because of their repetitive nature [79, 91, 92]. The mismatch repair (MMR) system recognizes and corrects these genomic alterations [76]. Whenever the DNA error cannot be repaired, apoptosis pathways are activated [77]. Thus, cells with MS alterations which escaped repair will not replicate and therefore in molecular studies should not become apparent among the large excess of the surrounding normal cells [93]. However, if deficient DNA repair is coupled with a failure to elicit an apoptotic response, this association may result in a growth advantage sufficient to generate a detectable clonal population of cells that share genetic alterations. Therefore, the detection of MSI in clinical samples indicates the presence of a cell population which i) was exposed to a factor which caused MSI, ii) failed to repair the genetic damage through their DNA repair mechanisms, iii) did not go to apoptosis through activation of DNA-damage checkpoints and finally iv) multiplied and perhaps acquired a growth advantage so as to create a detectable clonal population (Figure 1).

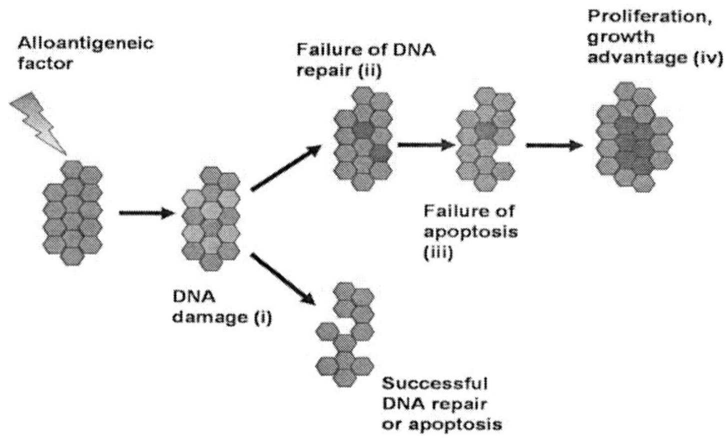

Figure 1. Emergence of genomic instable clones after allogeneic HCT. (i) A cell population is constantly exposed to an allogeneic factor which causes DNA damage (ii) Some cells fail to repair DNA damage through DNA repair mechanisms. (iii) Failure of apoptosis of damaged cells through DNA-damage checkpoints activation. (iv) Proliferation of damaged cells and perhaps acquisition of growth advantage so as to create a detectable clonal population.

i) Factors Inducing GI in the Allotransplanted Recipients

As mentioned before, MSI in non-neoplastic epithelial tissues has been found only in patients treated with myeloablative or reduced-intensity chemotherapy and allogeneic HCT but not in patients after myelosuppressive chemotherapy or myeloablative chemotherapy combined with autologous HCT. In addition, MSI was found also many years after HCT [90]. It is very likely that the alloantigeneic GvH reactions and the following tissue stress could be the the driving force in producing detectable MSI in the allografted patients. Several hypotheses could be made on which of the elements of this inflamed environment could be responsible for causing MSI and by which mechanism. During GvHD, donor activated lymphocytes and macrophages are recruited in the patient's tissues [6, 88]. These activated cells produce mediator molecules such as cytokines (IFN-γ, TNF-α, IL-1 etc) and reactive oxygen species (ROS) such as H_2O_2, $OH^{\cdot}$, $O_2^{\cdot}$. These factors have been shown to cause DNA damage in various experimental systems[94].

ROS can cause base pair mutations, deletions and insertions among other DNA structural alterations through different mechanisms [94]. Oxidants have been shown to induce mutations directly by chemical modification of DNA bases or conformational change of DNA that diminishes the accuracy of DNA polymerases [94]. *In vitro* experiments demonstrated that H_2O_2 can cause induction of MSI not only in MMR-deficient but also at higher concentrations in MMR-proficient human colorectal cancer cell lines [95]. Thus, even with an intact MMR system free radicals produced in inflamed tissues could cause such direct DNA damage which overwhelms the capacity of repair pathways. Oxidants may also facilitate the accumulation of mutations and the creation of MSI indirectly by oxidative damage of DNA repair proteins [96] or through DNA methylation and silencing of DNA repair genes [97]. Besides the effect of oxidants in the DNA repair machinery, ROS may also alter the DNA-damage checkpoints such as p53, facilitating this way the survival of cells with genomic alterations [98].

Inflammatory cytokines may also induce DNA damage in epithelial cells [99, 100]. A nitric oxide (NO) pathway is mainly involved in the cytokine-induced DNA damage. Cytokines such as TNF-α and IFN-γ, which are released in increased amounts in GvHD areas, may cause activation of nuclear factor κB (NFκB) which induces the expression of iNOS (inducible NO synthase) in the epithelial cells. NO produced by cytokine activated cells can be auto-oxidized leading to the formation of reactive radicals called reactive nitrogen species (RNS) which, like ROS, are mutagenic agents with the potential to chemically modify DNA bases by deamination, nitration or oxidation. In addition, NO may affect DNA repair processes by inhibiting DNA repair enzymes through sulfhydryl-nitrosylation of cystein residues of their DNA binding sites [94, 99]. Therefore, NO might be another key player in the induction of MSI after allo-HCT. NO may indeed be the link between chronic alloantigeneic stimulation, relaxation of DNA repair mechanisms and GvHD induced genomic instability. NO has been shown to be an important mediator in GvHD pathology [88]. Increased levels of circulating NO characterize GvHD and iNOS inhibition leads to decreased GvHD severity in animal models [101, 102]. In addition, plasma levels of NO have been associated with GvHD severity in humans [103].

Taken together, oxidative stress like the one produced in the biological chimera due to the interaction between donor T cells and host epithelium may lead to accumulation of genomic alterations in the recipient cells either by overwhelming the capacity for DNA repair or by directly inactivating DNA repair pathways.

ii) Failure of DNA Repair

The presence of MSI in non-neoplastic tissues after allo-HCT means that a replication error occurred and escaped from the DNA repair mechanisms. As mentioned before, oxidative stress may influence the function of the DNA repair machinery. The normal function of the MMR system has been identified as crucial to MS stability [76, 91]. It consists of several proteins (MSH2, MSH3, MSH6, MLH1, PMS2) with different functions who recognize base-base mismatches or insertion-deletion loops and correct them [104]. It has been shown that mutation rates of MS are increased in MMR deficient cell lines compared to MMR proficient ones [105]. MMR deficiency could be attributed to mutations, epigenetic changes or post-translational modifications, as mentioned previously. MSI in HNPCC has been correlated to mutations within MMR genes [81] and suppressed expression of MMR proteins has been found in several types of characterized as MSI-high cancers and cancer cell lines [106-108]. Suppressed expression of MMR could also be due to epigenetic changes as many MSI-high sporadic cancers have been found to lack hMLH1 expression because of methylation of hMLH1 gene promoter [109, 110]. Although mutations and silencing of MMR genes are usually responsible for high levels of MSI, low levels of MSI have been observed in some cancers with no known MMR mutations or promoter hypermethylation [81]. MMR deficiency can be attained also without mutation or epigenetic change, through a deregulation of expression of one of its subunits. MSH2 forms two different complexes with MSH3 and MSH6 with different activity. MSH3 and MSH6 compete each other for binding with MSH2. Thus, overexpression of either of MSH3 or MSH6 can lead to decreased activity of the other's complex with MSH2 [76]. In the subset of chronic tissue stress, ROS (reactive oxygen species) or RNS (reactive nitrogen species) may impair MMR function by post-translational modifications of MMR proteins [94].

Although the MMR system is responsible for correcting DNA strand loops typical for MSI, recent studies suggest that the different DNA repair systems do not act independently and that MSI may be attributable to alterations in DNA repair pathways distinct from MMR [111, 112]. In addition, since all the types of DNA repair mechanisms use the same types of polymerases for final DNA synthesis [104], excess activity of one repair mechanism may result in reduction of the activity of the other. Hofseth et al. demonstrated in an elegant study that the chronic inflammation in ulcerative colitis leads to MSI through excessive activity of BER enzymes and therefore insufficient MMR activity [111]. It has been also shown that imbalanced expression of Polβ can be associated with MSI and chromosome instability [112, 113]. The exact DNA repair defect behind the observed genomic instability found in allotransplanted patients needs to be elucidated.

iii) Failure of DNA Damage Checkpoints

Besides the DNA repair proteins, cells are equipped with additional DNA protective mechanisms (ATM, p53 etc.) which detect unrepaired DNA and lead the cell to cycle arrest or apoptosis [77]. So, even in the case of repair mechanisms failure to correct DNA damage, cells which exhibit genomic instability (GI) will not further proliferate and thus they shouldn't be detected among the rest of the normal cells which proliferate normally. Inactivation of p53 and the failure of cellular demise has been suggested as playing a mechanistic role in the occurrence of MSI in sporadic tumors and in chronically inflamed tissue [81, 86, 114-116]. Furthermore, it is interesting that solid tumours post-transplant exhibit p53 mutations [89, 117]. The pattern of p53 expression in GvHD-affected and genome instable epithelium in allotransplanted patients needs further evaluation.

iv) Growth Advantage of GI Clones in the Allotransplanted Recipients

Another interesting hypothesis is whether cells with instable MS gain an immunologic survival advantage in contrast to normal cells and thus, they can be detected after allo-HCT. In vitro experiments have shown that cells which display MSI can escape T-cell mediated destruction through inhibition of HLA antigen expression and abnormal presentation of peptide fragments [118, 119]. The inhibition of HLA expression can be caused by mutations in HLA transcriptional areas or by instability of MS located near the HLA gene complex. After allogeneic HCT the recipient's epithelial cells stimulate through HLA system the new immune system which derives from the donor. This could lead to immune mediated epithelial cell destruction, which we recognize clinically as GvHD. Therefore, if genomic instable cells reduce expression of HLA genes then they will acquire an immunologic survival advantage. Whilst the normal cells will undergo destruction by the donor derived immune system, the MSI displaying cells will not be recognized by the donor's T-cells. This hypothesis is surely challenging and should be further investigated.

Clinical Significance of GI in Allotransplanted Patients

MSI has been shown to be an indicator of genomic instability [79]. It is very likely that mutations occur not only in non-transcribed MS but also in coding regions of the genome [120]. Mutations in coding genes might be responsible for the protean post-transplant GvHD-related clinical syndromes and phenotypes such as scleroderma, Sjögren syndrome, musculoskeletal or pulmonary disease and many others. In addition to serving as an indicator for genomic instability, mutations of MS may directly contribute to evolution of post-transplant diseases. Although MS were thought to consist "junk" DNA dispersed in non-coding regions throughout the genome, there is evidence that MS distribution is not random and that there are MS within genes which play a regulatory role in gene expression [91]. TGFRII, IGFIIR and BAX genes are paradigms of transcribed genes which contain MS within their coding regions [81, 120]. Changes in the lengths of these repetitive sequences when found within coding regions of specific genes have been shown to result in gene inactivation or modification of function of the gene and cause disease in humans like Huntington's disease and myotonic dystrophy [120].

MSI has been mainly associated with cancer [81] or cancer risk in chronic inflammatory diseases [87]. In hereditary nonpolyposis colorectal carcinoma the MMR deficiency plays an aetiological role in the development of MSI and carcinogenesis [81]. MS alterations are also common in various sporadic cancers such squamous cancers [81]. It is interesting that squamous cell carcinomas are the most common secondary tumours after allogeneic HCT [121] and are associated with chronic alloantigeneic stimulation through GvHD. Therefore, the hypothesis that MSI may characterize a precancerous state of the epithelial cell seems logical. Our preliminary results in the analysis of nearly 70 allogeneic recipients suggest such an association (unpublished data). Genome analyses in allografted recipients may indeed identify specific genomic alterations which might be responsible for, or used as molecular biomarkers of post-transplant diseases, including secondary cancer.

Taken together, it seems that in the GvHD tissue environment cytokines, ROS and NO induce genomic alterations in epithelium by acting through several different but communicating pathways. The oxidative stress damages the DNA causing mutations such as MS length alterations. The induction of mutations is facilitated by a relaxation of DNA repair system mediated by NO or ROS. The cells may survive due to a possible inactivation of the DNA-checkpoint apoptotic mechanisms. Furthermore, the donor-derived immune system in an allogeneic setting may attack the recipient-derived, normal epithelial cells, yet spare cells with an MSI phenotype, providing in this way a selective growth advantage for the cells with novel repeat lengths. Elucidating the ultimate mechanisms underlying the genomic instability following alloantigeneic reactions in the chimeric organism is a major challenge. Findings may provide more information about GvHD pathology and pathogenesis of post transplantation clinical outcomes such as secondary malignancies and GvHD related syndromes. Focusing on the pathways through which the alloantigeneic reaction causes genomic instability may bring up novel therapeutic targets for the protection of the epithelium during GvHD and the prevention of malignant transformation.

CONCLUSION

Although allogeneic HCT has been a part of clinical practice for more than 30 years, the consequences of the unphysiological creation of these biological chimeras are still not fully explored. Development of epithelial cells with donor-derived genotype and accumulation of genomic alterations in the epithelial tissues are only two newly recognized phenomena caused by the co-existence of two genetically distinct populations in the transplant recipient. The ultimate mechanisms and the clinical consequences of these are still under investigation. It is unclear whether these two phenomena, which are both presented in the host epithelium, occur independently or are indeed aetiologically linked. A possible scenario which needs further experimental proof is the following. The transplanted and engrafted bone marrow produces continuously hematopoietic cells, like leukocytes and lymphocytes, in the recipient. Since these cells have a limited life span, they undergo apoptosis and charge constantly the host environment with donor DNA. The donor-derived apoptotic DNA fragments are than taken up and cleared by the recipient's mesenchymal and epithelial cells. It is possible that part of the donor-derived DNA is incorporated into recipient nucleus through horizontal gene transfer leading to occurrence of epithelial cells with donor-derived genome. Induction of genomic DNA damage through the conditioning for the allogeneic HCT leads to an increased frequency of illegitimate DNA integration [122-124].

On the other side, the incorporation of the foreign DNA in the host genome may result extensive physical rearrangements at the site of integration including deletions, duplications and translocations [125-128] leading this way to the detected genomic instability of the chimeric epithelium. Lymphocyte-epithelial interactions between the two genetically distinct cell populations in the transplant recipient should be investigated more precisely not only in cellular but also in molecular level.

ACKNOWLEDGMENTS

We would like to thank all our colleagues from the Department of Hematology in Patras University Medical Center, Patras, Greece and the Department of Hematology-Oncology in Albert-Ludwigs University Medical Center, Freiburg, Germany. We especially thank Miguel Waterhouse (Freiburg) and Eleni Lagadinou (Patras) for critical discussions and helping by preparing the manuscript. This work was supported by Landesstiftung Baden Württemberg.

REFERENCES

[1] Bizzazero, Sulla functione hemapoetica del midollo delle ossa. *Gaz Med. Ital Lomb*, 1868. 28: p. 381.

[2] Neumann, ứber die Bedeutung des Knochenmarks fớr die Blutbildung. *Zbl Med. Wiss,* 1868. 6: p. 689-672.

[3] Lorenz E, C.D., Uphoff D, Modification of acute irradiation injury in mice and guinea pigs by bone marrow injection. *Radiology,* 1951. 58: p. 863-877.

[4] Little, M.T. and R. Storb, History of haematopoietic stem-cell transplantation. *Nat. Rev. Cancer,* 2002. 2(3): p. 231-8.

[5] Bolan, C.D., et al., Prospective evaluation of cell kinetics, yields and donor experiences during a single large-volume apheresis versus two smaller volume consecutive day collections of allogeneic peripheral blood stem cells. *Br. J. Haematol*, 2003. 120(5): p. 801-7.

[6] Zeiser, R., et al., Immunopathogenesis of acute graft-versus-host disease: implications for novel preventive and therapeutic strategies. *Ann. Hematol*, 2004. 83(9): p. 551-65.

[7] Ferrari G, C.-D.A.G., Coletta M, Paolucci E, Stornaiuolo A, Cossu G, Mavilio F., Muscle regeneration by bone marrow-derived myogenic progenitors. *Science,* 1998. 279: p. 1528-30.

[8] Jang, Y.Y., et al., Hematopoietic stem cells convert into liver cells within days without fusion. *Nat. Cell Biol.*, 2004. 6(6): p. 532-9.

[9] Ianus A, H.G., Theise ND, Hussain MA, In vivo derivation of glucose- competent pancreatic endocrine cells from bone marrow without evidence of cell fusion. *J. Clin. Invest*, 2003. 111: p. 843- 850.

[10] Mezey, E., et al., Turning blood into brain: cells bearing neuronal antigens generated in vivo from bone marrow. *Science,* 2000. 290(5497): p. 1779-82.

[11] Camargo FD, G.R., Capetenaki Y, Jackson KA, Goodell MA, Single hematopoietic stem cells generate skeletal muscle through myeloid intermediates. *Nat. Med.,* 2003. 91: p. 1520- 1527.

[12] Korbling, M., et al., Recombinant human granulocyte-colony-stimulating factor-mobilized and apheresis-collected endothelial progenitor cells: a novel blood cell component for therapeutic vasculogenesis. *Transfusion,* 2006. 46(10): p. 1795-802.

[13] Alison MR, P.R., Jeffrey R, Dhillon AP, Quaglia A, Jacob J, Novelli M, Prentice G, Williamson J, Wright NA, Hepatocytes from nonhepatic adult stem cells. *Nature,* 2000. 406: p. 257.

[14] Theise, N.D., et al., Derivation of hepatocytes from bone marrow cells in mice after radiation-induced myeloablation. *Hepatology*, 2000. 31(1): p. 235-40.

[15] Anderlini, P., et al., Long-term follow-up of normal peripheral blood progenitor cell donors treated with filgrastim: no evidence of increased risk of leukemia development. *Bone Marrow Transplant*, 2002. 30(10): p. 661-3.

[16] Castro RF, J.K., Goodell MA, Robertson CS, Liu H, Shine HD., Failure of bone marrow cells to transdifferentiate into neural cells in vivo. *Science,* 2002. 297: p. 1299.

[17] Wagers, A.J., et al., Little evidence for developmental plasticity of adult hematopoietic stem cells. *Science,* 2002. 297(5590): p. 2256-9.

[18] Ono, K., et al., Preservation of hematopoietic properties in transplanted bone marrow cells in the brain. *J. Neurosci. Res.,* 2003. 72(4): p. 503-7.

[19] Holden C, V.G., Stem cells. Plasticity: time for a reappraisal? *Science*, 2002. 296: p. 2126-9.

[20] Wagers, A.J., Sherwood R.I., Christensen J.L., Weissman I.L., Response to comment on "Little evidence for developmental plasticity of adult hematopoietic stem cells". *Science,* 2003. 299: p. 1317.

[21] Theise, N.D., D.S. Krause, and S. Sharkis, Comment on "Little evidence for developmental plasticity of adult hematopoietic stem cells". *Science*, 2003. 299(5611): p. 1317; author reply 1317.

[22] Spyridonidis, A., R. Mertelsmann, and J. Finke, Hematopoietic stem cell transplantation: more than just hematopoietic? *J. Cancer Res. Clin. Oncol.*, 2004.
[23] Spyridonidis, A., et al., Epithelial tissue chimerism after human hematopoietic cell transplantation is a real phenomenon. *Am. J. Pathol*, 2004. 164(4): p. 1147-55.
[24] Bianchi DW, Z.G., Weil GJ, Sylvester S, DeMaria MA, Male fetal progenitor cells persist in maternal blood for as long as 27 years postpartum. *Proc. Natl. Acad. Sci. USA*, 1996. 93: p. 705- 708.
[25] Cogle, C.R., et al., Bone marrow transdifferentiation in brain after transplantation: a retrospective study. *Lancet,* 2004. 363(9419): p. 1432-7.
[26] Okamoto, R., et al., Damaged epithelia regenerated by bone marrow-derived cells in the human gastrointestinal tract. *Nat Med*, 2002. 8(9): p. 1011-7.
[27] Mattsson, J., et al., Lung epithelial cells and type II pneumocytes of donor origin after allogeneic hematopoietic stem cell transplantation. *Transplantation*, 2004. 78(1): p. 154-7.
[28] Tran SD, P.S., Dutra A, Barrett AJ, Brownstein MJ, Key S, Pak E, Leakan RA, Kingman A, Yamada KM, Baum BJ, Mezey E, Differentiation of human bone marrow-derived cells into buccal epithelial cells in vivo: a molecular analytical study. *Lancet,* 2003. 361: p. 1084- 1088.
[29] Metaxas Y, Z.R., Schmitt-Graeff A, Waterhouse M, Faber P, Follo M, Bertz H, Finke J, Spyridonidis A, Human hematopoietic cell transplantation results in generation of donr-derived epithelial cells. *Leukemia,* 2005. 19: p. 1287-1289.
[30] Lagasse E, C.H., Al-Dhalimy M, Reitsma M, Dohse M, Osborne L, Wang X, Finegold M, Weissman IL, Grompe M., Purified hematopoietic stem cells can differentiate into hepatocytes in vivo. *Nat. Med.*, 2000. 6: p. 1229-34.
[31] Willenbring, H., et al., Myelomonocytic cells are sufficient for therapeutic cell fusion in liver. *Nat. Med.*, 2004. 10(7): p. 744-8.
[32] Camargo FD, F.M., Goodell MA, Hematopoietic myelomonocytic cells are the major source of hepatocyte fusion partners. *J. Clin. Invest*, 2004. 113: p. 1266-1270.
[33] Hess, D., et al., Bone marrow-derived stem cells initiate pancreatic regeneration. *Nat. Biotechnol.*, 2003. 21(7): p. 763-70.
[34] Rafii, S. and D. Lyden, Therapeutic stem and progenitor cell transplantation for organ vascularization and regeneration. *Nat. Med.,* 2003. 9(6): p. 702-12.
[35] Wang Xiuli, S.G., McNamara G, Hao QL, Crooks GM, Nolta JA, Albumin- expressing hepatocyte- like cells develop in the livers of immune- deficient mice that received transplants of highly purified human hematopoietic stem cells. *Blood*, 2003. 101: p. 4201- 4208.
[36] Almeida-Porada, G., et al., Formation of human hepatocytes by human hematopoietic stem cells in sheep. *Blood,* 2004. 104(8): p. 2582-90.
[37] Stamm, C., Westphal B, Kleine HD, et al., Autologous bone-marrow stem-cell transplantation for myocardial regeneration. *Lancet*, 2003. 361: p. 45-46.
[38] Bolli R, J.H., Dawn B, Bone marrow cell-mediated cardiac regeneration: A veritable revolution. *J. Am. Coll Cardiol*, 2005. 46: p. 1659-1661.
[39] Houghton, J., et al., Gastric cancer originating from bone marrow-derived cells. Science, 2004. 306(5701): p. 1568-71.

[40] Roth K, K.S., Martin S, Lorenz R, Cellular immune responses are essential for the development of Helicobacter felis-associated gastric pathology. *J. Immunol*, 1999. 163: p. 1490-1497.
[41] Cogle CR, T.N., DongTao F, Ucar D et al, Bone marrow contributes to epithelial cancers in mice and humans as developmental mimicry. *Stem Cells*, 2007. online ahead publish.
[42] Abedi, M., et al., Tissue injury in marrow transdifferentiation. *Blood Cells Mol Dis*, 2004. 32(1): p. 42-6.
[43] Spyridonidis A, T.T., Zeiser R et al, Stem cell plasticity: The debate begins to clarify. *Stem Cell Reviews*, 2005. 1(1): p. 37-43.
[44] Idilman R, K.I., Erden E, et al, Evaluation of the effect of transplant-related factors and tissue-injury on donor-derived hepatocyte and gastrointestinal epithelial cell repopulation following hematopoietic cell transplantation. *Bone Marrow Transplant*, 2006. 37: p. 199-206.
[45] Herzog, E.L., Van Arnam J, Hu BuQu, Krause DS, Threshold of lung injury required for the appearance of marrow-derived lung epithelia. *Stem Cells*, 2006. 24: p. 1986-1992.
[46] Vieyra DS, J.K., Goodell MA, Plasticity snd tissue regenerative potential of bone marrow-derived cells. *Stem Cell Reviews*, 2005. 1(1): p. 65-69.
[47] Bruscia, E., Ziegler EC, Price JE et al, Engraftment of donor-derived epithelial cells in multiple organs following bone marrow transplantation into newborn mice. *Stem Cells*, 2006. 24: p. 2299-2308.
[48] Muller-Borer, B.J., et al., Adult-derived liver stem cells acquire a cardiomyocyte structural and functional phenotype ex vivo. *Am. J. Pathol.*, 2004. 165(1): p. 135-45.
[49] Jang, Y.Y., Sharkis SJ, Stem cell plasticity: A rare cell, not a rare event. *Stem Cell Reviews,* 2005. 1(1): p. 45-51.
[50] Krause DS, T.N., Collector MI, Henegariu O, Hwang S, Gardner R, Neutzel S, Sharkis SJ., Multi-organ, multi-lineage engraftment by a single bone marrow-derived stem cell. *Cell,* 2001. 105: p. 369-77.
[51] Brockes JP, K.A., Plasticity and reprogramming of differentiated cells in amphibian regeneration. *Nat. Rev. Mol. Cell Biol.*, 2002. 3: p. 566- 574.
[52] Takahashi K, Y.S., Induction of pluripotent stem cells from mouse embryonic and adult fibroblast cultures by defined factors. *Cell,* 2006. 126: p. 663-676.
[53] Okita, K., Ichisaka T, Yamanaka S, Generation of germline-competent induced pluripotent stem cells. *Nature*, 2007. 448: p. 313-317.
[54] Wernig M, M.A., Foreman R et al, In vitro reprogramming of fibroblasts into a pluripotent ES-cell-like state. *Nature,* 2007. 448: p. 318-324.
[55] Avital I, I.D., Aoki T, Tyan DB, Cohen AH, Ferraresso C, Rozga J, Arnaout WS, Demetroiu A, Isolation, characterization, and transplantation of bone marrow- derived hepatocyte stem cells. *Biochem. Biophys. Res. Commun*, 2001. 288: p. 156- 164.
[56] Ratajczak, M.Z., et al., Stem cell plasticity revisited: CXCR4-positive cells expressing mRNA for early muscle, liver and neural cells 'hide out' in the bone marrow. *Leukemia,* 2004. 18(1): p. 29-40.
[57] Jiang Y, J.B., Reinhardt RL, Schwartz RE, Keene CD, Ortiz- Gonzalez XR, Reyes M, Lenvik T, Lund T, Blackstad M, Du J, Aldrich S, Lisberg A, Low WC, Largaespada

DA, Verfaillie CM, Pluripotency of mesenchymal stem cells derived from adult marrow. *Nature*, 2002. 418: p. 41- 49.

[58] Check, Stem-cell paper corrected. *Nature,* 2007. 447: p. 763.

[59] Jiang Y, J.B., Reinhardt RL, Schwartz RE, Keene CD, Ortiz- Gonzalez XR, Reyes M, Lenvik T, Lund T, Blackstad M, Du J, Aldrich S, Lisberg A, Low WC, Largaespada DA, Verfaillie CM, Pluripotency of mesenchymal stem cells derived from adult marrow. *Nature,* 2007. 447: p. 880-881.

[60] Kucia M, R.R., Campbell FR, Zuba-Surma E, Majka M, Ratajczak J, Ratajczak Z, A population of very small embryonic-like (VSEL) CXCR4+SSEA-1+Oct-4+ stem cells identified in adult bone marrow. *Leukemia,* 2006. 20: p. 857-869.

[61] Kucia M, H.M., Wysoczynski M, et al, Morphological and molecular characterization of novel population of CXCR4+ SSEA-4+ Oct-4+ very small embryonic-like cells purified from human cord blood- preliminary report. *Leukemia,* 2007. 21: p. 297-303.

[62] Anjos-Afonso F, B.D., Nonhematopoietic/endothelial SSEA-1+ cells define the most primitive progenitors in the adult murine bone marrow mesenchymal compartment. *Blood,* 2007. 109: p. 1298-1306.

[63] Ratajczak MZ, M.B., Wojakowski W, Ratajczak J, Kucia M, A hypothesis for an embryonic origin of pluripotent Oct-4+ stem cells in adult bone marrow and other tissues. *Leukemia,* 2007. 21: p. 860-867.

[64] Gurtner GC, C.M., Longaker MT, Progress and potential for regenerative medicine. *Annu. Rev. Med.*, 2007. 58: p. 299-312.

[65] Vassilopoulos, G., P.R. Wang, and D.W. Russell, Transplanted bone marrow regenerates liver by cell fusion. *Nature,* 2003. 422(6934): p. 901-4.

[66] Wang, X., et al., Cell fusion is the principal source of bone-marrow-derived hepatocytes. *Nature*, 2003. 422(6934): p. 897-901.

[67] Metaxas, Z., Schmitt-Graeff, Waterhouse, Faber, Follo, Bertz, Finke, Spyridonidis, Human hematopoietic cell transplantation results in generation of donor-derived epithelial cells. *Leukemia*, 2005. 19: p. 1287-1289.

[68] Vogel G, Developmental biology. More data but no answers on powers of adult stem cells. *Science,* 2004. 305: p. 27.

[69] Quesenberry, P.J., Colvin G, Dooner G, Dooner M, Aliotta JM, Johnson K, The stem cell continuum: Cell cycle, injury, and phenotype lability. *Ann. NY Acad Sci.*, 2007. online pre-publication.

[70] Bergsmedh, A., et al., Horizontal transfer of oncogenes by uptake of apoptotic bodies. *Proc. Natl. Acad. Sc. USA*, 2001. 98(11): p. 6407-11.

[71] Jain, R., M.C. Rivera, and J.A. Lake, Horizontal gene transfer among genomes: the complexity hypothesis. *Proc. Natl. Acad. Sci. USA*, 1999. 96(7): p. 3801-6.

[72] Holmgren, L., et al., Horizontal transfer of DNA by the uptake of apoptotic bodies. *Blood,* 1999. 93(11): p. 3956-63.

[73] Schubbert, R., et al., Foreign (M13) DNA ingested by mice reaches peripheral leukocytes, spleen, and liver via the intestinal wall mucosa and can be covalently linked to mouse DNA. *Proc. Natl. Acad. Sci USA,* 1997. 94(3): p. 961-6.

[74] Mezey E, K.S., Vogelsang G, Szalayova I, Lange GD, Crain B, Transplanted bone marrow generates new neurons in human brains. *Proc. Natl. Acad. Sci. USA*, 2003. 100: p. 1364- 1369.

[75] Verfaillie, C.M., M.F. Pera, and P.M. Lansdorp, Stem cells: hype and reality. *Hematology* (Am Soc Hematol Educ Program), 2002: p. 369-91.

[76] Jiricny, J., Replication errors: cha(lle)nging the genome. *Embo. J.,* 1998. 17(22): p. 6427-36.

[77] Zhivotovsky, B. and G. Kroemer, Apoptosis and genomic instability. *Nat. Rev. Mol Cell Biol,* 2004. 5(9): p. 752-62.

[78] Sieber, O.M., K. Heinimann, and I.P. Tomlinson, Genomic instability--the engine of tumorigenesis? *Nat. Rev. Cancer*, 2003. 3(9): p. 701-8.

[79] Ellegren, H., Microsatellites: simple sequences with complex evolution. *Nat. Rev. Genet*, 2004. 5(6): p. 435-45.

[80] Spyridonidis, A., et al., Capillary electrophoresis for chimerism monitoring by PCR amplification of microsatellite markers after allogeneic hematopoietic cell transplantation. *Clin. Transplant*, 2005. 19(3): p. 350-6.

[81] Boland, C.R., et al., A National Cancer Institute Workshop on Microsatellite Instability for cancer detection and familial predisposition: development of international criteria for the determination of microsatellite instability in colorectal cancer. *Cancer Res,* 1998. 58(22): p. 5248-57.

[82] Sood, A.K., et al., Application of the National Cancer Institute international criteria for determination of microsatellite instability in ovarian cancer. *Cancer Res*, 2001. 61(11): p. 4371-4.

[83] Xu, L., et al., Microsatellite instability at AAAG repeat sequences in respiratory tract cancers. *Int. J. Cancer*, 2001. 91(2): p. 200-4.

[84] Danaee, H., et al., Microsatellite instability at tetranucleotide repeats in skin and bladder cancer. *Oncogene,* 2002. 21(32): p. 4894-9.

[85] Chen, S.H., X. Li, and X.J. Huang, Effect of recombinant human granulocyte colony-stimulating factor on T-lymphocyte function and the mechanism of this effect. *Int. J. Hematol.*, 2004. 79(2): p. 178-84.

[86] Sohn, S.K., et al., Harvesting peripheral blood stem cells from healthy donors on 4th day of cytokine mobilization. *J. Clin. Apher,* 2003. 18(4): p. 186-9.

[87] Willenbucher, R.F., et al., Genomic instability is an early event during the progression pathway of ulcerative-colitis-related neoplasia. *Am. J. Pathol.*, 1999. 154(6): p. 1825-30.

[88] Teshima, T. and J.L. Ferrara, Understanding the alloresponse: new approaches to graft-versus-host disease prevention. *Semen. Hematol.*, 2002. 39(1): p. 15-22.

[89] Deeg, H.J. and G. Socie, Malignancies after hematopoietic stem cell transplantation: many questions, some answers. *Blood,* 1998. 91(6): p. 1833-44.

[90] Faber, P., et al., Frequent genomic alterations in epithelium measured by microsatellite instability following allogeneic hematopoietic cell transplantation in humans. *Blood*, 2006. 107(8): p. 3389-96.

[91] Li, Y.C., et al., Microsatellites: genomic distribution, putative functions and mutational mechanisms: a review. *Mol. Ecol.*, 2002. 11(12): p. 2453-65.

[92] Mirkin, S.M., Expandable DNA repeats and human disease. *Nature*, 2007. 447(7147): p. 932-40.

[93] Mao, L., et al., Microsatellite alterations as clonal markers for the detection of human cancer. *Proc. Natl. Acad. Sci. USA*, 1994. 91(21): p. 9871-5.

[94] Wiseman, H. and B. Halliwell, Damage to DNA by reactive oxygen and nitrogen species: role in inflammatory disease and progression to cancer. *Biochem. J.,* 1996. 313 (Pt 1): p. 17-29.

[95] Gasche, C., et al., Oxidative stress increases frameshift mutations in human colorectal cancer cells. *Cancer Res.*, 2001. 61(20): p. 7444-8.

[96] Chang, C.L., et al., Oxidative stress inactivates the human DNA mismatch repair system. *Am. J. Physiol. Cell Physiol.*, 2002. 283(1): p. C148-54.

[97] Seril, D.N., et al., Oxidative stress and ulcerative colitis-associated carcinogenesis: studies in humans and animal models. *Carcinogenesis,* 2003. 24(3): p. 353-62.

[98] Cerutti, P.A., Oxy-radicals and cancer. *Lancet,* 1994. 344(8926): p. 862-3.

[99] Jaiswal, M., et al., Inflammatory cytokines induce DNA damage and inhibit DNA repair in cholangiocarcinoma cells by a nitric oxide-dependent mechanism. *Cancer Res,* 2000. 60(1): p. 184-90.

[100] Seidelin, J.B. and O.H. Nielsen, Continuous cytokine exposure of colonic epithelial cells induces DNA damage. *Eur. J. Gastroenterol. Hepatol.*, 2005. 17(3): p. 363-9.

[101] Drobyski, W.R., et al., Inhibition of nitric oxide production is associated with enhanced weight loss, decreased survival, and impaired alloengraftment in mice undergoing graft-versus-host disease after bone marrow transplantation. *Blood*, 1994. 84(7): p. 2363-73.

[102] Flanagan, D.M., et al., Nitric oxide participates in the intestinal pathology associated with murine syngeneic graft-versus-host disease. *J. Leukoc. Biol.,* 2002. 72(4): p. 762-8.

[103] Choi, I.C., et al., Plasma nitric oxide is associated with the occurrence of moderate to severe acute graft-versus-host disease in haemopoietic stem cell transplant recipients. *Haematologica*, 2001. 86(9): p. 972-6.

[104] Christmann, M., et al., Mechanisms of human DNA repair: an update. *Toxicology*, 2003. 193(1-2): p. 3-34.

[105] Boyer, J.C., et al., Sequence dependent instability of mononucleotide microsatellites in cultured mismatch repair proficient and deficient mammalian cells. *Hum. Mol. Genet*, 2002. 11(6): p. 707-13.

[106] Boyer, J.C., et al., Microsatellite instability, mismatch repair deficiency and genetic defects in human cancer cell lines. *Cancer Res*, 1995. 55(24): p. 6063-70.

[107] Liu, J., et al., Microsatellite instability and expression of hMLH1 and hMSH2 proteins in ovarian endometrioid cancer. *Mod. Pathol*, 2004. 17(1): p. 75-80.

[108] Yao, Y., et al., Alterations of DNA mismatch repair proteins and microsatellite instability levels in gastric cancer cell lines. *Lab. Invest*, 2004. 84(7): p. 915-22.

[109] Kane, M.F., et al., Methylation of the hMLH1 promoter correlates with lack of expression of hMLH1 in sporadic colon tumors and mismatch repair-defective human tumor cell lines. *Cancer Res.,* 1997. 57(5): p. 808-11.

[110] Fleisher, A.S., et al., Hypermethylation of the hMLH1 gene promoter in human gastric cancers with microsatellite instability. *Cancer Res.*, 1999. 59(5): p. 1090-5.

[111] Hofseth, L.J., et al., The adaptive imbalance in base excision-repair enzymes generates microsatellite instability in chronic inflammation. *J. Clin. Invest*, 2003. 112(12): p. 1887-94.

[112] Yamada, N.A. and R.A. Farber, Induction of a low level of microsatellite instability by overexpression of DNA polymerase Beta. *Cancer Res,* 2002. 62(21): p. 6061-4.

[113] Bergoglio, V., et al., Deregulated DNA polymerase beta induces chromosome instability and tumorigenesis. *Cancer Res*, 2002. 62(12): p. 3511-4.

[114] Ahrendt, S.A., et al., Microsatellite instability at selected tetranucleotide repeats is associated with p53 mutations in non-small cell lung cancer. *Cancer Res*, 2000. 60(9): p. 2488-91.
[115] Hussain, S.P., et al., Increased p53 mutation load in noncancerous colon tissue from ulcerative colitis: a cancer-prone chronic inflammatory disease. *Cancer Res*, 2000. 60(13): p. 3333-7.
[116] Inazuka, M., et al., Analysis of p53 tumour suppressor gene somatic mutations in rheumatoid arthritis synovium. *Rheumatology* (Oxford), 2000. 39(3): p. 262-6.
[117] Zouvelou C, B.H., Faber P, Spyridonidis A, p53 mutations in secondary malignancies after allogeneic hematopoietic cell transplantation. *Biology of Blood and Marrow Transplantation,* 2007. 13(2): p. 53.
[118] Hirata, T., et al., Characterization of the immune escape phenotype of human gastric cancers with and without high-frequency microsatellite instability. *J. Pathol*, 2007. 211(5): p. 516-23.
[119] Kloor, M., et al., Immunoselective pressure and human leukocyte antigen class I antigen machinery defects in microsatellite unstable colorectal cancers. *Cancer Res*, 2005. 65(14): p. 6418-24.
[120] Li, Y.C., et al., Microsatellites within genes: structure, function, and evolution. *Mol. Biol. Evol.*, 2004. 21(6): p. 991-1007.
[121] Curtis, R.E., et al., Impact of chronic GVHD therapy on the development of squamous-cell cancers after hematopoietic stem-cell transplantation: an international case-control study. *Blood,* 2005. 105(10): p. 3802-11.
[122] Bode, J., et al., Fatal connections: when DNA ends meet on the nuclear matrix. J Cell *Biochem. Suppl*, 2000. Suppl 35: p. 3-22.
[123] Shcherbakova, O.G. and M.V. Filatov, Camptothecin enhances random integration of transfected DNA into the genome of mammalian cells. *Biochim. Biophys Acta*, 2000. 1495(1): p. 1-3.
[124] Bennett, C.L., et al., Haematological malignancies developing in previously healthy individuals who received haematopoietic growth factors: report from the Research on Adverse Drug Events and Reports (RADAR) project. *Br. J. Haematol*, 2006. 135(5): p. 642-50.
[125] Covarrubias, L., Y. Nishida, and B. Mintz, Early postimplantation embryo lethality due to DNA rearrangements in a transgenic mouse strain. *Proc. Natl. Acad. Sci. USA*, 1986. 83(16): p. 6020-4.
[126] Covarrubias, L., et al., Cellular DNA rearrangements and early developmental arrest caused by DNA insertion in transgenic mouse embryos. *Mol Cell Biol*, 1987. 7(6): p. 2243-7.
[127] Kato, S., R.A. Anderson, and R.D. Camerini-Otero, Foreign DNA introduced by calcium phosphate is integrated into repetitive DNA elements of the mouse L cell genome. *Mol. Cell Biol.,* 1986. 6(5): p. 1787-95.
[128] Robins D, R.S., Henderson A, Axel R, Transforming DNA integrates into the host chromosome. *Cell*, 1981. 23: p. 29-39.

In: Stem Cell Research: New Developments
Editors: Hiroshi Tanaka and Michael C. F. Chang
ISBN: 978-1-61942-081-6

Chapter 5

TGF-B1 AND ITS ROLE IN CELL PROLIFERATION

***K. J. Rolfe*[1] *and A. O. Grobbelaar*[2]**
[1]The RAFT Institute, Mount Vernon Hospital, UK
[2]Department of Plastic Surgery, The Royal Free Hospital,
Pond Street Hampstead London, UK

ABSTRACT

Transforming growth factor-beta 1 (TGF-β1) is part of a large family of proteins which control a number of cellular responses in cells derived from a variety of tissues. TGF- β1 and its signalling pathways can inhibit proliferation in a number of cell types (e.g. non-transformed epithelial and endothelial cells) but causes proliferation in a number of transformed cells and immortalised fibroblasts. TGF-β1 binds to its heterodimeric receptors, of which there are a number and in some cell types such as endothelial derived cells it appears that the receptor can determine whether the cells undergo proliferation. Further, the signalling pathways involved in TGF-β appear to play a role in determining if cells proliferate. Aberrant TGF- β1 and its signalling is known to play a role in a number of diseases; this review will discuss the pathways involved in a number of cell types and discuss the effect of abnormal TGF-β1 and its signalling in a number of diseases.

INTRODUCTION

Transforming growth factor beta (TGF-β) is part of a large family of proteins which includes: TGF-β, activins, inhibins, bone morphometric proteins (BMPs), myostatin, Müllerian inhibiting substance and growth/differentiation factors. They are all known to play a diverse role in many physiological processes including tissue differentiation, chemotaxis, wound healing, cell cycle control and homeostasis. The majority of the ligands exist as either homo or heterodimers, which signal through ligand induced heteromeric complex formation of serine/threonine kinase receptors.

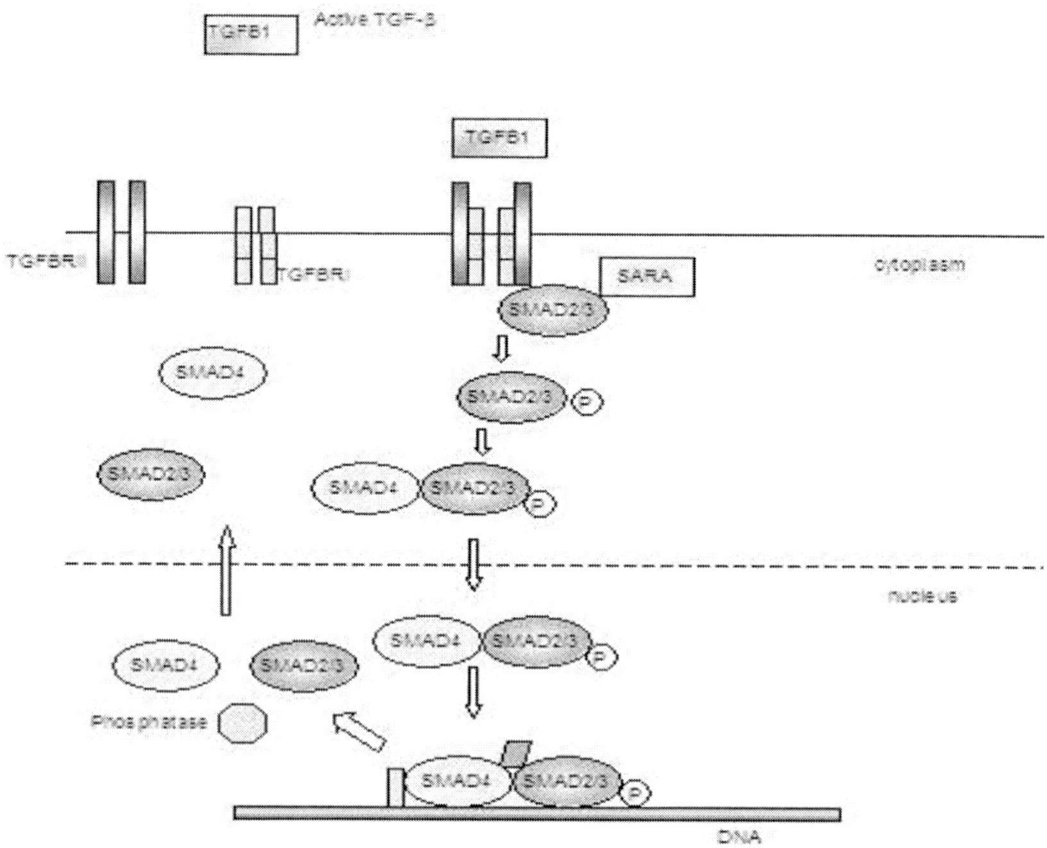

Figure 1. TGF-β signalling via the Smad pathway.

TGF-β consists of three mammalian isoforms (TGF-β1, -β2, -β3) each encoded by a distinct gene but with a 70-80% homology [1]. The isoforms are known to regulate multiple biological effects in a number of cell types such as extra cellular matrix synthesis, angiogenesis, immune response, cell differentiation and, can cause cell proliferation in some mesenchymal derived cells but inhibit proliferation in most including epithelial derived cells and, can induce apoptosis [2]. Aberrant expression of any part of the TGF-β signalling pathway can result in a number of human diseases: cancer, vascular disorders, diabetes, fibrosis and some autoimmune disorders.

All three TGF-β isoforms are secreted as latent precursors, which undergo proteolytic changes. Many proteins have been identified which can 'activate' TGF-β, including proteases, matrix-metalloproteinase –2 and –9, thrombospondin –1 and the integrin αvβ6. Activated TGF-β binds to the transmembrane serine/threonine kinase receptor TGFβRII which is constitutively phosphorylated and which in turn phosphorylates TGFβRI. The activated type one receptor (TGFβRI) is phosphorylated in a Gly-Ser region that is highly conserved in all TGFβRI. The TGF-β receptor (TGFβRI) propagates the intracellular signals and it is thought it may play a role in determining the specificity of the intracellular signalling by causing the phosphorylation (activation) of receptor-Smads (R-Smads: Smad 2, Smad3). These R-Smads (Smad 2 and 3) are bound to SARA (Smad anchor for receptor activation; Figure one) and on phosphorylation of the R-Smads (on two serine residues at the extreme C termini) they become dissociated from SARA. It has been proposed that internalisation of the TGF-β receptors is required for Smad presentation by SARA to the receptors [3]. R- Smads form a heteromeric complex with Smad 4 (common-partner; Co-Smad). This complex translocates into the nucleus via nucleoporins within the nuclear pore complex [4] and the Smad complex regulates gene transcription through interaction with a number of transcription factors.

The R-Smads and Co-Smad share two conserved domains MH1 and MH2, separated by a proline rich linker region, it is the MH1 domain of the R-Smad and Co-Smad which binds to the DNA, with the exception of Smad2 which has been found to have two extra peptide inserts [5]. Smads regulate gene expression by a variety of mechanisms, including transcriptional co activators such as CREB binding protein (CBP0/p300 [6], transcriptional co repressors such as Ski and SnoN and, R-Smads have been found to stabilise a number of proteins involved in gene transcription. The time that R-Smads (Smad 2/Smad3) are within the nucleus is transitory depending on their phosphorylation status. The R-Smads are de-phosphorylated via phosphatases within the nucleus [7,8] and are then redistribution back into the cytoplasm. If the receptors remain active the R-Smads will be re-phosphorylated and the cycle will continue [9].

The specificity of signalling may also be determined by the presence of accessory transmembrane proteins. Betaglycan (also known as TGFβRIII) is proteoglycan-containing membrane glycoprotein which is required for a subset of ligands to bind and activate TGFβRII. TGF-β2 has been found in some cell types to have a low binding affinity to TGFβRII and therefore requires betaglycan for high affinity binding [10,11]. TGFβRIII can form oligomeric complexes with TGFβRII and TGFβRI to positively or negatively modulate TGF-β induced responses depending on cell type [12]. Betaglycan has also been shown to be phosphorylated by TGFβRII and once phosphorylated interacts with β-arrestin which causes the internalization of both betaglycan and TGFβRII [13] and results in the down regulation of TGF-β signalling. Endoglin, which is structurally related to betaglycan, can also play a role in inhibiting TGF-β signalling [14]. Further, betaglycan and endoglin can be shed by cells and sequester TGF-β and therefore inhibit TGF-β signalling [15].

TGF-β can also cause the phosphorylation of other non-Smad signalling pathways the GTPase Ras and the Mitogen-activated protein kinases (c-Jun N-terminal kinases (JNK), Extra-cellular receptor kinase (ERK), and p38), though it remains unclear how, these non-Smad pathways link between an activated receptor and the effector molecules [16,17]. However, there is increasing evidence that a number of these pathways can interact with the Smad pathways causing different cellular outcomes depending on the circumstances. For instance the phosphorylation of the R-Smad's linker region (the area which connects MH1 DNA binding domain with the MH2 transcriptional domain) by ERK can negatively regulate the Smad pathway. Over expression of constitutively active members of Ras/MEK/ERK cascade can block nuclear accumulation of Smads and therefore may be a reason why transformed epithelial cells are no longer responsive to TGF-β [18] however, in other cell types it can promote Smad dependent processes [19]. In untransformed epithelial derived cells and mesenchymal derived cells transient expression of Ras/MEK/ERK pathway is required for the induced expression of some proteins [20,21], further ERK may enhance Smad3 dependent activation of a number of genes [22,23] but, conversely it has been shown that ERK can repress a subset of TGF-β responsive genes though its mechanism has yet to be elucidated [24].

TGF-β signalling is regulated by the induction of the inhibitory Smads: Smad 6 (inhibits bone morphometric proteins), and Smad 7 (inhibits activin, TGF-β and bone morphometric protein signalling), which cause signal termination [25]. The inhibitory Smads are induced by TGF-β, activin and BMP through phosphorylated R-Smads [26] and therefore inhibitory Smads act in a negative feedback loop to regulate duration and intensity of signalling. Inhibitory Smads are structurally similar in the MH2 region to receptor and co-Smads but lack a C-terminal SSXS motif, which prevents their phosphorylation. Inhibitory Smads can inhibit signalling by a number of mechanisms: competitive binding to TGFβRI [27], interacting with Smurfl (Smad specific E3 ubiquitin ligase) and Smurf2 causing the degradation of active receptors [28-30], Smad 7 can target the protein phosphatase-1 (PP1) to the active receptors causing their dephosphorylation and therefore their inactivation [31]. Further, Smad 7 can bind via its MH2 domain to Smad responsive elements on promoters and prevent gene activation [32]. Inhibitory Smads however, are themselves regulated by Arkadia an E3-ubiquitin ligase that regulates Smad 7 levels [33], causing a potential amplification of TGF-β signalling.

TGF-β and Cell Cycle Arrest

Stimulation with TGF-β1 causes a number of cell types to undergo growth arrest at G1 phase of the cell cycle [34]. This cell cycle arrest is through the activation of cyclin dependent kinase inhibitors $p15^{INK4B}$ in epithelial derived cells (thyroid, lung and breast and keratinocytes,) [35-38] and $p21^{CIP1}$ in keratinocytes and ovarian derived epithelial cells [37, 39-41] inactivating cdk2 and cdk4. $p21^{CIP}$ and $p15^{INK4B}$ Both these cyclin dependent kinase inhibitors are up regulated in a Smad dependent manner though a recent study also suggests that for $p21^{CIP1}$ other Smad independent signalling pathways may also be involved, such as protein kinase C [42]. A number of transcription factors (for instance FoxO, Spi/Sp3) associated with TGF-β signalling have been shown to be required for the up regulation of cyclin dependent kinase inhibitors [43,44]. TGF-β1 in epithelial-derived cells is known to cause the down regulation of Cdc25A, which belongs to a group of phosphatases that activate cyclin dependent kinases by the removal of an inhibitory phosphate group [45]. TGF-β therefore causes cdk4 and cdk6 to increase their level of phosphorylation preventing cell cycle progression [45]. A recent study has also indicated that TGF-β has a direct inhibitory effect on G2 checkpoint kinases amplifying TGF-β cell cycle arrest [46].

It has been further proposed that TGF-β can inhibit proliferation in a number of cell types via the down regulation of c-myc in the early G1 phase of the cell cycle by complexes containing Smad 3 [47] and P107 [48] which results in an up regulation of cyclin dependent kinase inhibitors. c-myc has a dual role in cell cycle progression by promoting both cyclin dependent kinase activity (for example CDK1, CDK2, CDK4) and, down regulating $p15^{INK4B}$ and $p21^{CIP1}$ [49]. However a down regulation of c-myc is required for the induction of both $p15^{INK4B}$ and $p21^{Cip1}$ [50,51] and this involves the transcription factor Miz-1 [52,53]. Therefore down regulation of c-myc and the inhibition of cyclin dependent kinases and the regulation of cyclin dependent kinase inhibitors results in the retinoblastoma protein (pRb) being maintained in its active hypophosphoylated forms [54] and therefore inhibiting progress into the S phase of the cell cycle. Therefore loss of pRb by various mechanisms (including viruses) can play a role in cells escaping from TGF-β growth inhibition and play a role in tumour development [55].

Id-1 is a member of the Id family of proteins, which are helix-loop-helix transcription factors and are therefore involved in a number of cellular processes [56,59]. Id proteins have been shown to be essential for proliferation in a number of cell types [57] while inhibiting cell differentiation. Aberrant expression of Id-1 can cause cell cycle progression in a number of cell types possibly through the suppression of cyclin dependent kinase inhibitors (p16, $p21^{cip1}$ and $p27^{KIP1}$) through a number of mechanisms [60-62]. TGF-β is an upstream regulator of Id-1 [63], TGF-β causes the repression of Id-1 resulting in an increase in cyclin dependent kinase inhibitors ($p21^{cip1}$, $p27^{KIP1}$) and therefore preventing cell cycle progression. The repression of Id-1 by TGF-β has been shown to require the transcriptional repressor ATF3. The phosphorylated (activated) R-Smad, Smad3, directly induces the expression of ATF3. ATF3 and Smad 3 then form a complex, which directly represses the expression of ATF3, therefore the repression of Id-1 is under control of the Smad signalling pathway [64].

TGF-β is also known to signal through non-Smad signalling pathway (as discussed previously) and cell cycle arrest can also occur independently of the phosphorylation of the R-Smads. $p21^{cip1}$ has been shown to be induced through non-Smad signalling pathways [65,66] and in Smad signalling pathways that lack the co-Smad (Smad4) [67]. Non-Smad signalling pathways such as protein kinase Cα can phosphorylate regulatory proteins (S100c/A11), which can translocate to the nucleus and aid in binding transcription factors, such as Sp-1, to the promoters of $p15^{INK4B}$ and $p21^{cip1}$ genes. Protein kinase Cα has also been shown to block Smad3's transcriptional activity [68]. Non-Smad signalling pathways have been shown to prevent cell proliferation through the: inhibition of p70 S6 Kinase by phosphatase 2 A (PP2A) [69], activation of ROCK1 by the GTPase RhoA which inactivates Cdc25A [70] in epithelial derived cells. Kamaraju and Roberts also showed that non-Smad signalling pathways (p38 MAP kinase and Rho/ROCK) can cooperate with Smad pathways and cause growth inhibition in epithelial derived cells [71] because Rho/ROCK are necessary for the down regulation of c-Myc and the up-regulation of $p21^{waf1}$ (in human breast carcinoma) [71]

TGF-β and Proliferation

TGF-β can cause the proliferation of mesenchymal derived cells such as fibroblasts and osteoblasts, whereas it inhibits proliferation in most cell types including epithelial, endothelial, myeloid, lymphoid and neuronal derived cells. Endothelial cells response appear to depend on the receptor and the activation of a specific intra-signalling pathway [72]. TGF-β inhibits proliferation at the G1 phase of the cell cycle through the inhibition or down regulation of a number of cell cycle regulators: retinoblastoma protein (pRb), c-Myc and, cyclin dependent kinases (CDKs), or stimulation and the activation of cyclin dependent kinase inhibitors such as $p15^{INK4B}$, $p21^{CIP1}$, $p27^{KIP1}$(as discussed previously) [35,39].

TGF-β and Fibroblast Cell Proliferation

In mesenchymal cells it appears that TGF-β activates a range of different signalling pathways, for instance Smad-independent activation of p21-activated kinase-2 (PAK2; a serine/ threonine protein kinase) and c-Abl non-receptor tyrosine kinase and phosphoinositide-3-kinase (PI3K) [73-76]. It appears that in a Smad independent manner, but dependent on Rho GTPase, Cdc42 and Rac1, TGF-β can activate PI3K/c-Abl/PAK-2, which appears to be required for proliferation and anchorage independent growth [76]. PAK2 belongs to a family of proteins of which there are two subfamilies [77]. PAK2 belongs to group I, which have been implicated in cell motility [78], clathrin –independent endocytic pathways [79], actin reorganisation [80], and apoptosis [81]. However Wilkes et al believe that both the Smad 2/3 and PAK2 dependent pathways are required for morphological transformation and cellular proliferation [74]. PI3K activity has been found to be required for the activation of PAK2 and Akt; PAK2 appears downstream of PI3K but upstream of c-Abl a non-receptor tyrosine kinase and appears essential for TGF-β stimulated proliferation in mesenchymal derived cells [73,74,82]. Spatial localisation of Abl, appears in some cell types to determine if the cells will undergo apoptosis or proliferation. Cytoplasmic Abl appears to result in cell survival and proliferation whereas activated nuclear Abl appears to induce apoptosis [83].

Other growth factors such as Hepatocyte growth factor (HGF) and Epidermal growth factor (EGF) can inhibit TGF-β induced growth inhibition [16]. These growth factors cause the activation of ERK and/or Ras, which can cause the phosphorylation of motifs in the linker regions of the R-Smads, which alters the nuclear translocation of Smads either preventing [17] or enhancing [18,84] translocation. Activated Ras has also been shown to promote the degradation of Smad 4 [85] and increase the expression of TGIF (TG-interacting factor)[86] TGIF has been found to be a transcriptional repressor, stabilisation of TGIF by the phosphorylation of Ras/ERK (by growth factors such as EGF) results in TGIF interacting with Smad2 and therefore regulating the transcription of TGF-β responsive genes [87]. *In vitro* studies on TGIF null fibroblasts have demonstrated a cell cycle progression defect which resulted in a slower proliferation rate and cells did not reach the same density as normal controls, this change in proliferation has also been identified in other cell types [88].

Fibroblasts have been shown to have important physiological functions, which include deposition of the extra cellular matrix (ECM) and cellular differentiation. Fibroblasts are known to play an important role in wound healing, they generate ECM and can modulate the immune responses for example. Aberrant fibroblast proliferation results in disorders in wound healing such as delayed healing or fibrosis. A number of mesenchymal cells (fibroblasts, osteoblasts, smooth muscle cells) have demonstrated a bi-directional proliferative response to levels of TGF-β1, which appears to play a role in wound healing. There have been a number of theories proposed for this mechanism [89,90], but a recent study suggests a role for c-Ski. Levels of TGF-β1 determining the expression of c-Ski which in turn alters Smad3 transcriptional activity. This alteration in transcription alters the expression of cdk inhibitors ($p21^{cip}$ and $p27^{kip1}$) and the levels, which are complexed with cyclins (cyclin D1 and E). These alterations in the complexes alter the phosphorylation of pRb, which in turn determines if the cell will proliferate [91].

TGF-β and Endothelial Cells and Angiogenesis

In endothelial cells TGF-β can activate two distinct TGFβRI pathways: ALK5, which causes the phosphorylation of Smad2/3 or through ALK1 activating the phosphorylation of Smad 1/5/8. Interestingly phosphorylation (activation) of ALK1 causes endothelial cell proliferation and cell migration, whereas ALK5 inhibits proliferation and cell migration [72, Figure 2]. Goumans et al demonstrated that ALK5 is required for ALK1 signalling though it appears that the ALK1 signalling cascade antagonizes ALK5 signalling [92,93]. ALK1 has been shown in endothelial cells [72], and hepatatic steallate cells [94] to cause the up regulation of Id1 gene expression.

Studies have suggested that an up regulation of endoglin is a marker for both angiogenesis and endothelial cell proliferation [95-100]. Endoglin appears to be required for ALK1 signalling [100]. Though others [101] suggest that this is not the case with a deletion of endoglin resulting in endothelial cells proliferating faster. This group suggested that this was through higher binding affinity of the receptors for TGF-β and that endoglin may suppress Smad 1 activation [101]. This discrepancy may be due to the different experimental methods resulting in a reduction of endoglin.

Endoglin cannot bind TGF-β in the absence of TGFβRII. Regulation in endothelial cells also appears to be through the levels of the ligand itself (TGF-β1), low extra cellular concentrations of TGF-β1 appear to promote cell proliferation and migration and therefore signalling through ALK1 [100]. However, the effect of TGF-β and ALK1 expression appears to depend on whether the endothelial cells are derived from microvascular or from a venous origin [102,103].

Epithelial Mesenchymal Transition

Epithelial mesenchymal transition (EMT) is involved in normal physiological processes including development, wound healing along with pathological processes such as fibrosis and malignancy. EMT is a complex process involving a number of signalling pathways and resulting in loss of the epithelial cell phenotype, dissolution of junctions containing ZO-1, E-cadherin and reorganisation of the actin cytoskeleton. TGF-β is known to play a prominent role in EMT in both normal physiological and pathological conditions and appears to require the Smad signalling pathways [104] and non-Smad pathways [70, 105-107]. Though other studies with a mutant TGFβR1 (ALK5) that was unable to activate receptor Smads but retained MAPK activity failed to induce EMT [108]. Further it remains unclear if indeed Smad signalling is required whether this is dependent [109] or independent [105] on the Co-Smad (Smad4).

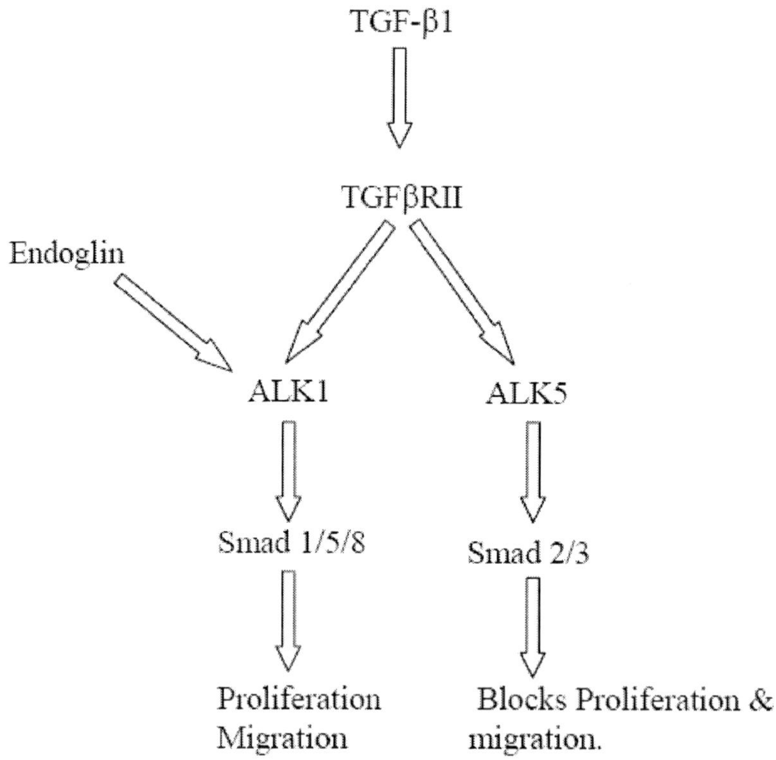

Figure 2. TGF-β1 can signal through two signalling pathways, depending on which TGFβRI is phosphorylated. ALK1 results in the phosophorylation of Smad 1/5/8 and results in proliferation. Whereas ALK5 will phosophorylate Smad2/3 and result in blocking proliferation and migration. An increase in the expression of endoglin results in ALK1 signalling whereas absence of endoglin present on cells will result in ALK5 signalling [100].

TGF-β1 and Cancer

TGF-β1 and its signalling components have been shown to suppress early carcinogenesis and therefore act as a tumour suppressor pathway [110,111]; however in later stages of tumour development TGF-β1 will enhance progression and acts as a tumour promoter [112]. In these late stage tumours TGF-β1 is often associated with malignant progression, metastases, reduced survival and the loss of sensitivity to the anti proliferative effects of TGF-β1 [113,114]. This lack of responsiveness to TGF-β1 is caused by either loss or reduced expression of parts of the TGF-β1 signalling pathways or through mutational changes found in a number of components of the signalling pathway (examples seen in Table 1).

In vitro studies have shown that TGF-β can stimulate proliferation and invasion in poorly differentiated and metastatic cell lines [115] , while a prolonged exposure of TGF-β1 in some cells will promote neoplastic transformation [116]. However TGF-β signalling can have both positive and negative effect on tumour development depending on the cell type involved and, the loss of regulation will have an effect on tumour progression and patient prognosis.

The TGFβRII is often mutated in areas of microsatellite sequences, which are prone to replication errors [117]. Loss of TGFβRII through a number of mutations in tumours results in pathway inactivation and this appears to result in a selective advantage during tumorigenesis. *In vivo* models have shown that animals that lack TGFβRII in the colon epithelium developed more colorectal adenocarcinomas and, showed increased proliferation compared to those with an intact functioning TGFβRII [118].

TGFβRI mutations have been associated with human cancers with TGFβRI*6A (deletion of three alanines within a 9-alanine stretch in the exon 1 coding sequence) [119] showed a significantly higher frequency in cancer patients compared to healthy controls [120]. Further mutational variants (TGFβRI*10A) of TGFβRI along with TGFβRI*6A show that these mutations can result in TGF-β stimulated proliferation [121]. Recent studies have indicated that TGFβRI*6A may contribute to cancer through a non-Smad signalling pathway (ERK and RhoA) [122].

Table 1. Examples of alterations in TGF-β signalling and the examples of the cancer which the alterations have been found

Component of TGF-βsignalling pathway either mutated or abnormally expressed	Examples of cancer	Reference
Activation of Latent TGF-β	Hepatocellular	[156,157]
TGFβRI	Breast, bladder, ovarian, T cell lymphoma, prostate	[158]
TGFβRII	Colorectal, liver, prostate	[159, 157,160, 161, 162]
Betaglycan (TGFβRIII)	Non small cell lung, prostate	[163, 164]
Endoglin	Pancreatic, oesophageal squamous cell carcinoma, hepatocellular carcinoma	[165-167]
Smad 4	Pancreatic, colorectal, head and neck squamous cell carcinoma, squamous cell carcinoma of the skin, lung	[123, 124, 168]
Smad 2	head and neck squamous cell carcinoma, squamous cell carcinoma of the skin, colorectal	[126, 160, 169]
Smad 3	Colorectal cancers (Smad3$^{-/-}$ mice)	[131]
Smad 7	pancreatic	[136,137]
E3 ubiquitin ligases: Smurf1 Smurf 2	Pancreatic P14ARF mutant melanoma	[170]
Co-repressors: Ski and SnoN TIEG1 Evi-1	Cell lines from neuroblastomas, carcinomas of the stomach, vulva and prostate Myeloid, ovarian,	[139,140] [171,172]
Adaptor proteins:ELF	Hepatocellular carcinoma	[173]
Others: P53	Hepatoma cell line (HepG2)	[174]

Both Smad 2 and Smad 4 mutations have been found in a number of human cancers and both are located on 18q21. Smad 4 has been found mutated in nearly half of all pancreatic carcinomas and in other cancers though less frequently [123-125]. Smad 2 mutations has also been identified in a number of tumour types [126,127] and have been suggested to disrupt

TGF-β signalling therefore resulting in the loss of growth inhibition by TGF-β. High Smad 2 activation has been associated with an increase in proliferation in some tumour types and a poor prognosis [128]. TGF-β1-knockout mice show the development of non-metastatic colon cancer [129] but not breast cancer [130]. While Smad 3 knockout mice will develop metastatic colon cancer and the tumours were hyperproliferative[131]. However in other studies colonic adenocarcinoma did not occur [132]. It has recently been proposed that chronic inflammation could explain this discrepancy [13]. To date Smad 3 mutations appear rare in human cancers though the level of Smad 3 may be altered during tumour progression [134,135].

Inhibitory Smads (Smad 6, 7) prevent the phosphorylation of R-Smads and therefore provide a negative feedback loop for TGF-β signalling. Over expression of inhibitory-Smads will therefore contribute to the loss of TGF-β anti-proliferative effects. Smad 6 and 7 have been found over expressed in both tumours, and cell lines [136,137] and appear in some tumours to play a role in metastasis [138]. Other proteins involved in TGF-β signalling appear to play a role in tumorigenesis for instance the transcriptional repressor Ski is known to repress the activated R-Smads from causing the transcription of TGF-β responsive genes possibly through competition with transcriptional co-activators p300 or CBP. The over expression of Ski has been found in a number of cancer cell lines [139,140]. Further Ski expression is up regulated in response to oestrogen in some tissues [141].

Other non-Smad signalling pathways may also be involved in causing the loss of TGF-β's anti proliferative response. Oncogenic Ras can negatively regulate TGF-β signalling via the phosphorylation of Smad 2 and Smad 3 at specific sites separate from the sites phosphorylated by TGFβR [18, 142]. Phosphorylation in these sites can result in reduced nuclear translocation and therefore cytoplasmic retention of Smad 2 and 3. Ras can also alter other TGF-β functions such as the up regulation of cyclin dependent kinases involved in the G1 phase of the cell cycle. Other signalling pathways which are over expressed (for example HER-2/Neu and EGF) have been hypothesised to phosphorylate the R-Smads through ERK and result in preventing the anti-proliferative effect of TGF-β [143].

TGF-β has been shown to down-regulate the transcription of the viral genes (E6 and E7) in the epithelial cell lines SiHa, CasK [144,145]. E6 and E7 are viral oncoproteins which exert effects over cell cycle control [146,147]. E7 is known to form complexes with members of the retinoblastoma family, pRb, p107, p130, and enhances pRB degradation which releases E2F allowing cell cycle progression [148,149]. E6 binds to p53 and mediates its degradation affecting cell cycle control [150]. However loss of other cell cycle control genes is required as E6/E7 is not sufficient for malignant transformation alone and this appears to include TGF-β signalling components. In HPV positive cervical cancer, progression is linked with loss of TGF-β sensitivity [151,152], this loss of sensitivity has been linked with a loss of TGFβRI [153] and some mutations and polymorphisms in TGFβRI have been shown to predispose the patient to cervical cancer [154]. The HPV viral oncoproteins have also been shown to prevent the R-Smad and Co-Smad binding to the DNA and therefore preventing gene transcription [155]. The viruses' hepatitis B and hepatitis C have also been shown to express oncoproteins that decrease expression or inhibit function of a number of cell cycle regulators (pRb, p53, p21; 14-22). Sheahan et al have demonstrated that loss of pRb function and $p21^{cip1}$, p53 may result in hepatocytes losing sensitivity to TGF-β cell cycle arrest [55].

Conclusion

TGF-β1 plays an important role in the regulation of fundamental cell homeostasis, which includes regulation of cellular proliferation. TGF-β1 signals through an intricate network of intracellular signalling proteins with a number of intracellular and extra cellular regulatory components. Aberrant expression of TGF-β1, its signalling components, and/or its regulators can result in aberrant proliferation leading to a number of human diseases. Studies are on-going to further understand the signalling pathways that are involved in this delicate balance.

References

[1] Massagué, J. TGF-Beta signal transduction. *Annu Rev Biochem* 1998; 67: 753-791.

[2] Roberts, A.B. Molecular and cell biology of TGF-beta. *Miner Electrolyte Metab.* 1998; 24: 111-9.

[3] Runyan, C.E., Schnaper, H.W., Poncelet, A.C. The role of internalization in transforming growth factor beta-1-induced Smad2 association with Smad anchor for receptor activation (SARA) and Smad2-dependent signaling in human mesangial cells. *J. Biol. Chem.* 2005; 280: 8300-8.

[4] Xu, L., Kang, Y., Cöl, S., Massagué, J. Smad 2 nucleocytoplasmic shuttling by nucleoporins CAN/Nup214 and Nup153 feeds TGFβ signaling complexes in the cytoplasm and nucleus. *Mol. Cell* 2002;10: 271-282.

[5] Dennler, S., Huet, S., Gauthier, J.M. A short amino-acid sequence in MH1 domain is responsible for functional differences between Smad2 and Smad 3. *Oncogene* 1999:18; 1643-1648.

[6] Janknecht, R. The versatile functions of the transcriptional coactivators p300 and CBP and their role in disease. *Histol. Histopath* 2002; 17: 657-668.

[7] Lin, X., Duan, X., Liang, Y-Y., et al. PPM1A functions as a Smad phosphatase to terminate TGFbeta signaling. *Cell* 2006; 125: 915-28.

[8] Chen, H.B., Rud, J.G., Lin, K., Xu, L. Nuclear targeting of transforming growth factor-β- activated Smad complexes. *J. Biol. Chem.* 2005; 22: 22139-21336.

[9] Inman, G.J., Nicolas, F.J., Hill, C.S. Nucleocytoplasmic shuttling of Smads 2,3, and 4 permits sensing of TGF-β receptor activity. *Mol. Cell* 2002; 10: 283-294.

[10] Esparaz-Lopez, J., Montiel, J.L., Vilchis-Landeros, M.M., et al Ligand binding and functional properties of betaglycan, a co-receptor of the transforming growth factor-β superfamily. Specialized binding regions for transforming growth factor-β and inhibin A. *J. Biol. Chem.* 2001;276: 14588-14596.

[11] Sankar, S., Mahooti-Brooks, N., Centella, M., et al. Expression of transforming growth factor type III receptor in vascular endothelial cells increases their responsiveness to transforming growth factor β2. *J. Biol. Chem.* 1995; 270: 13567-13572.

[12] Eickelberg, O., Cenrella, M., Reiss, M., et al. Betaglycan inhibits TGF-β signaling by preventing type I-type II receptor complex formation. Glycosaminoglycan modification alters β glycan function. *J. Biol. Chem.* 2002; 277: 823-829.

[13] Chen, W. Kirkbride, K.C., How, T. et al. Beta-arrestin 2 mediates endocytosis of type III TGF-beta receptor and down-regulation of its signaling. *Science*. 2003; 301: 1394-7.

[14] Letamendia, A., Lastres, P. Botella, L.M., et al. Role of endoglin in cellular responses to transforming growth factor-β. A comparative study with betaglycan. *J. Biol. Chem.* 1998; 273, 33011-33019.

[15] Lopez-Casillas F, Payne HM, Andres JL, Massagué J. Betaglycan can as a dual modulator of TGF-β access to signalling receptors: mapping of ligand binding and GAG attachment sites. *J Cell Biol* 1994; 124: 557-568.

[16] Moustakas, A., Heldin, C-H. Non-Smad TGF-beta signals. *J Cell Science* 2005; 117: 3573-3584.

[17] Massagué, J., Chen, Y-G. Controlling TGF-β signaling. *Genes Dev* 2000:14: 627-644.

[18] Kretzschmar, M., Doody, J., Timokhina, I., Massagué, J. A mechanism of repression of TGFbeta/Smad signaling in oncogenic Ras. *Genes Dev.* 1999; 13, 804-816.

[19] Hayashida, T., De Caestecker, M., Schnaper, H.W. Cross-talk between ERK MAP kinase and Smad signaling pathways enhances TGFbeta dependent responses in human mesangial cells. *FASEB J.* 2003; 17, 1576-1578.

[20] Yue, J., Buard, A., Mulder, K.M. Blockade of TGFbeta3 upregulation by $p27^{Kip1}$ and $p21^{Cip1}$ by expression of RasN17 in epithelial cells. *Oncogene* 1998; 17, 47-55.

[21] Yue, J., Mulder, K.M. Requirement of Ras/MAPK pathway activation by transforming growth factor beta for transforming growth factor beta1 production in Smad dependent pathways. *J. Biol. Chem.* 2000; 275: 30765-30773.

[22] De Caestecker, M.P., Parks, T.W., Frank, C.J.T., et al. Smad2 transduces common signals from receptor serine-threonine and tyrosine kinaes. *Genes Dev* 1998; 12: 1587-1592.

[23] Zhang, Y., Feng, X.H., Derynck, R. Smad3 and Smad4 cooperate with c-Jun/c-Fos to mediate TGF-beta –induced transcription. *Nature* 1998;394: 909-13.

[24] Yang, Y-C., Piek, E., Zavadil, J., et al. Hierarchical model of gene regulation by transforming growth factor-β. *PNAS* 2003; 100: 10269-10274.

[25] Itoh, S., Itoh, F., Goumans, M.J., Ten Dijke, P. Signaling of transforming growth factor- beta family members through Smad proteins. *Eur. J. Biochem.* 2000; 267: 6954-6967.

[26] von Gersdorff, G., Susztak, K., Rezvani, M., et al. Smad3 and Smad4 mediate transcriptional activation of the human Smad7 promoter by transforming growth factor beta. *J. Biol. Chem.* 2000; 275: 11320-6.

[27] Hayashi H, Abdollah S, Qiu Y et al. The MAD related protein Smad7 associates with the TGFbeta receptor and functions as an antagonist of TGF beta signaling. *Cell* 1997; 89: 1165-1173.

[28] Kavsak, P., Rasmussen, R.K., Causing, C.G. et al. Smad7 binds to Smurf2 to form an E3 ubiquitin ligase that targets the TGF beta receptor for degradation. *Mol. Cell* 2000; 6: 1365-75.

[29] Ebisawa, T., Fukuchi, M., Murakami, G., et al. Smurf 1 interacts with transforming growth factor beta type I receptor through Smad7 and induces receptor degradation. *J. Biol Chem* 2001; 276: 12477-80.

[30] Ogunjimi, A.A., Briant, D.J., Pece-Barbara, N. et al. Regulation of Smurf2 ubiquitin ligase activity by anchoring the E2 to the HECT domain. *Mol Cell* 2005; 19: 297-308.

[31] Shi, W., Sun, C., He, B., et al. GADD34-PP1c recruited by Smad7 dephosphorylates TGF beta type I receptor. *J. Cell Biol.* 2004; 164: 291-300.

[32] Zhang, S., Fie, T., Zhang, L., et al. Smad7 antagonizes transforming growth factor β signaling in the nucleus by interfering with functional Smad-DNA complex formation. *Mol. Cell Biol.* 2007; 27: 4488-4499.

[33] Koinuma, D., Shinozaki, M. Komuro, A., et al. Arkadia amplifies TGF-beta superfamily signalling through degradation of Smad 7. *EMBO J.* 2003; 22: 6458-6470.

[34] Massagué, J., Gomis, R.R. The logic of TGF-β signaling. *FEBS Lett* 2006; 580: 2811-2820.

[35] Carneiro, C. Alvarez, C.V., Zalvide, J., et al. TGFbeta 1 actions on FRTL cells provide a model for the physiological regulation of thyroid growth. *Oncogene* 1998; 16 1455-1465.

[36] Hannon, G.J. , Beach, D. p15INK4B is a potential effector of TGF-β induced cell cycle arrest. *Nature* 1994; 371: 257-261.

[37] Reynisdóttir, I., Polyak, K., Iavarone, A., Massagué, J. Kip/Cip and Ink4 Cdk inhibitors cooperate to induce cell cycle arrest in response to TGF-β. *Genes Dev* 1995; 9: 1831-1845.

[38] Sandhu, C., Garbe, J., Bhattacharya, N., et al. Transforming growth factor beta stabilises p15 INK4B protein increases p15INK4B-cdk4 complexes and inhibits cyclin D1-cdk4 association in human mammary epithelial cells. *Mol Cell Biol* 1997; 17: 2458-2467.

[39] Elbendary, A., Berchuck, A., Davis, P., et al. Transforming growth factor β1 can induce CIP1/WAF1 expression independent of the p53 pathway in ovarian cancer cells. *Cell growth Diff* 1994; 5: 1301-1307.

[40] Datto, M.B., Li, Y., Panus, J.F., et al. Transforming growth factor beta induces the cyclin-dependent kinase inhibitor p21 through a p53-independent mechanism. *Proc. Natl. Acad. Sci. USA* 1995; 92: 5545-9.

[41] Li, C.Y., Suardet, L., Little, J.B. Potential role of WAF1/Cip1/p21 as a mediator of TGF-beta cytoinhibitory effect. *J. Biol. Chem.* 1995; 270: 4971-4.

[42] Kim, Y.K. TGFbeta 1 induction of p21WAF1/cip1 requires Smad-independent protein kinase c signaling pathway. *Arch. Pharm. Res.* 2007; 30: 739-42.

[43] Tvrdik, D., Dundir, P., Povysil. C., et al. Up-regulation of p21WAF1 expression is mediated by Sp1/Sp3 transcription factors in TGF-β1 arrested malignant B cells. *Med. Sci. Monit* 2005; 12: BR227-34.

[44] Gomis, R.R., Alarcón, C., He, W., et al. A FoxO-Smad expression group in human keratinocytes. *Proc. Natl. Acad. Sci. USA* 2006; 103: 12747-52.

[45] Iavarone, A., Massagué, J. E2F and histone deacetylase mediate transforming growth factor β repression of cdc25A during keratinocyte cell cycle arrest. *Molec. Cell Biol.* 1999; 19: 916-922.

[46] Hu, X., Cui, D., Moscinski, L.C., et al. TGFbeta regulates the expression and activities of G2 checkpoint kinases in human myeloid leukaemia cells. *Cytokine* 2007; 37: 155-62.

[47] Frederick, J.P., Liberati, N.T., Waddell, D.S., et al. Transforming growth factor- beta mediated transcriptional repression of c-myc is dependent on direct binding of Smad3 to a novel repressive Smad binding element. *Mol. Cell Biol* 2004; 24: 2546-2559.

[48] Kowalik, T.F. Smad about E2F. TGFbeta repression of c-Myc via a Smad3/E2F/p107 complex. *Mol Cell.* 2002; 10: 7-8.

[49] Vermeulen, K., Berneman, Z.N., van Bockstaele, D.R. Cell Cycle and apoptosis. *Cell Prolif.* 2003; 36: 165-175.

[50] Warner, B.J., Blain, S.W., Seoane, J., Massagué, J. Myc down regulation by transforming growth factor beta required for activation of the p15(INK4B) G(1) arrest pathway. *Mol. Cell Biol.* 1999; 19: 5913-5922.

[51] Claassen, G.F., Hann, S.R. A role for transcriptional repression of p21Cip1 by c-Myc in overcoming transforming growth factor beta induced cell cycle arrest. *Proc. Natl Acad. Sci. USA* 2000; 97: 9498-503.

[52] Staller, P., Peukert, K., Kiermaier, A., et al. Repression of p15INK4b expression by Myc through association with Miz-1. *Nat. Cell Biol.* 2001; 3: 392-399.

[53] Seaone, J., Pouponnot, C., Staller, P., et al. TGFβ influences Myc, Miz-1 and Smad to control the CDK inhibitor p15INK4b. *Nat. Cell Biol* 2001; 3: 400-408.

[54] Laiho, M., DeCaprio, J.A., Ludlow, J.W., et al. Growth inhibition by TGF-beta linked to suppression of retinoblastoma protein phosophorylation. *Cell* 1990; 62: 175-185.

[55] Sheahan, S., Bellamy, C.O., Dunbar, D.R., et al. Deficiency of G1 regulators p53, p21 cip1 and /or pRb decreases hepatocyte sensitivity to TGFβ cell cycle arrest. *BMC Cancer* 2007; 7: 215.

[56] Ruzinova, M.B., Benezra, R. Id proteins in development, cell cycle and cancer. *Trends Cell Biol* 2003; 13: 410-418.

[57] Norton, J.D. ID helix-loop-helix proteins in cell growth , differentiation and tumorigenesis. *J. Cell Science* 2000; 113: 3897-3905.

[58] Benezra, R., Davis, R.L., Lockshon, D., et al. The protein Id: a negative regulator of helix –loop-helix DNA binding proteins. *Cell* 1990; 61: 49-59.

[59] Zebedee, Z., Hara, E. Id proteins in cell cycle control and cellular senescence. *Oncogene* 2001; 20: 8317-8325.

[60] Nickoloff, B.J., Chaturvedi, V., Bacon, P., et al. Id-1 delays senescence but does not immortalize keratinocytes. *J. Biol. Chem.* 2000; 275: 27501-27504.

[61] Tang, J., Gordon, G.M., Nickoloff, B.J., Foreman, K.E. The helix-loop-helix protein Id-1 delays onset of replicative senescence in human endothelial cells. *Lab. Invest* 2002; 82: 1073-1079.

[62] Prabhu, S., Ignatova, A., Park, S.T., Sun, X.H. 1997 Regulation of the expression of cyclin dependent kinase inhibitor p21 by E2A and Id proteins. *Mol. Cell Biol.* 1997; 17: 5888-5896.

[63] Ling, M.T., Wang, X., Tsao, S.W. Wong, Y.C. Down-regulation of Id-1 expression is associated with TGF beta 1- induced growth arrest in prostate epithelial cells. *Biochem. Biophys Acta.* 2002; 1570: 145-52.

[64] Kang, Y., Chen, C.R., Massagué, J. A self enabling TGF-beta response coupled to stress signaling: Smad engages stress response factor ATF3 for Id1 repression in epithelial cells. *Mol. Cell* 2003; 11: 915-926.

[65] Hu, P.P., Shen, X., Huang, D., et al. The MEK pathway is required for stimulation of p21WAF1/CIP1 by transforming growth factor-β. *J. Biol. Chem.* 1999; 274: 35381-35387.

[66] Kivinen, L., Laiho, M. Ras and mitogen activated protein kinase kinase-dependent and independent pathways in p21WAF1/CIP1 induction by fibroblast growth factor-2, platelet derived growth factor and transforming growth factor-β1. *Cell Growth Differ* 1999; 10: 621-628.

[67] Ijichi, H., Otsuka, M., Tateishi, K., et al. Smad4 independent regulation of p21/WAF1 by transforming growth factor-β. *Oncogene*. 2004; 23: 1043-1051.

[68] Yakymovych, I., ten Dijke, P., Heldin, C-H., Souchelnytskyi, S. Regulation of Smad signalling by protein kinase c. *FASEB J.* 2001; 15: 553-555.

[69] Petritsch, C., Beug, H., Balmain, A., Oft, M. TGF-β inhibits p70S6 kinase via protein phosphatase 2A to induce G1 arrest. *Genes and Dev.* 2000; 14: 3903-3101.

[70] Bhowmick, N.A., Ghiassi, M., Aakre, M. et al. TGF-beta-induced RhoA and p160ROCK activation is involved in the inhibition of Cdc25A with resultant cell-cycle arrest. *Proc. Natl. Acad. Sci. USA* 2003; 100: 15548-53.

[71] Kamaraju, A.K., Roberts, A.B. Role of Rho/ROCK and p38 MAP kinase pathways in transforming growth factor- beta-mediated Smad-dependent growth inhibition of human breast carcinoma cells in vivo. *J. Biol. Chem.* 2005; 280: 1024-36.

[72] Goumans, M-J., Valdimarsdottir, C., Itoh, S, et al. Balancing the activation state of the endothelium via two distinct TGF-β type I receptors. *EMBO J.* 2002; 21: 1743-1753.

[73] Wilkes, C., Mitchell, H., Gulati-Penheiter, S., et al. Transforming growth factor beta activation of phosphatidylinosital 3-kinase is independent of Smad2 and Smad3 and regulates fibroblast responses via p21 activate kinase-2. *Cancer Res.* 2005; 65: 10431-40.

[74] Wilkes, M.C., Leof, E.B. TGF-β activation of c-Abl is independent of receptor internalization and regulated by PI3K and PAK2 in mesenchymal cultures. *J. Biol. Chem.* 2006; 281: 27846-54.

[75] Wilkes, M.C., Murphy, S.J., Garamszegi, N., Leof, E.B. Cell-type specific activation of PAK2 by transforming growth factor beta independent of Smad2 and Smad3. *Mol. Cell Biol.* 2003; 23: 8878-89.

[76] Suzuki, K., Wilkes, M.C., Garamszegi, N. et al. Transforming growth factor beta signaling via Ras in mesenchymal cells requires p21-activated kinase 2 for extra cellular signal-regulated kinase-dependent transcriptional response. *Cancer Res.* 2007; 67: 3673-82.

[77] Jaffer, Z.M., Chernoff, J. p21 activated kinases: three more join the Pak. *Int. J. Biochem Vell Biol* 2001; 34: 713-717.

[78] Guo D, Tan YC, Wang D, et al.A Rac-cGMP signaling pathway. *Cell* 2007; 128 341-355.

[79] Grassart A, Dujeancourt A, Lazarow PB, et al. Clathrin-independent endocytosis used by the IL-2 receptor is regulated by Rac1, Pak1 and Pak2. *EMBO Rep.* 2008; 9:356-62.

[80] Turner, C.E., Brown, M.C., Perrotta, J.A., et al. Paxillin LD4 motif binds PAK and PIX through a novel 95 kD ankyrin repeat, ARF-GAP protein: A role in cytoskeletal remodelling. *J. Cell Biol.* 1999; 145: 851-63.

[81] Rudel, T., Bokoch, G.M. Membrane and morphological changes in apoptotic cells regulated by caspase-mediated activation of PAK2. *Science* 1997; 276 1571-1574.

[82] Daniels, C.E., Wilkes, M.C., Edens, M., et al. Imatinib mesylate inhibits the profibrogenic activity of TGFβ and prevents belomycin-mediated lung fibrosis. *J. Clin. Invest* 2004; 114: 1303-16.
[83] Yoshida, K. Regulation for nuclear targeting of the Abl tyrosine kinase in response to DNA damage. *Adv. Exp. Med. Biol.* 2007; 604: 155-65.
[84] Roelen, B.A., Cohen, O.S., Raychowdhury, M.K., et al. Phosphorylation of threonine 276 in Smad4 is involved in transforming growth factor-β- induced nuclear accumulation. *Am. J. Physiol. Cell Phsyiol.* 2003; 285: C823-30.
[85] Saha, D, Datta, P.K., Beauchamp, R.D. Oncogenic Ras represses transforming growth factor-β/Smad signaling by degrading tumor suppressor Smad4. *J. Biol. Chem.* 2001; 276: 29531-29537.
[86] Lo, R.S., Wotton, D., Massagué, J. Epidermal growth factor signaling via Ras control Smad transcriptional co-repressor TGIF. *EMBO J* 2001; 20 128-136.
[87] Wotton, D., Lo, R.S., Lee, S., Massagué, J. A Smad transcriptional co repressor. *Cell* 1999; 97: 29-39
[88] Mar, L., Hoodless, P.A. Embryonic fibroblasts from mice lacking TGIF were defective in cell cycling. *Mol. Cell Biol.* 2006; 26: 4302-4310.
[89] Battegay, E.J., Raines, E.W., Seifert, R.A., et al. TGF-β induces bimodal proliferation of connective tissue cells via complex control of an autocrine PDGF loop. *Cell.* 1990; 63: 515-524.
[90] Zhang, D., Jacobberger, J.W. TGF-β1 perturbation of the fibroblast cell cycle during exponential growth: switching between negative and positive regulation. *Cell Prolif.* 1996; 29: 289-307.
[91] Liu, X., Li, P., Liu, P., et al. The essential role of c-Ski in mediating TGF-β1 induced bi-directional effects on skin fibroblast proliferation during a feedback loop. *Biochem J.* 2008; 409: 289-297.
[92] Goumans, M.J., Valdimarsdottir, G., Itoh, S. et al. Activin receptor like kinase (ALK) 1 is an antagonistic mediator of lateral TGFβ/ALK signalling. *Mol. Cell* 2003; 12: 817-828.
[93] Oh, S.P., Seki, T., Goss, K.A., et al. Activin receptor-like kinase 1 modulates transforming growth factor-β1 signalling in the regulation of angiogenesis. *Proc. Natl. Acad. Sci.* 2000; 97: 2626-2631.
[94] Wiercinska, E., Wickert, L., Denecke, B., et al. Id1 is a critical mediator in TGF-β - induced transdifferentiation of rat hepatic stellate cells. *Hepatology* 2006; 43: 1032-1041.
[95] Burrows, F.J., Derbyshire, E,J., Tazzari ,O.L., et al. Up-regulation of endoglin on vascular endothelial cells in human solid tumors: implications for diagnosis and therapy. *Clin Cancer Res.* 1995; 1: 1623-1634.
[96] Bodey, B., Bodey, B., Sigel, S.E., Kaiser, H.E. Over-expression of endoglin (CD105): a marker of breast carcinoma- induced neo-vascularization. *Anticancer Res.* 1998; 18 1485-1500.
[97] Miller, D.W., Graulich, W., Karges, B., et al. Elevated expression of endoglin, a component of the TGF-beta-receptor complex, correlates with proliferation of tumor endothelial cells. *Int. J. Cancer* 1999; 81: 568-572.

[98] Duff SE, Li C, Garland JM, Kumar S CD105 is important for angiogenesis: evidence and potential applications. *FASEB J.* 2003; 17: 984-992.

[99] Fonsatti, E., Altomonte, M., Arslan, P., Maio, M. Endoglin (CD105): a target for anti-angiogenic cancer therapy. *Curr. Drug Targets* 2003; 4: 291-296.

[100] Lebrin, F., Goumans, M.J., Jonker, L., et al. Endoglin promotes endothelial cell proliferation and TGF-β / ALK1 signal transduction. *EMBO J.* 2004; 23: 4018-4028.

[101] Pece-Barbara, N., Vera, S., Kathirkamathamby, K., et al. Endoglin null endothelial cell proliferate faster and are more responsive to transforming growth factor β1 with higher affinity receptors and an activated Alk1 pathway. *J. Biol. Chem.* 2005; 280: 27800-27808.

[102] Lamouille, S., Mallet, C., Feige, J.J., Baily, S. Activin receptor like kinase 1 is implicated in the maturation phase of angiogenesis. *Blood* 2002; 100: 4495-4501.

[103] Ota, T., Fujii, M., Sugizak,i T., et al. Targets of transcriptional regulation by two distinct type I receptors for transforming growth factor beta in human umbilical vein endothelial cells. *J Cell Physiol* 2002; 193: 299-318.

[104] Piek, E., Moustakas, A., Kurisaki, A. et al. TGF-beta type I receptor/ALK5 and Smad proteins mediate epithelial to mesenchymal transdifferentiation in NmuMG breast epithelial cell. *J. Cell Sci.* 1999; 112: 4557-4568.

[105] Peinado, H., Quintanilla, M., Cano, A. Transforming growth factor beta 1 induces snail transcription factor in epithelial cell lines. *J. Biol. Chem.* 2003; 278: 2113-21123.

[106] Bakin, A.V., Tomlinson, A.K., Bhowmick, N.A. et al. Phosphatidylinositol 3-kinase function is required for transforming growth factor- beta mediated epithelial to mesenchymal transition and cell migration. *J. Biol. Chem.* 2000; 12: 27-36.

[107] Grände, M., Franzen, A., Karlsson, J. et al. Transforming growth factor-beta and epidermal growth factor synergistically stimulate epithelial to mesenchymal transition (EMT) through a MEK-dependent mechanism in primary cultured pig thyrocytes. *J. Cell Sci.* 2002; 115 4227-4236.

[108] Yu, L., Hébert, C., Zhang, Y.E. TGF-β receptor –activated p38 MAP kinase mediates Smad-independent TGF-β responses. *EMBO J.* 2002; 21: 3749-3759.

[109] Valcourt, U., Kowanetz, M., Nimi ,H. et al. TGF-beta and the smad signaling pathway support transcriptomic reprogramming during epithelial –mesenchymal cell transition. *Mol. Biol. Cell* 2005; 16: 1987-2002.

[110] Pierce, D.F. Gorska, A.E., Chytil, A., et al. Mammary tumor suppression by transforming growth factor- beta1 transegene expression. *Proc. Natl. Acad Sci. USA* 1995; 92: 4254-8.

[111] Siegel, P.M., Shu, W., Cardiff, R.D. et al. Transforming growth factor beta signaling impairs Neu-induced mammary tumorigenesis while promoting pulmonary metastasis. *Proc. Natl. Acad. Sci. USA* 2003; 100: 8430-5.

[112] Welch, D.R. Fabra, A., Nakajima, M. Transforming growth factor beta stimulates mammary adenocarcinoma cell invasion and metastatic potential. *Proc. Natl. Acad. Sci. USA* 1990; 87: 7678-82.

[113] Tsushima, H., Kawata, S., Tamura, S., et al. High levels of transforming growth factor beta 1 in patients with colorectal cancer: association with disease progression. *Gastroenterology* 1996; 110: 375-82.

[114] Wilkström, P., Stattin, P., Franck-Lissbrant, I., et al. Transforming growth factor beta 1 is associated with angiogenesis, metastasis and poor clinical outcome in prostate cancer. *Prostate* 1998; 37: 19-29.
[115] Schroy, P., Rifkin, J., Coffey, R.J., et al. Role of transforming growth factor beta 1 in induction of colon carcinoma differentiation by hexamethylene bisacetamide. *Cancer Res.* 1990; 50: 261-265.
[116] Sheng, H., Shao, J., O'Mahony, C.A., et al. 1999 Transformation of intestinal epithelial cells by chronic TGF-β1 treatment results in down-regulation of the type II TGF-beta receptor and induction of cyclooxygenase-2 *Oncogene* 1999; 18: 855-867.
[117] Ilyas, M., Efsathiou, J.A., Straub, J., et al. Transforming growth factor beta stimulation of colorectal cancer cell lines: type II receptor bypass and changes in adhesion molecule expression. *Proc. Natl. Acad. Sci. USA* 1999; 96: 3087-3091.
[118] Biswass, S., Chytil, A., Washington, K., et al. Transforming growth factor beta receptor II inactivation promotes the establishment and preogression of colon cancer. *Cancer Res*. 2004; 64: 4687-4692.
[119] Pasche, B., Luo, Y., Rao, P.H., et al. Type I transforming growth factor beta receptor maps to 9q22 and exhibits a polymorphism and a rare variant within a polyalanine tract. *Cancer Res.* 1998; 58: 2727-2732.
[120] Pasche, B., Kolachana, P., Nafa, K. et al. TβR-I (6A) is a candidate tumour susceptibility allele. *Cancer Res.* 1999; 59: 5678-5682.
[121] Pasche, B., Knobloch, T.J., Bian, Y. et al Somatic acquisition and signalling of TGFβR1*6A in cancer *JAMA* 2005; 294: 1634-1646.
[122] Rosman, D.S., Phukan, S., Huang, C.C., Pasche, B. TGFβR1*6A enhances the migration and invasion of MCF-7 breast cancer cells through RhoA activation. *Cancer Res* 2008; 68: 1319-28.
[123] Hahn, S.A., Schutte, M., Hoque, A.T. et al. DPC4, a candidate tumor suppressor gene at human chromosome 18q21.1. *Science* 1996; 271: 350-353.
[124] Nagatake, M., Takagi, Y., Osada, H., et al. Somatic in vivo alterations of the DPC4 gene at 18q21 in human lung cancers. *Cancer Res*. 1996; 56: 2718-2720.
[125] Kim, S.K., Fan, Y., Papadimitrakopoulou, V., et al. DPC4, a candidate tumor suppressor gene is altered infrequently in head and neck squamous cell carcinoma *Cancer Res* 1996; 56: 2519-2521.
[126] Takagi, Y., Koumura, H., Futamura, M. et al. Somatic alterations of the SMAD-2 gene in human colorectal cancers. *Br. J. Cancer* 1998: 78: 1152-1155.
[127] Eppert, K., Schere, S.W., Ozcelik, H., et al MAPR2 maps to 18q21 and encodes a TGFβ- regulated MAD related protein that is functionally mutated in colorectal carcinoma. *Cell* 1996; 86: 543-552.
[128] Bruna, A., Darken, R.S., Rojo, F., et al. High TGFβ-smad activity confers poor prognosis in glioma patients and promotes cell proliferation depending on the methylation of the PDGF-B gene. *Cancer Cell* 2007; 11: 147-160.
[129] Engle, S.J., Hoying, J.B., Boivin, G.P., et al. Transforming growth factor beta 1 suppresses nonmetastatic colon cancer at an early stage of tumorigenesis. *Cancer Res.* 1999; 59: 3379-3386.
[130] Boivin, G.P., Molina, J.R., Ormsby, I., et al. Gastric lesions in transforming-growth factor beta-1 heterozygous mice. *Lab. Invest* 1996; 74: 513-518.

[131] , Y., Richardson, J.A., Parada, L.F., Graff, J.M. Smad3 mutant mice develop metastatic colorectal cancer. *Cell* 1998; 9: 703-714.

[132] Yang, X., Letterio, J.J., Lechleider, R.J., Chen, L., et al. Targeted disruption of SMAD3 results in impaired mucosal immunity and diminished T cell responsiveness to TGF-beta. *EMBO J.* 1999; 18: 1280-1291.

[133] Maggio-Price, L., Treuting, P., Zeng, W., et al. Helicobacter infection is required for inflammation and colon cancer in SMAD3 deficient mice. *Cancer Res.* 1006; 66: 828-838.

[134] Han, S.U., Kim, H.T., Seong, D.H., et al. Loss of the Smad 3 expression increases susceptibility to tumorigenecity in human gastric cancer. *Oncogene* 2004; 23: 1333-41.

[135] Xu, G., Chakraborty, C., Lala, P.K. Reconstitution of Smad 3 restores TGF-beat response of tissue inhibitor of metalloproteinase-1 upregulation in human choriocarcinoma cells. *Biochem Biophys Res Commun* 2003; 300: 383-90.

[136] Kleef, J., Ishiwata, T., Maruyama, H. et al. The TGF-β signaling inhibitor Smad 7 enhances tumorigenicity in pancreatic cancer. *Oncogene* 1999; 18: 5363-5372.

[137] Kleef, J., Maruyama, H., Fries, H., et al. Smad6 suppresses TGF-β induced growth inhibition in COLO-357 pancreatic cancer cells and is over expressed in pancreatic cancer. *Biochem. Biophys. Res. Commun.* 1999; 255: 268-273.

[138] Halder, S.K., Rachakonda, G., Deane, N.G., Datta, P.K. Smad7 induces hepatic metastasis in colorectal cancer. *Br. J. Cancer* 2008; 99: 957-65.

[139] Fumagalli, S., Doneda, L., Nomura, N., Larizza, L. Expression of the c-ski proto-oncogene in human melanoma cell lines. *Melanoma Res.* 1993; 3: 23-27.

[140] Nomura, N., Sasamoto, S., Ishii, S., et al. Isolation of human cDNA clones of ski and the ski-related gene sno. *Nucleic Acid. Res.* 1989; 17: 5489-5500.

[141] Yamanouchi, K., Soeta, C., Harada, R., et al. Endometrial expression of cellular protooncogene c-ski and its regulation by estradiol -17β. *FEBS Lett* 1999; 449: 273-276.

[142] Calonge, M.J., Massagué, J. 1999 Smad4/DPC4 silencing and hyperactive Ras jointly disrupt transforming growth factor-β antiproliferative responses in colon cancer cells. *J. Biol. Chem.* 1999; 274: 33637-33643.

[143] Kretzschmar, M. Transforming growth factor- β and breast cancer: Transforming growth factor-β/SMAD signaling defects and cancer. Review. *Breast Cancer Res* 2000; 2: 107-115.

[144] Kang, S.H., Won, K., Chung, H.W. et al Genetic integrity of transforming growth factor-β receptors in cervical carcinoma cell lines: loss of growth sensitivity but conserved transcriptional response to TGF-β. *Int. J. Cancer* 1998; 77: 620-5.

[145] Lee, S., Cho, Y.S., Shim, C. et al. Aberrant expression of Smad4 results in resistance against the growth inhibitory effect of transforming growth factorβ in the SiHa human cervical carcinoma cell line. *Int. J. Cancer* 2001; 94: 500-7.

[146] Zur Hausen P. Papillomavirus infections: a major cause of human cancers. *Biochem Biophys. Acta* 1996; 1288: F55-78.

[147] Brandsma, J.L., Abramson, A.L. Association of papillomavirus with cancers of the head and neck. *Arch. Otolaryngol Head Neck Surg* 1989; 115: 621-62.

[148] Dyson, N., Howley, P.M., Műnger, K., Harlow E. The human papilomavirus 16 E7 protein is able to bind the retinoblastoma gene product. *Science* 1989; 243: 934-7.

[149] Boyer, S.N., Wazer, D.E., Band, V. E7 protein of human papillomavirus-16 induced degradation of retinoblastoma protein through ubiquitin-proteasome pathway. *Cancer Res* 1996; 56: 4620-4.

[150] Scheffner, M., Huibregtse, J.M., Vierstra, R.D., Howley, P.M.. The HPV-16 E6 and E6-AP complex functions as a ubiquitn-protein ligase in the ubiquitintion of p53. *Cell* 1993; 75: 495-505.

[151] Hasskarl, J., Butz, K., Whitaker, N. et al. Differential cell cycle response of nontumorigenic and tumorigenic human papilomavirus- positive keratinocytes towards transforming growth factor-β1. *J. Mol. Med.* 2000; 78: 94-101.

[152] Creek, K.E., Geslani, G., Batova. A., Pirisi, L. Progressive loss of sensitivity to growth control by retinoic aid and transforming growth factor-β at late stages of human papillomavirus type 16 initiated transformation of human keratinocytes. *Adv Exp Med Biol* 1995; 375: 117-35.

[153] Mi, Y-D., Borger, D., Fernandes, P.R., et al. Loss of transforming growth factor-β receptor type 1 mediates TGF-β resistance in human papillomavirus type 16 transformed human keratinocytes at late stages of in vitro progression. *Virology* 2000; 270: 408-16.

[154] Chen, T., deVries, E.G., Hollema, H., et al. Structural alterations of transforming growth factor beta receptor genes in human cervical carcinoma. *Int. J. Ca*ncer 1999; 82: 43-51.

[155] Lee, D.K., Kim, B.C., Kim, I.Y., et al. The human papillomavirus E7 oncoprotein inhibits transforming growth factor beta signalling by blocking binding of the Smad complex to its target sequence. *J. Biol. Chem.* 2002; 277: 38557-64.

[156] De Souza, A.T., Hankins, G.R., Washington, M.K., et al. M6P/IGF2R gene is mutated in human hepatocellular carcinomas with loss of heterozygosity. *Nat. Genet* 1995; 11: 447-449.

[157] Sue, S.R., Chari, R.S., Kong, F-M., et al. Transforming growth factor-beta receptors and mannose 6-phosphate/insulin like growth factor –II receptor expression in human hepatocellular carcinoma. *Ann. Surg.* 1995; 222: 171-178.

[158] Guo, Y., Jacobs, S.C., Kyprianou, N. Down regulation of protein and mRNA expression for transforming growth factor-β (TGF-β1) type I and II receptors in human prostate cancer. *Int. J. Cancer* 1997; 71: 573-9.

[159] Takayama, T., Miyanishi, K., Hayashi, T., et al. Colorectal cancer: genetics of development and metastasis. *J Gastroenterol* 2006;41: 185-192.

[160] Bedossa, P., Peltier, E., Terris, B., et al. Transforming growth factor- beta 1 (TGF-β1) and TGF-β1 receptors in normal, cirrhotic and neoplastic human livers. *Hepatology* 1995; 21: 760-766.

[161] Williams, R.H., Stapleton, A.M., Yang, G., et al. Reduced levels of transforming growth factor β receptor type II in human prostate cancer tissues. *Clin. Cancer Res.* 1996; 2: 1255-61.

[162] Finger, E.C., Turley, R.S., Dong, M., et al. TGFbeta RIII suppresses non-small cell lung cancer invasiveness and tumorigenicty. *Carcinogenesis* 2008; 29: 528-35.

[163] Turley, R.S., Finger, E.C., Hempel, N., et al. The type III transforming growth factor-β receptor as a novel tumor suppressor gene in prostate cancer. *Cancer Res.* 2007; 67: 1090-8.

[164] Yoshitomi, H., Kobayashi, S., Ohtsuka, M., et al. Specific expression of endoglin (CD105) in endothelial cells of intratumoral blood and lymphatic vessels in pancreatic cancer. *Pancreas.* 2008; 37: 275-81.

[165] Li, S.L., Gao, D.L., Zha, Z.H., et al. Correlation of marix metalloproteinase suppressor genes RECK, VEGF, and CD105 with angiogenesis and biological behavior in esophageal squamous cell carcinoma. *World J. Gastroenterol.* 2007; 13: 6076-81.

[166] Yu, D., Zhuang, L., Sun, X., et al. Particular distribution and expression of endoglin (CD105) in the liver of patients with hepatocellular carcinoma *BMC Cancer* 2007; 7:122.

[167] Howe, J.R., Roth, S., Ringold, J.C., et al. Mutations in the SMAD/DPC4 gene in juvenile polyposis. *Science* 1998; 280: 1086-1088.

[168] Lazzereschi, D., Nardi, F., Turco, A., et al. A complex pattern of mutations and abnormal splicing of Smad4 is present in thyroid tumours. *Oncogene.* 2005; 24: 5344-54.

[169] Hoot, K.E., Lighthall, J., Han, G., et al. Keratinocyte- specific Smad2 ablation results in increased epithelial-mesenchymal transition during skin cancer formation and progression. *J. Clin. Invest* 2008 ; 118: 2722-32.

[170] Packer, L.M., Pavey, S.J., Boyle, G.M., et al. Gene expression profiling in melanoma identifies novel downstream effectors of p14ARF. *Int J Cancer.* 2007; 121: 784-90.

[171] Kurokawa, M., Mitani, K., Imai, Y., et al. The t(3:21) fusion product, AML/Evi-1 interacts with Smad3 and blocks transforming growth factor-β mediated growth inhibition of myeloid cells. *Blood.* 1998; 92: 4003-4012.

[172] Brooks, D.J., Woodward, S., Thompson, F.H., et al. Expression of the zinc finger gene EVI-1 in ovarian and other cancers. *Br. J. Cancer* 1996; 74: 1518-1525.

[173] Kitisin, K., Ganesan, N., Tang, Y., et al. Disruption of transforming growth factor-beta signaling through beta-spectrin ELF leads to hepatocellular cancer through cyclin D1 activation. *Oncogene* 2007; 26: 7103-10.

[174] Cordenonsi, M., Dupont, S., Maretto, A., et al. Links between tumor suppressors:p53 is required for TGF-β gene responses by cooperating with Smads. *Cell* 2003; 113: 301-314.

In: Stem Cell Research: New Developments
Editors: Hiroshi Tanaka and Michael C. F. Chang
ISBN: 978-1-61942-081-6

Chapter 6

ORAL CANCER: BIOMARKERS, HALLMARKS, STEM CELL ORIGIN AND CLINICAL IMPLICATIONS

Athanassios Kyrgidis and Konstantinos Antoniades
Aristotle University of Thessaloniki, Greece

ABSTRACT

Oral Squamous Cell Carcinoma (OSCC) is the sixth most common malignant tumor and its incidence is increasing worldwide. The overall five-year survival rate in patients with OSCC is still lower than 50%. The classification and prognostic assessment of oral cancer is currently based on clinical and histopathologic biomarkers. Availability of an increasing number of molecular biomarkers provides with the potential for redefining diagnostic and prognostic categories and utilizing pharmacogenomics for the treatment of patients. The aim of the present chapter is to provide a basis that will allow the reconstruction of future oral cancer research. We critically review the common medical databases (PubMed, EMBASE, Scopus and Cochrane CENTRAL) for studies reporting on molecular biomarkers for oral carcinoma. In this chapter we will try to focus on oral cancer biomarkers through a cell cycle perspective. For this, the hallmarks proposed by Hanahan and Weinberg offer a good basis for segregation of various biomarkers. We further discuss the genetic basis of oral cancer with regard to the possible stem cell origin of cancer cells and the role of alcohol and tobacco in carcinogenesis.

Substantial evidence points to genomic instability as a cause rather than as a consequence of malignant transformation. In cell cycle reality, molecular and genetic changes interplay to give birth to a population of cells with enhanced properties. Cancer may be considered a process of "natural selection." If these new cells acquired properties that give them advantage over the remainder of cells in a multicellular organism, they would proliferate. Once these cells reach a significant number (clinically manifesting as cancer) they could attempt a "mutiny" and subsequently destroy the host organism-cell community.

Oral cancer will eventually end being a "black box" for researchers. Cancer precursor cells -stem cells more likely- undergo several genome changes. These changes could be either mutations or epigenetic. These changes provide the stem cells with the ability to self-invoke growth signals, the ability to suppress anti-growth signals, to avoid apoptosis, to replicate without limit, to invade, proliferate and sustain blood supply. Stem cells are able to collect progressively these changes in their genome. Mutations, epigenetic changes, nemosis, neosis and meiomitosis all have roles in the machinery that moves precursor stem cells round the hallmarks of cancer. Contemporary use of biomarkers although limited, is a reality, with HPV tumor discrimination, EGFR targeted therapy and aneuploidy being the most well documented.

INTRODUCTION

Epidemiology

Worldwide, more than 300,000 new cases of oral squamous cell carcinoma (OSCC, for abbreviations list, see Table 1) are being diagnosed annually. OSCC is the sixth most common malignant tumor and its incidence is increasing worldwide. [1] In the US, oral cancer accounts for 2.4% of new cancers while oral cancer case fatality accounts for 1.4% of total cancer case fatality.[2]

Morbidity

The overall five-year survival rate in patients with OSCC is still lower than 50%.[14] Being an aggressive epithelial malignancy, oral cancer is associated with severe morbidity despite advances in the application and combination of the major treatment modalities, namely surgery, radiation, and chemotherapy.[3] The poor prognosis of oral cancer has not improved significantly over the last four decades.[4] Locoregional failures include second primary tumors (this is oftenly termed "field cancerization") in those patients with early stage disease (American Joint Committee on Cancer, AJCC stages I and II) and local recurrence and/or regional metastases in those patients with locally advanced disease (AJCC stages III and IV).[5-6] Oral cancer is usually diagnosed only after becoming locally advanced in the majority of cases. [3, 5] It has been proposed that the ability to detect patients at an earlier stage may improve treatment results. [3, 5]

According to histopathological grading, OSCC displays variable metastatic potentials, and highly differentiated OSCC (G1) displays slow growth and destruction to adjacent muscle and the jawbone. By contrast, high invasiveness, early spread to regional and cervical lymph nodes, and poor prognosis are hallmarks of poorly differentiated OSCC. OSCC frequently shows local recurrence after the initial surgical or radiological treatment at the primary site and, unfortunately, even after complete resection (R0-treatment) [14-15] Despite all attempts, no significant progress has been achieved by combining surgery and radiotherapy, as ''traditional'' ways of treatment, with chemotherapy (neo-adjuvant strategies). Furthermore, there are no standardized protocols or common therapeutic strategies currently available, and the identification of relevant cellular and molecular markers primarily involved in oral pre-cancerous lesions and OSCC is imperative.[16]

Table 1. List of abbreviations

AJCC	AMERICAN JOINT COMMITTEE ON CANCER
AKT	V-AKT MURINE THYMOMA VIRAL ONCOGENE HOMOLOG 1
APAF-1	APOPTOTIC PROTEASE ACTIVATING FACTOR 1
ASIP	AGOUTI SIGNALING PROTEIN
BCC	BASAL CELL CARCINOMA
Bcl-2	B-CELL CLL/LYMPHOMA 2
BRAF	V-RAF MURINE SARCOMA VIRAL ONCOGENE HOMOLOG B1
CAF	CANCER ASSOCIATED FIBROBLASTS
CCND1	CYCLIN D1
CDK4	CYCLIN-DEPENDENT KINASE-4
CDKN2A	CYCLIN-DEPENDENT KINASE INHIBITOR 2A
c-Jun	MITOGEN-ACTIVATED PROTEIN KINASE 9
c-KIT	KIT HARDY-ZUCKERMAN 4 FELINE SARCOMA VIRAL ONCOGENE HOMOLOG
COX	CYCLOOXYGENASE
CPDs	CYCLOBUTANE PYRIMIDINE DIMERS
CSCs	CANCER STEM CELLS
CTNNB	BETA-CATENIN
DNMT	DNA METHYLTRANSFERASE
DPAGT1	DOLICHYL - PHOSPHATE N - ACETYLGLUCOSAMINE PHOSPHOTRANSFERASE
ECAD	E-CADHERIN
ECM	EXTRACELLULAR MATRIX
EGF	EPIDERMAL GROWTH FACTOR
EGFR	EPIDERMAL GROWTH FACTOR RECEPTOR
EMT	EPITHELIAL TO MESENCHYMAL TRANSITION
HPV	HUMAN PAPILLOMA VIRUS
INOS	NITRIC OXIDE SYNTHASE, INDUCIBLE
Ki-67	PROLIFERATION-RELATED KI-67 ANTIGEN
MAPK	MITOGEN-ACTIVATED PROTEIN KINASE
Mcl-1	MYELOID CELL LEUKEMIA 1
Mcm2	MINICHROMOSOME MAINTENANCE, S. CEREVISIAE, HOMOLOG OF, 2
MEK	MITOGEN-ACTIVATED KINASE
MITF	MICROPHTHALMIA-ASSOCIATED TRANSCRIPTION FACTOR
MMP	MATRIX METALLOPROTEINASE
MN/PGs	MULTINUCLEATE/POLYPLOID GIANT CELLS
MSH	MELANOCYTE-STIMULATING HORMONE
MYC	MYC AVIAN MYELOCYTOMATOSIS VIRAL ONCOGENE HOMOLOG
NAE1	NEDD8-ACTIVATING ENZYME E1
NBI	NARROW BAND IMAGING
NEDD9	NEURAL PRECURSOR CELL EXPRESSED, DEVELOPMENTALLY DOWNREGULATED 9
NER	NUCLEOTIDE EXCISION REPAIR
NGF	NERVE GROWTH FACTOR
NOTCH	DROSOPHILA, HOMOLOG OF
NRAS	NEUROBLASTOMA RAS VIRAL ONCOGENE HOMOLOG
OSCC	ORAL SQUAMOUS CELL CARCINOMA
p21	CYCLIN-DEPENDENT KINASE INHIBITOR 1A
P53	TRANSFORMATION-RELATED PROTEIN 53
PDGF	PLATELET-DERIVED GROWTH FACTOR
PPAR	PEROXISOME PROLIFERATOR-ACTIVATED RECEPTOR
PTEN	PHOSPHATASE AND TENSIN HOMOLOG
RB	RETINOBLASTOMA
SAC	S-ALLYLCYSTEINE
SCF	STEM CELL FACTOR
SHH	SONIC HEDGEHOG
SMN1	SURVIVAL OF MOTOR NEURON 1
SNP	SINGLE NUCLEOTIDE POLYMORPHISM
SRC	V-SRC AVIAN SARCOMA SCHMIDT-RUPPIN A-2
TGF	TRANSFORMING GROWTH FACTOR
TKI	TYROSINE KINASE INHIBITOR
TNC	TENASCIN C
TSG	TUMOUR STEM CELL
Wnt	WNT PROTEINS ARE A LARGE FAMILY OF SECRETED GLYCOPROTEINS THAT PLAY ESSENTIAL ROLES IN EMBRYONIC AND FETAL DEVELOPMENT, AND TISSUE MAINTENANCE. THEY BIND TO FRIZZLED RECEPTORS AND ACT AS PARACRINE PROTEIN FACTORS TO INITIATE A VARIETY OF SIGNAL TRANSDUCTION PATHWAYS.

Risk Factors and Biomarkers

Several models have been proposed to elucidate risk factors, such as smoking and alcoholic beverages. Genetic and epidemiological markers are involved in the generation and progress of OSCC. [1]

It has been reported that oral cancer develops as a result of the accumulation of genetic errors in the same tissue [7-8], with the activation of oncogenes and the inactivation of tumour suppressor genes also being involved [9]. The same apply for other types of gastrointestinal cancer [10] and melanomas [11]. Statistical studies of molecular aspects suggest that between six and ten genetic alterations (hits) are required to produce a malignant transformation of the oral mucosa. [12]

According to the multi-step carcinogenesis concept, OSCC develops in a series of more or less defined intermediate stages through the accumulation of molecular changes and progression from a pre-cancerous leukoplakia to pre-invasive (erythroplakia) and finally to the invasive cancer disease with lympho-nodal outspread and severe local destruction. [13] There are a large number of cell and tissue biomarkers that, may provide additional information to that obtained from the clinical examination and histopathological study.[9]

Knowledge Context

Oral Cancer Precursor Lesions

White patches (leukoplakias) of the oral mucosa are frequently encountered in the oral cavity and have been proposed as precancerous lesions. [17-19] Importantly leukoplakia is an entirely different entity compared to oral cancer in terms of prognosis and treatment. Five to 15% of oral white patches are histologically classified as epithelial dysplasias. [18] Of these, a substantial part (15–20%) is reported to progress to carcinomas. [19, 20]

However, the clinical problem of identifying the subgroup of oral leukoplakias that would progress into oral carcinoma has continued to challenge researchers. Accurate prognostication in patients with oral leukoplakia would ensure that they receive appropriate treatment necessary to prevent occurrence and dissemination of malignant disease. [13, 21-22]Furthermore, the identification of patients with particularly aggressive white patches may translate into more efficient primary preventive measures toward well-known risk factors as tobacco and alcohol. [13, 21]

Although the diagnosis of precancerous lesions begins with the clinical examination and the diagnosis of leukoplakia (which is a clinical sign) it is the histopathological study which determines the presence and degree of epithelial dysplasia (a term covering various alterations of the normal development and maturation of tissue). Thus, information is provided about the potential or risk (to varying degrees) of the lesion in question becoming malignant. However, the data obtained from the clinical examination and routine histopathological study are not entirely satisfactory. Therefore, several researchers have been studying the possibility of using (selectively) other more specific examinations that enable cell alterations to be evaluated. [9]

Convetional Prognostic Markers

The traditional prognostic marker of typing and grading of oral epithelial dysplasia is still extensively used but is of limited prognostic value. One important cause for this is the fact that both the intra- and interobserver reproducibility in typing and grading of oral epithelial dysplasia is poor. [23] Although many centers will perform preventive resection of leukoplakia showing mild or moderate dysplasia, there is no consensus on this approach, and surgical excision is only uniformly performed in cases with histologically proven transition to carcinoma in situ or carcinoma. Notably, the discrimination between severe dysplasia and carcinoma in situ is a difficult one. This most likely is a contributing factor to oral cancer being diagnosed at a late clinical stage. Therefore, reliable predictive markers that may be used to make a treatment decision at an early stage of disease development is badly needed. A number of such markers have evolved during the past decade. [24-25]

The Need for Oral Cancer Biomarkers

Improvement in oral cancer mortality has been pursued through in vivo and ex vivo strategies. [27-28] In vivo tactics seek to differentiate normal, precancerous, and cancerous epithelial cells using novel imaging instruments. Significant advances have been achieved in viewing oral tissue in situ with diverse strategies. Examples of the schemes that have proven useful feature technologies that use fluorescence spectroscopy, photodynamic imaging of tumors[29] and multiphoton microscopy of healthy tissue versus malignant lesions as defined in studies of carcinogen-induced tumors. [30] Another approach, introduced in the 1980s was the application of different tissue dyes. For example, toluidine blue has been used as a mouth stain for identifying high-risk primary oral premalignant lesions [31-32] Recently, this dye has been used successfully in clinical studies that have correlated histologic progression with high-risk clinicopathologic molecular patterns (i.e., loss of chromosomal heterozygosity; [31]). The use of advanced optical devices has further implemented such techniques. Such an example is Narrow Band Imaging (NBI), an optical technique in which filtered light enhances superficial neoplasms based on their neoangiogenic pattern.[33]

In ex vivo strategies, biopsies of normal and malignant tissues, or scrapings containing exfoliated buccal cells, have been long employed. [28] These strategies are intended to identify the precise location of an oral cancer in an early stage and thus enhance the prognosis through a variety of biomarkers. [31-32] *Biomarkers* are tumour- or host-related factors that correlate with tumour biological behaviour and patient prognosis. Practically, a biomarker is any measurable diagnostic indicator that is used to assess the risk or presence of disease.[26]

Both schemes are not without limitations and challenges. For example, screening for premalignant oral tissues by visual examinations with the naked eye, or facilitated with a scope, may be complicated by the presence of surrounding non-neoplastic tissue with inflammation or fibrosis [31]. Likewise, ex vivo assays may identify cellular or genetic changes; however, these alterations (biomarkers) may not correlate with true neoplasia and therefore may not be effectively used for tumor diagnosis. [34-35]

Genomic Instability in Oral Carcinogenesis

Substantial evidence points to genomic instability (as indicated by the finding of aneuploidy) as a cause rather than as a consequence of malignant transformation. [10, 36-37] Several studies indicate that mutations in genes controlling chromosome segregation during mitosis and centrosome abnormalities play a critical role in causing chromosome instability in cancer, [37-39] and chromosomal aberrations consistent with impaired fidelity of chromosome segregation during mitotis have been shown to occur exclusively in aneuploid tumor cell lines. These observations point to a key role of aberrant DNA content in carcinogenesis. Ploidy analysis has also been shown to predict, with a considerable degree of certainty, which non-dysplastic oral epithelial lesions will progress into carcinomas. [40-41]

The Processes Involved in Malignant Transformation

Apoptosis is the process of programmed cell death that occurs in multicellular organisms. Programmed cell death involves a series of biochemical events leading to a characteristic cell morphology and death. Apoptosis occurs via two interconnected pathways: the extrinsic(death receptor) and intrinsic(mitochondrial-dependent) pathways, both of which ultimately lead to the activation of effector-caspases(caspases-3, -6, -7), the final mediators of cell death,[42] PTEN, CDKN2A and APAF-1.[43]

Epigenetics refer to changes in phenotype(appearance) or gene expression caused by mechanisms other than changes in the underlying DNA sequence, hence the name *epi-*(Greek:over;above)-*genetics*. These changes may remain through cell divisions for the remainder of the cell's life and may also last for multiple generations. However, there is no change in the underlying DNA sequence of the organism;instead, non-genetic factors cause the organism's genes to behave differently. Epigenetic alterations include both DNA modification(methylation of CpG islands) and alteration in DNA packaging(histones). Over the past 10 years, more than 20 genes in oral have been shown to be dysregulated through epigenetic changes. [8, 44-47]

Nemosis is a novel term referring to fibroblast activity. Nemosis involves an increased production of growth factors and proinflammatory and proteolytic proteins, while at the same time cytoskeletal proteins are degraded. The cells that produce these cytokines are cancer associated fibroblasts (CAF), in plain English these are peritumoral fibroblasts. The expression of CAF markers differs between normal fibroblasts and CAFs in nemosis. This emphasizes the heterogeneity of fibroblasts and the evolving tumor-promoting properties of CAFs. [48]

Senescence is a characteristic of normal cells that refers to their limited proliferative potential, that is, they permanently cease proliferating ('senesce') after about 50 population doublings. During normal cell proliferation the ends of chromosomes (telomeres) become progressively shortened due to a phenomenon known as the 'end replication problem'. Senescence is thought to be triggered by signals generated by one or more telomeres reaching a critical length. It has been reported that only about 40% of primary OSCCs and about 60% of dysplasias are mortal and undergo senescence. [49] The remainder 60% and 40% respectively might owe its development partially to breaking the senescence barriers.

*Neosis*is a novel type of cell division, characterized by karyokinesis via nuclear budding followed by asymmetric, intracellular cytokinesis, producing several small mononuclear cells, termed the Raju cells, with extended mitotic life span. Normally, multinucleate/polyploid giant cells (MN/PGs) formed due to DNA damage are supposed to die via mitotic catastrophe. Before they die, some MN/PGs may undergo neosis. In the latter case, mitotic derivatives of Raju cells would give rise to transformed cell lines, which inherit may genomic instability, display a phenotype and transcriptome different from the maternal cell population, and anchorage-independent growth.[47, 50] Sundaram et al suggested that stemness may be a transient, cyclic property afforded by de-polyploidisation of senescing cells which have undergone polyploidisation. Furthermore, it has been suggested that mitotic catastrophe may represent a mechanism through which the cell can switch from the usual mitotic cell-cycle to this novel but evolutionarily conserved life cycle. Intriguingly, some most recent data suggest that cell senescence may be reversible and that stem cells are tolerant to polyploidy caused by genotoxic stress. [51] Senescence phenotype can be induced by i) telomere attrition-induced senescence at the end of the cellular mitotic life span and ii) also by replication history-independent, accelerated senescence due to inadvertent activation of oncogenes or by exposure of cells to genotoxins. Tumor suppressor genes p53/RB/p16INK4A and related senescence checkpoints are involved in effecting the onset of senescence. However, senescence as a tumor suppressor mechanism is a leaky process and senescent cells with mutations or epigenetic alterations in these genes escape mitotic catastrophe-induced cell death by becoming polyploid cells. These polyploid giant cells, before they die, give rise to several cells with viable genomes via neosis and the immediate neotic offsprings are the Raju cells. The latter inherit genomic instability and transiently display stem cell properties in that they differentiate into tumor cells and display extended, but, limited mitotic life span, at the end of which they enter senescent phase and can undergo secondary/tertiary neosis to produce the next generation of Raju cells. Neosis could be repeated several times during tumor growth in a non-synchronized fashion, is the mode of origin of resistant tumor growth and contributes to tumor cell heterogeneity and continuity. The main event during neosis might be the production of mitotically viable daughter genome following epigenetic alterations from the non-viable polyploid genome of neosis maternal cell. This could allow for the growth of resistant tumor cells. Because spindle checkpoint is not activated during neosis, aneuploidy can result. [47] Thus, tumor cells may also be destined to die due to senescence, but may be able to escape senescence due to mutations or epigenetic alterations in the senescent checkpoint pathway.

*Meiomitosis*is a mitotic division of cancer cells where these cells also express meiotic machinery during their division(Figure 1). Normal meiosis is a cellular division pathway in germ cells that promotes the recombination of large expanses of chromosomal DNA, potentially similar in size to those lost or gained in cancers. A major charactreristic of meiosis is chiasma or sister chromatid exchange. In this process, homologous chromosomes are held together by cohesions, and after resolution of chiasma (the recombination crossover points with the other chromosome pair), the homologous chromosomes are segregated together. In normal mitosis, there are no chiasma and sister chromatids are directly separated. In meiomitosis, the presence of chiasma, cohesins, and an aberrantly assembled mitotic spindle would be expected to result in significant shearing and/or mis-segregation of DNA sequences. Cells surviving this event would likely be aneuploid. [52] In the future we may come to understand that meiomitosis plays a role in genomic instability.

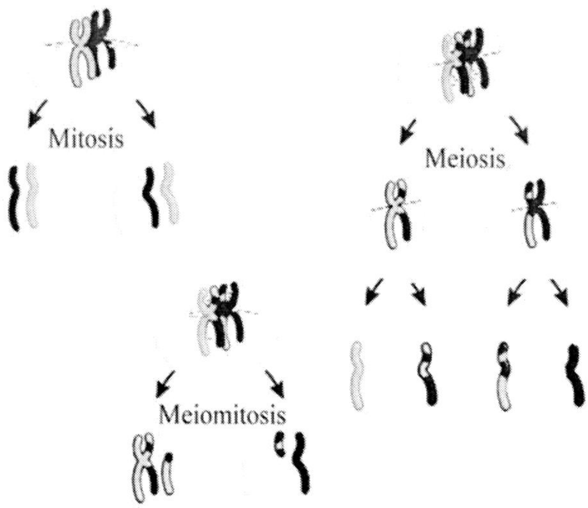

Figure 1. Mitosis, Meiosis and Meiomitosis. During normal Mitosis sister chromatids are simply separated into different cells. During normal Meiosis in germ cells, homologous chromosomes are held parallel to each other with similar regions facing each other. Chiasma is the point in meiosis where two homologous non-sister chromatids exchange genetic material during chromosomal crossover (sister chromatids also form chiasmata between each other, but because their genetic material is identical, it does not cause any change in the resulting daughter cells). After resolution of chiasma (recombined DNA at crossover points) chromosomes are segregated. A second meiotic cycle separates the sister chromatids. In Meiomitosis, mitotic cells express meiotic machinery. In these cells, chiasmata occur and homologous non-sister chromatids are partially linked together with cohesions. During chromosome segregation, shearing and/or mis-segregation of DNA sequences occurs that results in aneuploidy.

The Hallmarks for Malignant Transformation

Back in 2000, Hanahan and Weinberg reported the hallmarks of cancer.[12] In recent years, cancer research is focussing on finding new biomarkers of potential prognostic value and on better understanding the pathophysiological processes of the disease, on improving current therapies or introducing novel treatment approaches.[10]

Human cells, in order to transform to cancer cells, need to 1)provide growth signals-obtain growth self-sufficiency, 2)ignore growth-inhibitory signals, 3)avoid apoptosis, 4)replicate without limit, 5)sustain angiogenesis and 6) invade and proliferate (Figure 2).[10]

In this chapter we will try to focus on oral cancer biomarkers through a cell cycle perspective. For this, the hallmarks proposed by Hanahan and Weinberg offer a good basis for segregation of various biomarkers. Of course, this segregation is only aimed to provide better understanding of the various mechanisms by researchers. In cell cycle reality, all these molecular and genetic changes interplay to give birth to a population of cells with enhanced properties. Cancer may be considered a process of "natural selection." If these new cells acquired properties that give them advantage over the remainder of cells in a multicellular organism, they would proliferate. Darwin's law states "survival of the fittest"; cancer cells are only fittest than normal cells and this gives them the advantage to proliferate. This proliferation takes place at the expense of the community. Once these cells reach a significant number (clinically manifesting as cancer) they could attempt a "mutiny" and subsequently destroy the host organism-cell community.

We systematically reviewed the common medical databases (PubMed, EMBASE, Scopus and Cochrane CENTRAL) for studies reporting on molecular biomarkers for oral cancer. Articles were not reviewed on the grounds of outcome or methodology. Rather, the systematic review process aimed to identify eligible articles to support the aim of this study. Results were critically appraised and classified according to the hallmarks for cell malignant transformation proposed by Hanahan and Weinberg, the genetic basis of cancer, the stem cell cancer theory and the role of alcohol and tobacco in carcinogenesis.

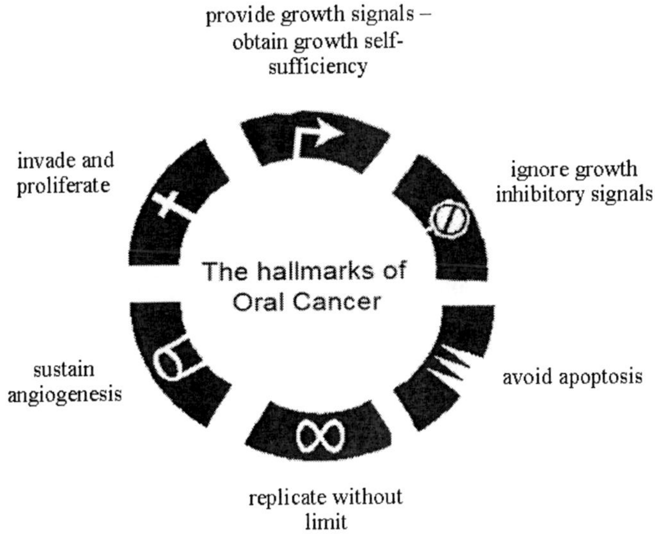

Figure 2. The hallmarks of oral cancer. See text for details.

Stem Cells

While extensive progress has been made on the molecular mechanics of cancer, the exact population of cancer cells where these changes will occur has not been defined. Along with the progress of stem-cell biology, the possible existence of "cancer stem-cells" that is rare cancer cells with indefinite potential for self-renewal that drive carcinogenesis has been proposed.[53]The recognition of a subpopulation of cancer stem cells (CSCs) in solid cancers has reinvigorated the field. These cells have the capacity for self-renew and give rise to more differentiated cell forms.[52] Importantly, these cells have the ability to survive long enough so that the required number of "hits" for malignant transformation occur. [11]

CSCs have access to embryologic developmental programs, including the capacity to differentiate along multiple cell lineages.[52] To sustain and repair tissue, a considerable number of daughter cells, CSCs must maintain significant plasticity into adulthood.[54] Carcinogenesis is currently considered to be an aberrant developmental process.[43]

According to the stem cell model, the initial mutations accumulate in a quiescent stem cell. When eventually, environmental signaling would activate the stem cell, due to these mutations, proliferation would not be appropriately controlled.[55] The neoplastic cells produced would attempt to follow normal differentiation pathways Although CSCs are likely to play a role in the cause of a variety of cancers, there have been no research reports proving the successful isolation of specific CSCs from OSCC lesions to date. Immuno-chistochemistry, transcriptional studies and micro-morphological data have all been employed to demonstrate or refute the CSC hypothesis in oral carcinomas. [53, 56]Treatment strategies of OSCC are based on the idea that oral cancer is generated by a population of cells of equal proliferative and aggressive potential [57] More recent reports suggest that the CSC hypothesis may likely also apply to OSCC [16, 56-58] OSCC CSCs could either originate directly from malignant stem cells or the tumorigenic potential may be promoted in the supra-basal compartment, where differentiating cells deviate from their predetermined differentiation route and transform into malignant intra-epithelial cells. The latter possibility is supported by the existence of the Tis-stage (carcinoma in situ) with the presence of typical malignant intraepithelial cells and an intact basal membrane. In Tis-lesions, malignant potential seems to develop in the stratum spinosum, but not in the stratum basale of the squamous epithelium. The dedifferentiation cascade in OSCC is typically associated with p53-mutations and loss of DNA-repair mechanisms [16, 59-60] In addition, oncogene activation, tumor suppressor gene inactivation, and the downregulation of cell-cell contact proteins, such as E-cadherin and β-catenin (which is also an intracellular mediator[11]), were described in OSCC [58, 60-65]. OSCC is comprised from malignant keratinocytes and their corresponding malignant stem cells might be found in the stratum basale of the oral and dermal epithelium, which has been identified in immunohistochemical studies to harbor epithelial stem cells. [56] The highest numbers of stem cells, which express β1-integrin and cytokeratin 15, are located adjacent to the dermal papillas and the basal membrane. [66] Several factors are involved in epidermal cell-cycle control and the regulation of normal differentiation pathways in keratinocyte formation. [66] Notch receptors are a family of conserved cell surface receptors that contain epidermal growth factor repeats in their extracellular domain and ankyrin repeats in their cytoplasmic domains. The cytoplasmic domain of notch receptors is released upon ligand binding and translocates to the cell nucleous where it acts as transcription factor. Notch genes encode large single transmembrane proteins and are crucial for normal epidermal integrity and function. In both skin and oral mucosa, Notch1 (NOTCH, DROSOPHILA, HOMOLOG OF, 1; NOTCH1, gene map locus 9q34.3) and Notch2 (NOTCH, DROSOPHILA, HOMOLOG OF, 2; NOTCH2, gene map locus 1p13-p11) signaling pathways induce and control the differentiation of keratinocytes. Notch2 is exclusively present in the basal epithelial layer while Notch1 is present in all epidermal layers. In skin, Notch1 and Notch2 have been proposed to act as tumor suppressors and regulate stem-cell maintenance, proliferation, and apoptosis. [67-68] Basal Cell Carcinoma (BCC) is the most common form of skin cancer and develops from basal epithelial cells of the skin which become malignant upon prolonged sunlight and/or UV--light exposure.[69] BCC is the result of a long-term process and this carcinoma usually grows much more slowly than squamous cell cancer or malignant melanoma. [70]BCC is believed to be an epidermal stem cell-derived carcinoma of the skin. For BCC, the increase in Sonic hedgehog (SHH) signal transfer and activation of the Wnt pathway were found to be the molecular cause for malignant transformation. [70] This imbalance is strongly connected to Notch deficiency and Notch1 and Notch2 expression are reduced in BCC [68-69] Experimental studies in mice reported that deletion of the Notch gene can lead to BCC development. [68-70] Furthermore, UV-light expo-sure triggers malignant basal cell transformation, especially in Notch1-defient skin areas. [68-69] BCC has an extremely low metastatic potential and is therefore considered a "semi-malignant" tumor. However, once ulcerated, BCC shows aggressive growth and deep local tissue invasion. [68-70]

The Quest for Stem-Cell Populations

Established OSCC cell lines would expectedly contain a small stem-cell fraction with high regenerative potential. When cultured at low densities, OSCC cell lines would generate cell aggregates with morphological and clonal features distinct from those of the rest of the tumor cells. These subpopulations that would be CD44+ vary in their morphological features, display different growth potential for each clonal subtype, and might be considered stem cell-like populations [16, 57-58] When cultured at low density in proper mediums, fibroblast-shaped cell lines derived from a highly differentiated OSCC will group into small clusters of cells with an epithelial phenotype and limited mitogenic activity. [16]. Currently, the origin of this CSC population remains to be determined, mainly due to the lack of stem-cell markers for head and neck cancers. One such promising candidate molecule is the EGF-7TM protein CD97. CD97 is highly expressed in bone marrow cells, undifferentiated thyroid carcinoma, and dedifferentiated (G3) OSCC [16, 58, 71-74] This surface molecule co-localizes within the basal cell layer of the oral squamous epithelium. It is currently not known whether these CD97 + β1-integrin-positive cells express other known stem-like markers or possess higher proliferative potential, as would be expected from stem/progenitor cells. The identification of specific stem cell-like markers for OSCC is most definitely challenging and might require the combined approach of high-end cell-separation techniques, such as laser dissection of cells, single-cell Q-RT-PCR, and DNA-fingerprinting. [53, 57-58, 75]

Tobacco and Oral Carcinogenesis

The frequency of oral cancer around the world is often indicative of the patterns of use of tobacco products.[76-77] A dose-response relationship between the amount of tobacco product used and the development of oral cancer has been established. [76] Every part of the oral cavity is susceptible to cancer from tobacco smoking or chewing, including the lip, tongue, palate, gum, and cheek.[78]

Besides these widely accepted statements, the contribution of different types of cigarettes consumed is yet to be defined. Nationally defined cigarette or tobacco categories and their relation to oral cancer have not been defined either. [79-80] It has been proposed that smokers need to be categorized by the Federal Trade Commission classification (regular, >14.5 mg tar; light, 6.5-14.5 mg; ultralight, <6.5 mg tar) in future studies. [81-82] Other unstudied cigarette features that might play a role in assessing buccal cell toxicity may include cigarette filtration (e.g., nonfilter versus filter), filter modification (e.g., charcoal filter), flavor (e.g., menthol), tobacco type (e.g., ''American'' blend), cigarette origin (e.g., Japan), and brand (e.g., Winston®).[35]

The mouth is the only body site that permits viewing with the naked eye the negative effects of smoked and smokeless (''chewing'') tobacco. For a given patient, it is often possible to view in the mouth during a clinical examination normal tissue, premalignant lesions (e.g., leukoplakia), and malignant tumors. [76] The need to identify biomarkers of oral cancer and their association with tobacco smoking is justified. [34, 83-84] When compared with other body sites, the oral cavity offers a unique opportunity for defining novel biomarkers since it allows noninvasive, repetitive examinations in longitudinal studies.

Thirty to eighty percent of oral cavity neoplasms arise from premalignant lesions, such as leukoplakia, erythroplakia, and oral submucous fibrosis. [85-86] Currently, the most common type of cancer detection is through visual inspection of the oral cavity with varied results. Sensitivity has been reported to be as low as 58%, and specificity as low as 76% [77] Moreover, there is scattered evidence that this type of visual screening helps to reduce the incidence or mortality from oral cancer. It is therefore commonsensical that such methods have not been recommended as screening tools by many government programs around the world [35, 77]

The preponderance of information identifies a positive association of tobacco smoking with buccal cell mutations. This conclusion is consistent with previous studies which reported on a positive association between tobacco smoking and mutations of lymphocytes [83, 87-88] and urinary bladder cells. [89] Buccal cell mutations might be useful biomarkers that could implement current clinical screening procedures.

The risk of developing oral cancer has been reported to be associated with both intensity and duration of exposure to alcohol in combination with smoking. A case-control study estimated that the risk of developing oral cancer was approximately 50-fold greater (odd ratio [OR] 50.65; 95% CI = 19–134) in heavy smokers and drinkers than those who never smoked and never drank. [90] In vitro studies have shown that alcohol enhances the penetration of tobacco associated carcinogens across oral mucosa. [91]

Alcohol and Oral Carcinogenesis

An extensive study of the association between nation-based alcohol-drinking profiles and oral cancer mortality of 20 countries in Europe, Northern America and Far Eastern Asia, reported that there were significant increases in male age standardized mortality rate associated with alcohol use, and that a high fraction of oral cancer deaths could be attributable to heavy alcohol consumption. [92 93]

A prospective study that assessed associations in the development of oral premalignant lesions using a cohort of over 50,000 United States male health professionals (58 per cent of whom were dentists) reported alcohol consumption as an independent risk factor for the development of these lesions, regardless of beverage type, drinking pattern or tobacco use. [94] The same study concluded that an interaction between alcohol drinking and smoking was apparent by their more- than-additive joint effects.

It has been reported that alcohol eliminates the lipid component of the oral mucosa barrier surrounding the granules of the epithelial spinous layer. [91] Another study reported that short-term exposure to 15% alcohol increased the permeability of human ventral tongue mucosa. [95] The authors postulated that this could be attributable to a disruption of the epithelial lipid molecules from their normal orderly arrangement, opening up the intercellular epithelial routes. Chronic exposure to alcohol has been known to cause epithelial atrophy and decreased basal cell size of the rat oesophageal mucosa. [96] Short-term alcohol exposure resulted in varying degrees of oral mucosa damage proportionate to alcohol concentrations; long-term use caused both macroscopic and microscopic changes to tissue, including dysplastic changes with keratosis, increased density of the basal cell layer and increased number of mitotic figures in a rabbit experimental model. [97] Another study assessed chronic alcohol consumption in an experimental rat model and reported oral mucosal atrophy with excessive regeneration, which could enhance susceptibility of the mucosal epithelium towards chemical carcinogens. [98] These data where in accordance with the results of another study in hamsters where the animals' cheeks were painted with a known carcinogen and those animals that were additionally administered alcohol developed earlier and larger epithelial tumors than with chemical treatment alone. [99] Sufficient experimental evidence supports an association between alcohol and oral cancer development.

Possible Mechanisms for Alcohol Induced Dysplasia and Carcinogenesis

Acetaldehyde is a primary metabolic product of alcohol and has been shown to be mutagenic. Alcohol metabolism is mainly carried out in the liver, however, some extrahepatic metabolism of alcohol to acetaldehyde, has been reported to occur in the oral cavity. [100] The authors further showed that there was differential expression of enzymes in the oral cavity, which could allow the accumulation of acetaldehyde in oral tissues. [100] Other studies reported that oral microflora produces considerable quantities of acetaldehyde during social alcohol consumption, a phenomenon more pronounced in individuals with a tendency to aerobic flora. [101] Activity of alcohol dehydrogenase enzyme has been documented in a range of oral bacteria. [102] This latter study showed significant variation among species in their ability to produce acetaldehyde with common oral bacteria, like Streptococcus salivarius, S. intermedius and S. mitis producing high amounts of acetaldehyde. Aerobic oral streptococci may contribute significantly to the normal individual variation of salivary acetaldehyde levels after alcohol drinking and thereby alter susceptibility to alcohol induced oral cancer. [102] The observation that individuals with poor oral hygiene have an increased risk of developing oral cancer might be explained by variations in oral bacteria [103] Warnakulasuriya et al in an immunohistochemistry study assessed specific alcohol-induced changes to the oral epithelium in patients with both oral cancer and dysplasia. [104] This study assessed the generation and sub-cellular distribution of ethanol-induced DNA-protein alterations, particularly the presence of covalently bound intra-cellular proteins with acetaldehyde, the first metabolite of ethanol, as well as end products of lipid peroxidation, phenomena which support ethanol-induced carcinogenesis.[104 93]

HPV Associated Oral Cancer

The association between OSCC and human papilloma virus (HPV) has drawn much light in the past decade. [105-106] The expression of the E6 and E7 oncogenes coupled with inactivation of RB and p53 proteins being the major molecular alterations associated with the presence of HPV-16. RB protein levels have been reported to be down regulated in HPV-16-positive OSCC, a fact clearly indicative of E7 activity. [107] With regard to E6 and p53 , the HPV-16-positive tumors could be classified into two groups. Those tumors i) exhibiting E6 gene expression and lacking p53 mutations and those ii) lacking E6 expression and carrying p53 mutations, the latter subgroup having a worse prognosis. [108] It is widely accepted that future HPV research needs to focus on developing a sensitive, validated laboratory test to detect HPV in oral exfoliated cells that would reflect HPV high risk types in head and neck tumors. [109] HPVs are small oncogenic viruses, which are implicated in epithelial carcinogenesis, and p53 is a tumor suppressor gene with a central role in the prevention of genomic injury. HPV infection and activation of the H-ras gene has been firstly reported in oral verrucous carcinomas. This fact is in accordance with the multiple hit carcinogenesis theory and suggest that in –at least- some cases, oral cancer may be a sequelae of the latter events. [49, 110] The E6 oncoproteins of these high risk HPVs are known to bind and induce degradation of p53 tumor suppressor protein through the ubiquitin pathway. [49] This degradation is largely controlled by a common polymorphism of the p53 gene encoding either a proline or an arginine at its codon 72 in exon 4.[110] However, no evidence suggests that TP53 codon 72 polymorphisms may be a risk factor for oral carcinoma. [111] It has been reported that HPV is not associated with the recent surge in the incidence of biologically aggressive oral cavity cancer in young populations[112] nor is HPV presence in oral leukoplakia is a prognostic indicator of malignant transformation.[113]

The most significant biomarker for HPV-related cancer is p16 or CDKN2A (reported below). Assessing both the expression level of the E6/E7 mRNAs and of CDKN2A in OSCC is required to detect active HPV infection. The loss of the chromosomal region 16q was reported to be a major genetic event in HPV-positive lesions. A cluster of genes located in 16q21-24 displayed decreased expression levels, notably NAE1 (NEDD8-ACTIVATING ENZYME E1, SUBUNIT 1, NAE1, AMYLOID BETA PRECURSOR PROTEIN-BINDING PROTEIN 1; APPBP1, gene map locus 16q22) that is involved in the modulation of the transcriptional activity of p53. [114].

Although tempting, the detection of HPV 16 and 18 in saliva from both oral cancer, oral leukoplakias and normal mucosa was not able to reveal any significant differences.[115] Other authors detected HPV significantly more frequently in patients than in controls and noted that HPV prevalence increased gradually with increasing severity of lesions along the oral lichen planus – leukoplakia - oral cancer sequence.[116]

A recent proteomic analysis detected thioredoxin (TRX) and epidermal-fatty acid binding protein to be upregulated in HPV related tumor tissue. [117] Further proteomic analyses are warranted to elucidate the molecular mechanisms of HPV-induced carcinogenesis. Despite the initial enthusiasm, it is becoming more and more evident that the use of HPV as a biomarker to early detect OSCC may be limited. On the contrary, its detection may allow for the segregation of a subset of tumors of better prognosis.

Hallmarks for Carcinogenesis

1. Provide Growth Signals – Obtain Growth Self-Sufficiency

The first hallmark cells need to acquire is generate their own growth signals in order to obtain self sufficiency from external autocrine or paracrine growth mediators.

NRAS

Marshall et al.[118] identified a gene with transforming activity in two different human sarcoma cell lines and identified this gene as a member of the RAS gene family and designated it NRAS(Figure 3). [119] Neuroblastoma RAS Viral Oncogene Homolog (NRAS;gene map locus 1p13.2) gene has been long reported to be mutated in OSCC. [120]

Given the sheer prevalence of RAS mutations in human cancer, direct and efficacious inhibition of RAS would be an ideal therapeutic goal. Currently, this might be more feasible in melanomas. However, inhibition of MEK kinase which is a downstream NRAS mediator via an investigational agent (ARRY-142886) is studied in oral cancer among others.[121]

MEK

MEK kinase(MITOGEN-ACTIVATED KINASE 1;MAP3K1;gene map locus 5q11.2), is a serine/threonine kinase that occupies a pivotal role in a network of phosphorylating enzymes integrating cellular responses to a number of mitogenic and metabolic stimuli, including insulin and many growth factors (Figure 3).[43, 122]

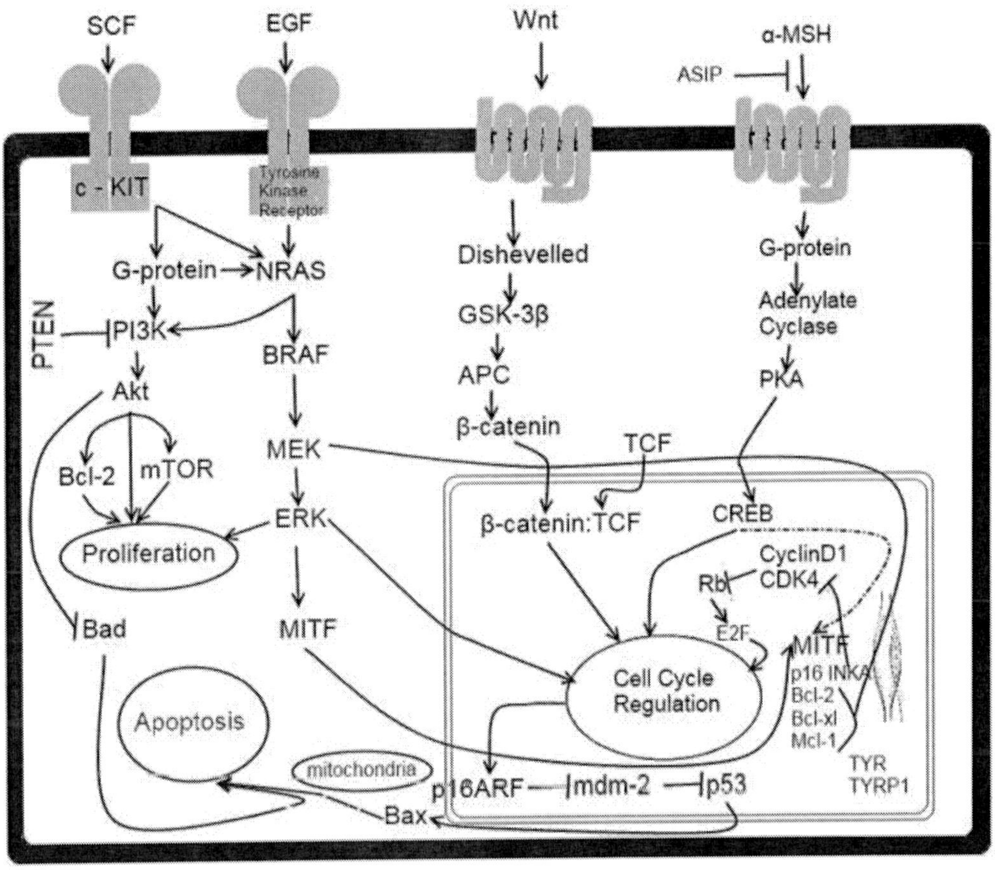

Figure 3. Oral cancer intracellular signalling pathways: A simplified diagram of three of the major genetic networks involved in carcinogenesis. The SCF/c-KIT signaling network(NRAS, MAPK and PI3 Kinase/AKT pathways), the Wnt/Frizzled signaling network(APC, β-catenin), and the Tyrosine Kinase Receptor signaling network (Ras, MEK, ERK) which have been implicated in oral cancer proliferation, apoptosis and cell cycle regulation. p16INKA and p14ARF are two separate tumor suppressors both of which are thought to contribute to senescence and tumor growth restriction. The p53 proapoptotic signaling network is also a major contributor to tumor cell apoptosis and chemosensitivity and is regulated by many of the oncogenic cancer pathways. →: designates a positive feedback.⊣ : designates a negative feedback.

MAPKs are located at downstream of a lot of growth factors (epidermal growth factor (EGF), nerve growth factor (NGF), platelet-derived growth factor (PDGF), etc.), the overexpressions and activation of which are frequently detected on a number of cancers including oral squamous cell carcinoma (OSCC).[123]

It has been reported that S-allylcysteine effectively inhibited the proliferation, up-regulated the expression of E-cadherin molecule and stabilized the E-cadherin/β-catenin adherent junction complex in human oral squamous cancer cells. The mechanism of action was reported to be at least partially through the suppression of MAPK/ERK signaling pathway and down-regulation of the SLUG repressor protein. [124]

OSU03012, a Celecoxib derivative, has been shown to inhibit proliferation and induce apoptosis in human cancer cell lines. Expression of constructively active MEK enhanced OSU03012-induced apoptosis. [125] OSU03012 has potent anti-proliferative and apoptotic activity against premalignant and malignant human oral cells through activation of Erk1/2, and Cdks and its results may be augmented by its administration in combination with a MEK activation treatment.

An experimental study in Syrian golden hamsters, reported that c-Jun (MITOGEN-ACTIVATED PROTEIN KINASE 9; MAPK9, C-JUN KINASE 2; JNK2, gene map locus 5q35) expression in oral cancer is increased through the EGFR-PLCγ-Raf-MEK-ERK pathway and not the H-ras-Raf-MEK-ERK/JNK pathway. [126] Bleomycin A5 is an anti-neoplastic glycoprotein antibiotic used for the treatment of various cancers. Previous work has shown that bleomycin A5 exerts its apoptotic effects on tumor cells. he apoptotic effect was associated with the sustained activation of c-Jun N-terminal kinases and the inhibition of extracellular signal-regulated kinases MAPK-3 (MITOGEN-ACTIVATED PROTEIN KINASE 3, MAPK3, EXTRACELLULAR SIGNAL-REGULATED KINASE 1, ERK1, gene map locus 16p11.2) and MAPK-2 (MITOGEN-ACTIVATED PROTEIN KINASE KINASE 2, MAP2K2, MAPK/ERK KINASE 2; MEK2 gene map locus 19p13.3) activities, suggesting that JNK2 plays a positive role in the death process. Upon bleomycin A5 treatment, cells expressing MEK1 exhibited significant delays in the onset of apoptosis, where the presence of MEK1 inhibitor enhanced cell death. [127]

In the leukocytes of patients with stage II and III SCC, the p38 MAPK pathway performs an essential role in the induction of iNOS expression, and the process of lipid peroxidation is not dependent on NO. In contrast, in patients with advanced-stage SCC, iNOS expression did not seem to be linked with the p38 MAPK pathway, and NO directly influenced the process of lipid peroxidation.[128]

Expression of MEK kinase may be a useful biomarker to discriminate subsets of patients that could benefit from celecoxib or bleomycin.

AKT

Phosphoinositide 3-kinases, or PI3Ks, generate specific inositol lipids implicated in the regulation of cell growth, proliferation, survival, differentiation, and cytoskeletal changes. One of the best characterized targets of PI3K lipid products is the protein kinase AKT(PKB; V-AKT MURINE THYMOMA VIRAL ONCOGENE HOMOLOG 1;PROTEIN KINASE B-ALPHA;gene map locus 14q32.3) (Figure 3). The Akt/PKB family of kinases is frequently activated in human cancers, include-ing oral squamous cell carcinoma (OSCC). [129 20]

The mitotic Aurora-A kinase (AURORA KINASE A, AURKA, gene map locus 20q13.2-q13.3) exerts crucial functions in maintaining mitotic fidelity. As an oncoprotein, AURKA aberrant overexpression leads to oncogenic transformation. AURKA, through Akt activation, stimulated nuclear factor-kappaB signaling pathway to promote cancer cell survival, and promised a novel combined chemotherapy targeting both Aurora-A and PI3K in cancer treatment. [130]

Inhibition of phosphoinositide-3 kinase (PI3K) increased EGF-induced COX-2 expression in the basaloid OSCC cell line (C12), suggesting a PI3K-controlled, inhibitory COX-2-regulating pathway [131].

Radiotherapy is the standard adjuvant treatment for OSCC and the Ras/PI3K/AKT pathway is the major mechanism associated with radioresistance. The methylation status of genes known to be involved in Ras/PI3K/AKT pathway were studied in 482 OSCCs. The Ras/PI3K/AKT pathway was activated in 140 primary OSCCs among 286 patients treated with radiotherapy after surgery and methylation of *RASSF1* (RAS ASSOCIATION DOMAIN FAMILY PROTEIN 1, gene map locus 3p21.3) (75.7%) was the most common mechanism. This study indicates that epigenetic silencing of tumor suppressor genes involved in the Ras/PI3K/AKT pathway plays an important role in OSCC radioresistance and this provides a rationale for exploring novel treatment strategies.[132]

Akt-induced epithelial-to-mesenchymal transition (EMT) involves downregulation of E-cadherin, which appears to result from upregulation of the transcription repressor Snail. Recently, it was proposed that carcinoma cells, especially in metastatic sites, could acquire the mesenchymal-to-epithelial reverting transition (MErT) in order to adapt the microenvironments and re-expression of E-cadherin be a critical indicator of MErT. Akt inhibition could induce the MErT through decreased NF-NB signaling and downregulation of Snail and Twist in OSCC cells. A strategy involving Akt inhibition might be a useful therapeutic tool in controlling cancer dissemination and metastasis in oral cancer patients.[129]

KIT

The tyrosine kinase receptor c-KIT (KIT HARDY-ZUCKERMAN 4 FELINE SARCOMA VIRAL ONCOGENE HOMOLOG;STEM CELL FACTOR RECEPTOR;SCFR; gene map locus 4q12) and its ligand, KITLG (KIT LIGAND;STEM CELL GROWTH FACTOR;SCF;gene map locus 12q22), are known to have multiple functions in hematopoiesis, melanogenesis, and gametogenesis (Figure 3).[133] In a series of 101 cases of salivary gland carcinoma lack of C-KIT was associated with worse prognosis. [134] However, not evidence exists to date that this oncogene has a role in oral cancer.

Ki-67

Ki-67 is a commercially available monoclonal antibody that reacts with a nuclear antigen (PROLIFERATION-RELATED Ki-67 ANTIGEN; KI67, gene map locus 10q25-qter) expressed in proliferating cells but not in quiescent cells. Expression of this antigen occurs preferentially throughout late G1, S, G2, and M phases of the cell cycle, while in cells in G0 phase the antigen cannot be detected. As a result, the antibody is used in tumor pathology to identify proliferating cells in neoplastic diseases. In cultured cells an antigen in the nucleolus of interphase cells stains with Ki-67, which, furthermore, reacts with an interchromatinous network during mitosis. [135]

In a clinical study of 28 patients with OSCC, Moota and colleagues, reported thatp53 and Ki67 expression analyzed together, were associated with tumor volume. The authors reported that with regard to OSCC, p53 and Ki-67 are related to larger tumors, metastasis to lymph nodes and very likely to a worse prognosis. [136]

Montebugnoliand colleagues examined the Ki67 expression in the opposite side of the lesion in OSCC patients. The mean Ki67 valuein the distant mucosa was statistically higher than that in controls. Abnormally high Ki67 values were detected in 23% OSCC patients. Multivariate analysis showed that Ki67 value in distant mucosa was a powerful independent prognostic factor, greater than tumour differentiation or clinical stage for the disease-free survival rate. Subsets of patients surgically treated for OSCC that have an abnormal proliferative status in areas distant from the primary tumour may benefit from the use of Ki67 value as a prognostic factor. [137]

Shpitzer and colleagues performed salivary analysis of oral cancer biomarkers. [138] They reported that five markers statistically significant increased in cancer patients by 39-246%: carbonyls, lactate dehydrogenase, metalloproteinase-9 (MMP-9), Ki67 and Cyclin D1. Three markers decreased by 16-29%: 8-oxoguanine DNA glycosylase, phosphorylated-Src and mammary serine protease inhibitor (Maspin). Sensitivity values of the eight analysed markers ranged from 58% to 100%; specificity values ranged from 42% to 100%. [138]

Torres-Rendonand colleagues immunostained paraffin sections of 41 oral epithelial dysplasia cases that progressed to carcinoma, 40 oral epithelial dysplasias without malignant progression, 38 OSCC and 15 normal mucosa controls, with antibodies against Mcm2 (MINICHROMOSOME MAINTENANCE, S. CEREVISIAE, HOMOLOG OF, 2; MCM2, gene map locus 3q21), geminin (GMNN)and Ki67. Labelling indices increased progressively from normal mucosa to epithelial dysplasia to OSCC (Mcm2, $P<0.001$; geminin, $P<0.001$ and Ki67, $P<0.001$). In all epithelial dysplasia cases (n=81) the levels of expression of Mcm2 gemininand Ki67 were elevated demonstrating a continuous cell-cycle re-entry. When the epithelial dysplasia groups were compared, Mcm2 protein expression was higher in the epithelial dysplasia with malignant progression ($P=0.04$), likewise there was a significant increase in the Mcm2/Ki67 and geminin/Ki67 ratios ($P=0.04$ and 0.02 respectively). Mcm2 and geminin proteins seem to be novel biomarkers of growth and may be useful prognostic tools for oral epithelial dysplasia. [139]

EGFR

The EGFR (EPIDERMAL GROWTH FACTOR RECEPTOR; EGFR, ONCOGENE ERBB, ERBB1, HER1, gene map locus 7p12.3-p12.1) and its ligands are cell signalling molecules involved in diverse cellular functions, including cell proliferation, differentiation, motility, and survival, and in tissue development (Figure 3). EGFR overexpression is reported to be present in up to 90% of OSCCs. Its presence is reported to be associated with nodal metastases and more rapid clinical course.

There is evidence supporting a role for the inhibition of cell cycling through blockade of EGFR-mediated signals via small-molecule tyrosine kinase inhibitors (TKIs) of the cytosolic kinase domain or antibody targeting of the extracellular portions of the EGFR. [140] It has further been shown that molecular blockade of EGFR with either an EGFR monoclonal antibody or an EGFR TKI enhances the radiosensitivity of human squamous cell carcinomas. [140] These observations have led to a series of clinical investigations that culminated in a phase III clinical trial for patients with locoregionally advanced OSCC, who were randomized to treatment with radiotherapy alone versus radiotherapy plus cetuximab/ [141] This clinical trial [141] showed statistically significant benefits in locoregional control and survival for patients who received the investigational agent, and subsequently led to the Food and Drug Administration approval of cetuximab for the treatment of locoregionally advanced OSCC.[140] In a subsequent large randomized phase III trial, the addition of cetuximab to platin-based chemotherapy [142] led to a significant prolongation of overall survival. The combination of cetuximab and platin/5-fluorouracil should be considered the current standard first-line regimen.[143]

A well designed study including 172 OSCCs [144] reported overexpression of EGFR in 27.9% (48 of 172) of the OSCCs analyzed. EGFR overexpression was associated with lymph node metastasis and extracapsular spread.[145] EGFR gene copies number is reported to be significantly associated with EGFR protein expression. Pretreatment EGFR staining intensity has been reported to be associated with non-pathological complete remission after preoperative radiotherapy for Stage II OSCC. Of note, no correlation was found between EGFR status and survival but EGFR FISH results were significantly higher in more advanced tumours (Stages II, III and IV) than in the tumours in Stage I. Non-smokers exhibited a significantly higher EGFR gene copy number and protein overexpression in Stages I and II OSCC than smokers. [144]

Both clinical and experimental data converge to the signifiacne of EGFR in oral carcinogenesis. Among the members of the erbB family, EGFR (HER1) was found to be the most frequently amplified and highly expressed gene in both human and mouse oral tumors. Genes for downstream effectors of EGFR, including KRAS, mitogen-activated protein kinase 1, and CCND1, were also found amplified or mutated, which resulted in activation of EGFR signaling in 55% of OSCC patients. Head and neck squamous cancer cells with different EGFR expression levels showed differential sensitivity to antitumor effects of AG1478, a potent EGFR inhibitor. AG1478-induced EGFR inactivation significantly suppressed tumor development and progression in a mouse oral cancer model[146]

Alphanubeta6 integrin, which is a marker for aggressive oral cancer, may regulate epidermal growth factor receptor expression. Targeting both alphanubeta6 and EGFR may provide additional benefits.[147]

EGFR is probably the most useable biomarker for oral cancer today, the administration of anti-EGFR cetuximab taking the merit. Since further study is logically expected, more prognostic and therapeutic uses of EGFR for oral cancer can be anticipated.

SRC

The SRC (V-SRC AVIAN SARCOMA (SCHMIDT-RUPPIN A-2) VIRAL ONCOGENE, gene map locus 20q12-q13) gene is homologous in sequence to the v-src gene of the Rous sarcoma virus (also called avian sarcoma virus, ASV). SRC oncogene has been associated with epithelial to mesenchymal transition, high-grade tumors, lymph node metastases and sarcomatous transformation in oral cancer. [148]

Immunohistochemistry revealed that, particularly in Bettel Quid chewing cases, the activity of Src family kinases was significantly higher in tumor-adjacent mucosa than that in solid tumor areas. These results suggest a possible role of Src family kinases in tumor-host interface and thus in early tumor invasion in vivo. Consistent with this is the observation that activation of Src family kinases is colocalized with invasive tumor fronts in oral squamous cell carcinoma [149]. Together, these data suggest that SRC may represent a potential biomarker of invasion and therapeutic target in oral cancer.

Radiation-Induced Bystander Effect

Irradiated fibroblasts adjacent to the tumor induce a response of non-irradiated neighboring cells that is called 'radiation-induced bystander effect'. [150] This phenomena is still unclear in non-irradiated OSCC cells. [151] Irradiated fibroblasts promoted the invasive growth of T3M-1 OSCC cells, but not their apoptosis, more greatly than non-irradiated fibroblasts, using collagen gel invasion assay, immunohistochemistry and Western blot in an experimental design. Following 1,6,12or 24 Gy cumulative dose, the numbers of irradiated fibroblasts was reported to decrease to about 30% when compared with non-irradiated fibroblasts. Still, irradiated fibroblasts increased the expression of Ki-67 proliferation marker of SCC cells more greatly than non-irradiated fibroblasts. Irradiated fibroblasts may promote invasion and growth of SCC cells by enhancinginvasive growth-related molecules through a TGF- b1-mediated bystander mechanism, in which irradiated fibroblast-induced genomic instability of SCC cells may be implicated. [151]

2. Ignore Growth Inhibitory Signals

The second hallmark cell need to obtain to progress to cancer is the ability to ignore inhibitory signals. This mainly occurs via loss of function mutations in tumour suppressor genes (TSGs). These mutations can be either true mutations or epigenetic alterations.

RB

The retinoblastoma gene RB(RETINOBLASTOMA;gene map locus 13q14.1-q14.2) was the first tumour suppressor gene cloned, and is a negative regulator of the cell cycle through its ability to bind the transcription factor E2F and repress transcription of genes required for S phase.[12] No studies have systematically examined the status of RB in oral cancer. Clinical studies report that RB loss is neither a frequent nor an early event in oral carcinogenesis. [152] Other clinical studies reported that disabling of the RB and p53 pathways were frequent events in oral carcinoma. [153] It has been supported that the Rb pathway proteins are comparatively more important than p53 pathway proteins for the prognostication of oral carcinoma patients.[153] Besides the inconsistency of clinical results, experimental results support the belief that the expression of RB is related to malignant transformation and conversion of the oral mucosa, being a reliable biomarker linked to oral cancer pathogenesis.[154]

CCND1

CCND1 (CYCLIN D1;B-CELL CLL/LYMPHOMA 1;BCL1;B-CELL LEUKEMIA 1;gene map locus 11q13) is the regulatory subunit of a holoenzyme that phosphorylates and inactivates the RB protein and promotes progression through the G1→S phase of the cell cycle in a manner dependent on CDKs (Figure 3). Furthemore, CCND1 is involved in a number of cell-cycle CDK-dependent and independent functions. CCND1regulates transcription factors, coactivators, and corepressors that govern histone-acetylating and chromatin-remodelling-proteins. CCND1 also has multiple roles in cellular growth, metabolism, and cellular differentiation. Amplification or overexpression of CCND1 plays pivotal roles in the development of several human cancers, including parathyroid adenoma, breast cancer, colon cancer, lymphoma, melanoma, and prostate cancer.[12, 155] Oncogenic RAS has been shown to positively impact the cell cycle by upregulating CCND1 through MAPK signaling[156] thereby serving as a link between the MAPK and p16-cyclin D/CDK4-RB pathways). The combined evaluation of p16 and cyclin D1 in oral carcinoma could identify a group of patients with the worst survival who might therefore need alternate or more intense treatment strategies. [153] Rb pathway proteins, Rb cyclin D1 and p16 showed significant association with disease-free survival, and p16 and cyclin D1 with the overall survival. [153] In cyclin D1 knockdown cells the down-regulation of cisplatin-induced NF-kB activity was independent of CDK4 function. In vivo tumor transplantation models also confirmed a cisplatin-sensitizing effect of cyclin D1 silencing RNA in OSCC. A TUNEL assay validated the increase in apoptosis as induced by cisplatin in cyclin D1 knockdown cells. Cyclin D1 may be an important target for future therapy in patients with OSCC. [157]

CDKN2A

The CDKN2A(CYCLIN-DEPENDENT KINASE INHIBITOR 2A; CDKN2A; CDKN2; gene map locus 9p21) gene encodes proteins that regulate two critical cell cycle regulatory pathways, the p53 pathway and the RB pathway. Through the use of shared coding regions and alternative reading frames, the CDKN2A gene produces 2 major proteins: p16INK4A, which is a cyclin-dependent kinase inhibitor, and p14ARF, which binds the p53-stabilizing protein MDM2(Figure 3).[158] p16INK4A inhibits Cdk4/6-mediated phosphorylation of the retinoblastoma protein. In the hypophosphorylated state, RB binds and represses the E2F transcription factor and prevents G1→S transition. Alternatively, p14ARF directly prevents MDM2 from accelerating the degradation of p53. Loss of the CDKN2A locus negatively impacts on both the RB and p53 pathways. In addition to its effects on the p53 pathway, there is emerging evidence to suggest that p14ARF also possesses tumour-suppressive effects that are independent of p53. The percentages of p16 positive cells in OSCC and oral leukoplakia without dysplasia were 89% and 17%, respectively while no significant difference in the percentage of positive keratinocytes was found. It has been reported that p16 is not a reliable biomarker for oral mucosal dysplasia and malignant transformation.[159] However, loss of Heterozygocity (LOH) at the 9p21 site was found to be over 30% in dysplasia and over 80% in cancer; furthermore the authors reported it was associated with increased risk for SCC.[148]

The transcriptional epigenetic silencing of some cell cycle inhibitors and tumor suppressors, such as p16 and retinoic acid receptor β, by DNA hypermethylation at CpG islands is commonly found in human oral squamous carcinoma cells. In a mouse model DNA methyltransferase inhibitor 5-Aza-2′-deoxycytidine, retinoic acid and the combination of 5-Aza and the low-dose RA on murine oral cavity carcinogenesis induced by the carcinogen 4-nitroquinoline 1-oxide (4-NQO) were reported to be effective treatments with the combination being the most potent. [160]

In aprospective cohort study which included one hundred one patients with histologically confirmed mild or moderate oral epithelial dysplasia were therate of progression to oral cancer in the group of patients withmethylated p16 oral epithelial dysplasia was significantly higher than that with the unmethylated p16 oral epithelial dysplasia (43.8% versus 17.4%; adjusted odds ratio, 3.7; = 0.013), especially for patients at the baseline age of ≥60 years (adjusted odds ratio, 12.0; = 0.003) and patients with moderate oral epithelial dysplasia (adjusted odds ratio, 15.6; = 0.022). This study with a 46 months follow-up period showed that methylation of p16 CpG Island is a frequent event in oral epithelial dysplasia. The overall sensitivity and specificity of prediction of malignant transformation of oral epithelial dysplasia by methylation were 63.6% and 67.9%, respectively. Thus p16 CpG island methylation is a potential biomarker for prediction of prognosis of mild or moderate oral epithelial dysplasia in humans.[161] Another study reported loss of p16 expression by promoter hypermethylation to be an early event in the development of oral cancer and that participants with positive molecular margins had a 6.3-fold increased risk of having local recurrence as compared to participants with negative margins. [162]

CDK4

Cyclin-dependent kinase-4(CDK4;gene map locus 12q14) is a protein-serine kinase involved in the cell cycle. Human cell division is regulated primarily at the G1→S or the G2→M boundaries within the cell cycle. The sequential activation of cyclin-dependent kinases and their subsequent phosphorylation of critical substrates promote orderly progression through the cell cycle. The complexes formed by CDK4 and the D-type cyclins are involved in the control of cell proliferation during the G1 phase. CDK4 is inhibited by p16INK4A. Given that p16INK4A needs to directly interact with the cyclin–CDK complex in order to inhibit its protein kinase activity, changes in CDK4 that render it resistant to p16INK4A mimic p16INK4A loss.

In OSCC, loss of CDK4 function has not been shown to play any role as a biomarker.

PTEN

Early loss-of-heterozygosity studies suggested the presence of a chromosome 10q locus lost early in tumor progression(Figure 3).[163] PTEN (PHOSPHATASE AND TENSIN HOMOLOG;gene map locus 10q23.31) was one of the putative TSGs on chromosome 10 and had been shown to be mutated in gliomas, breast, prostate, and kidney cancers and melanomas.[43] Immunohistochemiistry showed statistically significant differences in the immunohistochemical scores for PTEN protein in normal tissues and in cancerous regions, suggesting that PTEN protein expression is down-regulated in OSCC. [164]

In a study which investigated a number of genes as potential biomarkers in 49 OSCCs, p16INK4a, p14ARF, 06-MGMT, RB1, PTEN, and p27Kip1 were found to be methylated in 34.7%, 20.4%, 12.2%, 10.2%, 6.1%, and 4.1% respectively.[165] Treatment of an OSCC cell line with the methyltransferase inhibitor 5-azacytidine showed a significant increase in the expression of TSG genes, suggesting methylation of their promoters.[166] Moreover, treatment with demethylating reagents restored PTEN mRNA expression in 4 OSCC cell lines in another study. [164] No genetic mutations were detected in these cell lines by polymerase chain reaction-single strand conformation polymorphism (PCR-SSCP) analysis. [164] Thus epigenetic changes are probably related to the down-regulation of PTEN expression. In this regard a low LOH rate of 13% at the PTEN locus has been reported in the study which included 49 tumours. [165] No significant correlations were reported to exist between the down-regulation of PTEN protein expression and the clinicopathological features of the tumor. [164] PTEN may play a role in the oncogenesis of oral squamous cell carcinoma, and PTEN may down-regulate the expression of cyclin D1, which leads to the suppression of cell growth.[167] Despite the fact that PTEN cannot be considered as useful biomarker for oral cancer as it is in melanoma, [11] it is plausible that reversal of its epigenetic silencing through methylation inhibitors may be a treatment option.

B-Catenin

Beta-catenin (CTNNB;gene map locus 3p22-p21.3) is an adherens junction protein and a transcriptional coactivator (Figure 3). Adherens junctions mediate adhesion between cells, communicate a signal that neighbouring cells are present, and anchor the actin cytoskeleton thus regulate normal cell growth and behaviour β-catenin is an important downstream mediator of the Wnt pathway.. Wnt proteins are a large family of secreted glycoproteins that play essential roles in EMBRYONIC AND FETAL DEVELOPMENT, and tissue maintenance. They bind to FRIZZLED RECEPTORS and act as PARACRINE PROTEIN FACTORS to initiate a variety of SIGNAL TRANSDUCTION PATHWAYS. It has been reported that WNT-5A may be an important marker during initial events of actinic cheilitis malignant transformation, in which non-canonical and canonical Wnt/beta-catenin signaling pathways could be involved. Additionally, WNT-5A might recruit other events in lip SCC, such as MMP-3 protein synthesis, as its presence is increased in established malignant processes even without beta-catenin dependency.[168] The canonical Wnt signaling pathway stabilizes β-catenin, with MITF as a critical downstream target. The expression of Wnt1 and Wnt5a is considered to be associated with malignant transformation and conversion of the oral mucosa.[169]

In a tongue cancer cell line the introduction of N-cadherin and beta-catenin silencing RNAs gave rise to proliferation suppression of the cells, accompanied with a cell cycle inhibition at the G0/G1 phase and cell apoptosis. The authors suggested that N-cadherin and beta-catenin are of vital importance in the invasion and metastasis of SCC of the tongue.[170]

Apart for its intracellular signalling role, b-catenin is implicated in carcinogenesis as a structural component of cells. A strong correlation between the ability of the WNT-1 gene to induce beta-catenin accumulation and its transforming potential in vivo, suggesting that the WNT-1 gene activates an intracellular signaling pathway that can induce the morphological transformation of cells has been described.[171] A statistically significant difference was found between the reduced expression of E-cadherin and β-catenin and high malignancy score. The reduced immunoexpression of E-cadherin and β-catenin in the membrane was attributed tohigh degree of cell indifferentiation in cases of oral squamous cell carcinoma.[172]

3. Avoid Apoptosis

Development as well as maintenance of many adult tissues is achieved by several dynamically regulated processes that include cell proliferation, differentiation, and programmed cell death. This alternative senescence barrier in epithelial cells is likely to involve p53.

p53

p53 (TRANSFORMATION-RELATED PROTEIN 53; TRP53, Gene map locus 17p13.1) is a nuclear oncosuppressor protein involved in the maintenance of genomic integrity: DNA damage results in increased expression of p53, which then causes G1 arrest in the actively cycling cells (Figure 3). It can then induce factors that either allow DNA repair to occur or, if the damage is too great, cause apoptosis. Indeed, in cases of significant, nonrepairable genomic damage, p53 levels continue to rise until the caspases cascade leading to apoptosis is triggered. Evidence suggests that p53 itself also exerts a direct role in accomplishing cell death at the mitochondria. [10]]Experiments in mice showed that wild-type p53 rapidly translocates to mitochondria in response to multiple death stimuli in cultured cells. Mitochondrial p53 physically interacts with antiapoptotic Bcl proteins, induces Bak oligomerization, permeabilizes mitochondrial membranes, and rapidly induces cytochrome (Cyt) C release. In the cytoplasm, Cyt C binds to apoptotic protease activating factor APAF-1, forming a complex that binds caspase 9 and induces its activation. Consecutively, activated caspase 9 activates other proteases, including caspase 3, thus inducing cleavage of various substrates that subsequently leads to cell death and phagocytosis. The transcriptional p53 program has a longer lag phase than the rapid mitochondrial p53 program. In mice thymus, the earliest apoptotic target gene products PUMA, Noxa, and Bax appear at 2, 4, and 8 h, respectively, while Bid, and p53 remain uninduced even after 20 h. [10] Target gene induction then leads to further increase in active caspase 3. Similar biphasic kinetics has been observed in cultured human cells. These results suggest that mitochondrial p53 accumulation in vivo occurs soon after a death stimulus, triggering a rapid first wave of apoptosis that is transcription independent and may precede a second slower wave that is transcription dependent.[10]

P53 mutations have been reported in up to 50% of OSCCs and they were associated with decreased overall survival. [148] P53 was expressed focally in normal epithelium adjacent to tumors, while expression was high in intra-epithelial neoplasia and moderate in OSCC. Immunostaining of p53 family members might be helpful in diagnosis and monitoring of high-risk pre-malignant lesions of oral epithelium.[173] Because no statistically significant differences between the expression of p53 in oral lichen planus and oral squamous cell carcinoma were observed, the potential of malignant transformation of oral lichen planus has been underlined.[174] Intraepithelial injections of recombinant human adenovirus-p53 have been proposed as a safe, feasible, and biologically active treatment for patients with dysplastic oral leukoplakia. Recombinant adenovirus-p53 could strongly inhibit cell proliferation, induce apoptosis, and arrest cell cycle in stage G(1) in OSCC cell lines by inducing p21(CYCLIN-DEPENDENT KINASE INHIBITOR 1A; CDKN1A, WILDTYPE p53-ACTIVATED FRAGMENT 1; WAF1, p21, gene map locus 6p21.2) and downregulating bcl-2 expression.[175]

Loss of function p53 mutations in OSCC patients have been reported to predict significant low pathologic complete remission rates and suboptimal response to cisplatin-based neoadjuvant chemotherapy. [176] Similarly, Perrone et al [176] reported the relation between *p53* functional statusand response to neoadjuvant chemotherapy in patients with locallyadvanced OSCC. They reported that few oral-cavity tumors lacking functional*p53* responded fully to cisplatin/fluorouracil chemotherapy, while 40% of patients whose tumors contained functional *p53*had a complete response by histopathology. This clinical use of *p53* functionalityas a biomarker provides a step toward risk stratification ofpatients, with a view toward personalizing therapy and maximizingorgan preservation. The authors nevertheless highlighted the limitationsof focusing solely on p53.[176-177] Mutated*p53*, found in about half of OSCC, has been associatedwith worse outcome not onlyafter chemotherapy but also after surgery. A crucial detail that is receiving increasedattention in such studies is how *p53*mutations are categorized, since not all p53 mutants behave similarly. For example, Poeta et al [178] found worse outcome for "disruptive" than for "nondisruptive"mutations, where "disruptive" mutations are those producing truncated proteinor changing the polarity of amino acids in the DNA-bindingdomains of p53.[177] It has been proposed that there is little benefit by subjectingpatients with non-functional *p53* to neoadjuvant cisplatin/fluorouraciltreatment. However, due to study limitations it has been noted that the current benefit/risk ratioof neoadjuvant chemotherapy might be greater for an increasedfraction of patients with mutant p53 and that simply viewing functional p53as a predictor of complete response when compared to non-functional p53 would be incorrect. Limitations likely arise from the complex roles of p53 both in tumor biology and in mediating treatment responses in OSCC.[177] In an effort to identify patients with advanced oral-cavity tumors who are most likely to benefit from neoadjuvant chemotherapy, Perrone et al [176] have found functional p53 status to be a potent and clinically useablebiomarkerTheir finding needsto be followed up in further clinical trials before they arewidely applied in clinical practice. Better understanding ofthe cellular networks involving p53, associated biomarkers, and their relations to responses to therapy might eventuallyreduce or eliminate surgical interventions in a subset of OSCCs. [177]

APAF-1

APAF-1(APOPTOTIC PROTEASE ACTIVATING FACTOR 1;gene map locus 12q23), plays an essential role in apoptosis (Figure 3). In the presence of cytochrome C and dATP, APAF1 assembles into an oligomeric apoptosome, which is responsible for activation of procaspase-9 and maintenance of the enzymatic activity of processed caspase-9.[179] APAF-1 expression has been shown to be altered in oral cancer cells. [180] The expression of the retinoic acid receptor beta (RARB, RETINOIC ACID RECEPTOR BETA, gene map locus 3p24), which is reported to be absent or down-regulated in oral squamous cell carcinomas may be related to APAF-1 expression. [181] Cisplatin, which is commonly used in the treatment of oral cancer has been reported to significantly augment APAF-1 expression. [182]

Bcl-2 Gene Family

The Bcl-2 network is thought to be one of the most crucial regulators of apoptosis(Figure 3).[183] At the core of the Bcl-2 network lives a family of anti- and proapoptotic proteins that function to regulate and execute the core mitochondrial pathway of apoptosis.[184] Proper regulation requires that a delicate balance is maintained between proapoptotic members of the Bcl-2 family(Bax, BAK, BAD, BID, Bim, NOXA, PUMA) and the antiapoptotic members(Bcl-2, Bcl-xL, Mcl-1, BCL-w, and A1).[43, 184] Many of the signalling pathways responsible for tumour growth and progression have also been shown to possess profound downstream effects on the regulation of the Bcl-2 apoptotic network.

3. Antiapoptotic Bcl-2 Members

Bcl-2

Both effector and repressor genes exist within each mammalian cell death pathway. Bcl-2 (B-CELL CLL/LYMPHOMA 2;ONCOGENE B-CELL LEUKEMIA 2;gene map locus 18q21.3) is one such mammalian gene that has been identified; it functions as a repressor of programmed cell death. Bcl-2 which is the founding member of the Bcl-2 family of proteins, was first identified at the chromosomal breakpoint of t(14;18) in follicular B-cell lymphoma and found to block cell death following a variety of toxic insults.[185-187]

No statistically significant differences between the expression of bax, and bcl-2 in oral lichen planus and oral squamous cell carcinoma were observed[174, 188], which may be an evidence of the potential of malignant transformation of oral lichen planus.[174] Bcl-2 expression was not found to be correlated with overall or disease free survival. [152] Celecoxib treatment induced significant changes in bcl-2 and bax expression in precancerous lesions in a rat carcinogenesis model. [189]

Aloe-emodin, one of the anthraquinones, has been shown to have anticancer activity in different kinds of human cancer cell lines, namely increase the Bax/Bcl-2 ratio and activate caspases -9 and -3. Aloe-emodin induced apoptosis in the SCC-cell lines through the Fas/death-receptor, mitochondria and caspase cascade. [190]

Bcl-x

Other antiapoptotic Bcl-2 members might serve as a substitute for Bcl-2 once it is lost. Boise et al.[191] isolated a Bcl-2-related gene, which they designated Bcl-X(Bcl-2-RELATED GENE; BCLX;BCLXL;BCLXS), and showed that it can function as a Bcl-2-independent regulator of programmed cell death (apoptosis). Alternative splicing resulted in 2 distinct Bcl-X mRNAs. The protein product of the larger mRNA (Bcl-xL) was similar in size and predicted structure to Bcl-2. When transfected into an IL3-dependent cell line, it inhibited cell death upon growth factor withdrawal at least as satisfactorily as Bcl-2.[191] Unexpectedly, the smaller mRNA species (Bcl-xS) was found to encode a protein that inhibited the ability of Bcl-2 to enhance the survival of growth factor-deprived cells. In vivo, Bcl-xS mRNA is expressed at high levels in cells that undergo a high rate of turnover, such as developing lymphocytes. In contrast, Bcl-xL is found in tissues containing long-lived post-mitotic cells, such as adult brain. These data suggested that Bcl-x plays an important role in both positive and negative regulation of programmed cell death.[191] Tumor cells are able to switch expression from Bcl-2 to Bcl-xL,[192] and in many cases Bcl-2 and Bcl-xL are expressed in a reciprocal fashion.[193]

Aurora-A overexpression upregulated Akt activity a change accompanied by nuclear translocation of nuclear factor-kappaB and increased expression of its target gene Bcl-xL.[130] The protein kinase C inhibitor safingol increased rounding and detachment of human oral squamous cell carcinoma (SCC) cells in monolayer cultures. During the induction of apoptosis in cell suspensions by safingol, there was an increase of the pro-apoptotic BH-3 only protein Bim and decrease of pro-survival Bcl-2 family proteins Bcl-xL and mitochondrial pro-apoptogenic factor endonuclease G translocated to the nucleus.[194] Apoptosis inhibitory proteins (such as Bcl-2, Bcl-xL, IL-6, etc.) were highly induced in non-functional p53 cells after heat treatment when compared to control wild-type p53 cells.[195] Two PI 3K inhibitors, wortmannin and LY294002, markedly suppressed the phosphorylation of Akt in OSCC cells. Expression of Bcl-2, and expression of Bax was up-regulated by PI3K inhibitors, while that of Bcl-xL, Bak and cIAP-2 was not attenuated.[195] All these remarks suggest that the bcl-family genes have pluripotent roles in cell proliferation and apoptosis and interact with a large number of intracellular pathways.

Reactive Oxygen Species (ROS) induce apoptosis by regulating the phosphorylation and ubiquitination of Bcl-2 family proteins, resulting in increased proapoptotic protein levels and decreased antiapoptotic protein expression. Mn-superoxide dis-mutase (SOD) antisense-transfected OSCC cells expressed high levels of Bax and Bak, but low levels of Bcl-2 and Bcl-XL when treated with CDDP, peplomycin, 5-fluorouracil or gamma-rays. The phosphorylation levels were very low in the antisense-transfected cells. Bcl-2 ubiquitination was increased, but ubiquitination of Bad and Bax was decreased in the antisense-transfected cells, although their ubiquitination was increased by the antioxidants.[196]

Mcl-1

Mcl-1(MYELOID CELL LEUKEMIA 1;gene map locus 1q21) is a potent multidomain antiapoptotic protein of the Bcl-2-family that heterodimerizes with other Bcl-2-family members to protect against apoptotic cell death(Figure 1).[197] Multiple studies have now demonstrated that resistance to a variety of traditional and targeted chemotherapeutic agents is largely mediated by Mcl-1 overexpression.[198] Mcl-1 possesses qualities that distinguish it from other antiapoptotic Bcl-2 members. Whereas most antiapoptotic Bcl-2 members show little selectivity in their inhibition of proapoptotic members BAK and Bax, Mcl-1 has been shown to have a uniquely high specificity for suppressing apoptosis induced by BAK but not Bax.[199] Although Mcl-1 inhibitors may generally increase tumour-cell sensitivity to a variety of traditional chemotherapeutic agents, their unique relationship with the proteasome inhibitor class of chemotherapeutic agents may prove especially beneficial.[43, 200] Like BAK, NOXA possesses a BH3 domain that has a high specificity for binding with Mcl-1. When activated by various stimuli, NOXA binds to Mcl-1, thereby freeing BAK from the BAK–Mcl-1 complex and promoting apoptosis.[200] Since bortezomib(Velcade®) simultaneously induces the proapoptotic Bcl-2 member, NOXA, and antiapoptotic Mcl-1, Mcl-1 inhibition is an attractive means for increasing the efficacy of bortezomib. Bortezomib led to increased MYC protein function and NOXA expression was only increased when c-Myc was bound to its recognition sites in the NOXA promoter.[198]

A high level expression observed in tumor cells of human primary SCC, lymph node metastasis tissues, and SCC cell lines. Combination therapy of Mcl-1 siRNA and anti-tumor drug drastically inhibited the cell growth in comparison to that in each single treatment. The cell growth inhibition caused by knockdown of Mcl-1 was suggested to be mainly a result of suppression of proliferation via the inhibition of intracellular FAK/MAPK signaling pathways.[201] In polymorphonuclear neutrophils (PMNs) of OSCC patients, a decreased expression of anti-apoptotic Mcl-1 protein was associated with an unchanged expression of pro-apoptotic Bax protein. There were no such changes in the patients' peripheral blood PMNs. Following surgical treatment, an increase in the expression of Mcl-1 in the PMNs was recorded.[202

Cytoplasmic Mcl-1 immunoreactivity is ubiquitously more prominent along the submucous fibrosis, leukoplakia and OSCC sequence when compared to normal mucosa. However, its expression was not correlated significantly with clinicopathological parameters. Since the majority of oral tumours associated with tobacco-chewing evolve from premalignant lesions, it has been suggested that the sustained expression of full-length anti-apoptotic Mcl-1 protein in these tissues denotes an important role for Mcl-1, early in oral cancer pathogenesis in protecting cells from apoptosis via neutralization of pro-apoptotic members and could be a potential therapeutic target for oral cancers.[203]

Proapoptotic Bcl-2 Members in Oral Cancer

Bak

The functional analysis of BAK(Bcl-2 ANTAGONIST KILLER 1;gene map locus 6p21.3-p21.2), which promotes cell death and counteracts the protection from apoptosis provided by Bcl-2 was described in 1995.[204-205] Chittenden et al.[205] found that enforced expression of BAK induced rapid and extensive apoptosis of serum-deprived fibroblasts. This suggested that BAK may be directly involved in activating the cell death machinery. Kiefer et al.[204] pointed out that, like Bax, the BAK gene product primarily enhances apoptotic cell death following an appropriate stimulus. Unlike Bax, however, BAK can inhibit cell death in an Epstein-Barr virus-transformed cell line.

Overexpression (64%) of Bak in the cytoplasm of epithelial cells in primary OSCCs and in (75%) lymph node metastasis as been recorded. Still, no statistically significant correlations were observed between Bak immunoreactivity and age, pT and G of the carcinoma in both primary OSCC or lymph node metastases.[206]

A clinical study compared Bak expression with previously investigated apoptosis-related parameters namely apoptotic index (AI), Bax and Bcl-2 expression, and p53 accumulation.[207] Bak expression correlated positively with Bcl-2 expression but not with Bax expression, AI, or p53 accumulation. Patients with Bak expression exceeding the mean value had poorer disease-specific survival when compared with those with values below the mean Bak expression. Cox proportional hazards regression analysis revealed that Bak expression was a significant, independent prognostic variable. A two-parameter combination of Bak expression and Bax expression, AI, or p53 accumulation revealed an enhanced prognostic potential ($p<0.0001$) when compared with single parameters. [207] Bak expression, particularly in combination with Bax expression, as well as in combination with AI, or p53 accumulation, has been reported to be of prognostic value in tongue SCC.

Bax

The proapoptotic Bax(Bcl-2-ASSOCIATED X PROTEIN; gene map locus 19q13.3-q13.4) protein, induces cell death by acting on mitochondria. Oltvai et al.[208] showed that Bcl-2 associates *in vivo* with Bax. Bax shows extensive amino acid homology with Bcl-2 and forms homodimers and heterodimers with Bcl-2 *in vivo*. When Bax predominates, programmed cell death is accelerated, and the death repressor activity of Bcl-2 is countered. The ratio of Bcl-2 to Bax has been suggested[208] to determine survival or death following an apoptotic stimulus.

Berberine-induced apoptosis was associated with a reduction of the mitochondrial membrane potential associated with changes in the Bax/Bcl-2 ratio, release of cytochrome c from mitochondria and activation of down stream caspase-3. [209] In an experimental model, Celecoxib treatment reduced tongue precancer lesions at week 8. Significant differences were noted in the average expression of Ki-67, c-erb-B2, bax, and bcl2. [189] Bax may be a useful biomarker of treatment response.

4. Replicate without Limit

Human telomeres consist of many kilobases of the “TTAGGG” sequence together with various associated proteins. Small amounts of these terminal sequences are lost from the tips of the chromosomes each S phase because of incomplete DNA replication, but de novo addition of TTAGGG repeats by the enzyme telomerase compensates for this loss. Many human cells progressively lose terminal sequence with cell division, a loss that correlates with the apparent absence of telomerase in these cells.[210]

TERT

Human telomerase(TERT; TELOMERASE REVERSE TRANSCRIPTASE;gene map locus 5p15.33) was recognized and reported to catalyze the addition of a 6 nucleotide repeating pattern "TTAGGG" to oligonucleotide primers containing human or telomeric repeat sequences.[211] Higher expression of human telomerase reverse transcriptase (hTERT) and subsequent activation of telomerase occur during cellular immortalization and are maintained in cancer cells. The identified proteins include MutS homolog 2 (MutS, E. COLI, HOMOLOG OF, 2; MSH2, gene map locus 2p22-p21), heterogeneous nuclear ribonucleoprotein D (HETEROGENEOUS NUCLEAR RIBON-UCLEOPROTEIN D; HNRNPD, gene map locus 4q21.1-q21.2), hnRNP K (HETER-OGENEOUS NUCLEAR RIBONUCLEOPROTEIN K; HNRNPK , gene map locus 9q21.32-q21.33)and grainyhead-like 2 (GRAINYHEAD-LIKE 2; GRHL2, gene map locus 8q22). We noticed a higher expression of these proteins in human oral squamous cell carcinoma (OSCC) cells than in normal cells, which do not exhibit telomerase activity. Knockdown of MSH2, hnRNP D and GRHL2 resulted in a notable reduction of the hTERT promoter activity in tested cancer cells.[212]

Increased hTERT protein expression was more frequently found in OSCC (71.1%, 155/218) than in pharyngeal / laryngeal SCC (36.0%, 35/89) ($P < 0.001$). By contrast, specific TERT amplifications were less common in OSCC (2.1%, 4/191) compared withpharyngeal / laryngeal SCC (9.9%, 8/81) ($P = 0.047$).[213]

A study used an immunohistochemical technique to examine the expression of hTERT protein in 82 specimens of OSCC, 116 specimens of oral epithelial dysplasia, and 21 specimens of normal oral mucosa. The mean cytoplasmic hTERT expression increased significantly from normal oral mucosa through oral epithelial dysplasia to OSCC samples ($p=0.000$). A significant correlation was recorded between the higher mean cytoplasmic hTERT labelling scores and OSCCs occurring in male patients ($p=0.023$), with larger tumor sizes (T3 and T4, $p=0.048$), with more advanced clinical stages (stages III and IV, $p=0.033$), or from patients with areca quid chewing ($p= 0.029$), cigarette smoking ($p=0.027$), or alcohol drinking habit ($p=0.025$). Furthermore, OSCC patients with nuclear hTERT labelling scores greater than 100% were prone to have a higher recurrence rate ($p=0.044$) and a lower 5-year survival rate ($p=0.011$). These results indicate that the increased expression of hTERT protein is an early event in oral carcinogenesis and hTERT may be a biomarker for OSCCs.[214]

MYC

The MYC(MYC AVIAN MYELOCYTOMATOSIS VIRAL ONCOGENE HOMOLOG;gene map locus 8q24.12-q24.13) proto-oncogene encodes an ubiquitous transcription factor involved in the control of cell proliferation and differentiation. Deregulated expression of MYC caused by gene amplification, retroviral insertion or chromosomal translocation is associated with carcinogenesis. Understanding of the function of MYC and its role in carcinogenesis was aided by the demonstration by Wu et al that MYC has a direct role in induction of the activity of telomerase.[215]

There was no significant difference between patients with OSCC and healthy controls. Patients with the L-MYC S allele and a positive family history of cancer were found to be 1.74 times more at risk for OSCC than those with any other genotype (95% confidence interval=0.88-3.45). Moreover, tumor recurrence was higher among individuals carrying a L-MYC S allele than those with any other allele type. L-MYC polymorphism may be a useful marker for identifying patient susceptibility to tumor recurrence and to developing OSCC, especially in individuals having a family history of cancer.[216] C-Myc has been reported not to be associated with survival. [152]

In a pilot study including ten OSCC patients, the Koehn et al we found 8 upregulated gene products to be linked to three main locus genes, p53, MYC, and MYCN, which they proposed to be candidate biomarkers for OSCC.[217]

A significant correlation between Bmi-1 (LEUKEMIA VIRAL BMI-1 ONCOGENE, MOUSE, HOMOLOG OF; BMI1, gene map locus 10p13) protein expression and recurrence (log-rank test, P=0.005) was detected. Snail (SNAIL, DROSOPHILA, HOMOLOG OF, 1; SNAI1, gene map locus 20q13.1) and c-myc expression did not correlate with prognosis. Snail expression correlated with histopathological grade and with the invasion depth of tumours. [218]

Aneuploidy

Aneuploidyrefers to the chromosome number being different for that species and indicates widespread DNA changes due to genomic instability. It is known that the assessment of the DNA content of cells can be accomplished with the use of a flow cytometer technique. [10] Aneuploidy has been reported to be a significant biomarker in a similar carcinogenesis process: from dysplasia to Barrett's oesophagus to oesophageal adenocarcinoma. [10]

Klanrit et al studied aneuploidy in six patients with leukoplakia and reported that the most frequently affected sites were alveolar ridge and/or gingiva (6/6), buccal mucosa (3/6), palate (3/6), tongue (2/6), buccal sulcus (2/6), and lip (1/6). During follow up, three patients developed multiple primary carcinomas, either invasive or verrucous. A ploidy anomaly at any oral site would have predicted malignant transformation in four cases and probably in a fifth for whom DNA ploidy failed to meet diagnostic criteria but was suspicious of aneuploidy. The site of transformation was predicted by ploidy and histopathology for all three carcinomas and a further carcinoma showed severe dysplasia and a suspicious ploidy result in adjacent tissue.[219]

Sudbo et al. [220] argued that DNA analysis constitutes an important advance in the evaluation of the risk of oral cancer in patients with leukoplakias. Therefore, DNA is a powerful predictor of the risk of a lesion's malignant transformation. Despite the well-recognized fact that the data where at least partially fabricated and therefore a series of articles supporting the author's hypothesis were retracted, one cannot be sure that his findings, which precisely identified people at high risk of the deadly disease, have not been accurate, even though data were faked. [221] DNA ploidy state reflects the risk of oral cancer: i) Aneuploidy: high risk, ii) Tetraploidy: intermediate risk, iii) Diploidy: low risk. [222] It has been proposed that32% of oral leukoplakias and 45% of squamous, cell carcinomas have aneuploid nuclei. Aneuploid nuclei are found, in 29% of leukoplakias without dysplasia, in 22% of leukoplakias with mild dysplasia, and in 67% of leukoplakias with severe dysplasia. Therefore, it can be said that molecular information enables the evaluation of the risk of oral cancer to be redefined and serves as a treatment guide in the case of lesions such as leukoplakia. In other words, aneuploid oral leukoplakias require more aggressive treatments in order to prevent them becoming more malignant [220]. Chromosomal polysomy determines genetic instability. [223] Kim et al. reported extensive chromosomal polysomy in areas classified as high risk of malignant transformation when compared with low-risk areas. These polysomies are much more numerous in dysplasic epithelia compared with hyperplasic epithelial cells. [223] Flow cytometry to determine ploidy status will be a useful adjunct to early detect in situ carcinomas arising in leukoplakias in the future.

5. Sustain Angiogenesis

One main etiology for oral squamous cell carcinoma (OSCC) is inflammation. Inducible nitric oxide synthase (iNOS), vascular endothelial growth factor (VEGF) and cyclooxygenase-2 (COX-2) are the important molecules showing close relation to not only inflammation but also carcinogenesis and angiogenesis. Angiogenesis is defined as the formation of new blood vessels from existing vasculature. It is necessary for tumor growth and progression and also involved in metastasis.

VEGF

Angiogenesis is essential for tumor growth and metastasis. An association between microvessel density, a measure of tumor angiogenesis, and conventional prognostic variables has been shown for many tumor entities. [10] VEGF (VASCULAR ENDOTHELIAL GROWTH FACTOR, Gene map locus 6p12) is a mitogen primarily for vascular endothelial cells which is structurally related to platelet-derived growth factor (PDGF). VEGF and PDGF have been implicated as one of the principal mitogens involved in cutaneous wound healing.[49]

Numerous past studies have suggested a critical role of the paracrine effect between tumor vascular endothelial growth factor (VEGF)-C and lymphatic FLT-4 in solid tumor-associated lymphangiogenesis. It has been suggested that the VEGF-C/FLT-4 autocrine loop in tumor cells is a potential enhancer system to promote cancer progression, and FLT-4 in tumor tissue might become an effective biomarker target for cancer therapy. [224] Along withFGF, VEGF mRNA levels were reported to be upregulated to variable degrees in nemosis. [48] The VEGFA + 936 T polymorphism is associated with increased risk of oral cancer. A meta-analysis indicated that individuals with the +936 T polymorphism had increased risk of oral cancer (OR = 1.39, 95% CI = 1.03-1.88). [225] In a clinical study which included tongue cancer patients, significant correlations were found between VEGF and Notch1 expression and cervical lymph node metastasis, tumor depth of invasion and microvessel density indicated by CD34 staining. Along with nodal metastasis and T stage, positive VEGF expression was statistically significant prognostic factor for disease-specific survival.[226]

Sugiura et al reported that VEGF-C and VEGF-D overexpression were significantly associated with lymph node metastasis. Overexpression of VEGF-C and VEGF-D significantly increased the lymphatic vessel density. Multivariate analysis showed that VEGF-C expression and lymphatic vessel density were significantly associated with lymph node metastasis. This study presented clinical evidence to support the important roles of

VEGF-C and VEGF-D in lymphangiogenesis and lymphatic metastasis in OSCC, and suggested that VEGF-C or lymphatic vessel density can effectively predict lymphatic metastasis of OSCC.[227]

VEGF is also a promoter of angiogenesis in many tumour types, and has therefore been subject to numerous studies in oral dysplasia and squamous cell carcinomas. The contribution of VEGF to the development of oral dysplasia and invasive carcinomas is currently disputed due to conflicting results within the literature. [228]

Expectedly, VEGF correlated with micro vessel density in OSCC. Micro vessel density was associated with T stage, tumor differentiation, and stage of invasion. VEGF expression also correlated with tumor differentiation and the stage of invasion.[229] A direct correlation of VEGF with tumor grading, tumor staging and angiogenesis has also been shown. [230] It has been recorded that iNOS gene silencing reduces VEGF expression levels in Tca8113 cells. Therefore a relationship has been suggested between iNOS and VEGF expression in tongue squamous cancer cells.[231]

PDGF

Human platelet-derived growth factor (PDFG, gene map locus 7p22) is a cationic glycoprotein consisting of homo- or heterodimers of polypeptide chains A (PDGFA) and/or B (PDGFB). It is a potent mitogen for connective tissue cells and exerts its function by interacting with 2 related receptor tyrosine kinases, PDGFRA and PDGFRB.ignificantly higher levels of expression of VEGF, PDGF were recordedin OSCC tissue compared to normal oral mucosal tissue. In OSCC samples, significant positive correlations, based on the Spearman correlation test, existed between the lymphovascular density and VEGF but also PDGF. These evidence point that several growth factors may promote lymphangiogenesis in OSCC.[232]

PDGF expression also correlated with microvessel density which was significantly increased in tumor tissues. Expression of angiogenic factors was not found in normal oral mucosa, but increased in association with increasing vascularity in OSCC tissue.[229]

iNOS

Nitric oxide (NO) is a messenger molecule with diverse functions throughout the body. In the brain and peripheral nervous system, NO displays many properties of a neurotransmitter; it is implicated in neurotoxicity associated with stroke and neurodegenerative diseases, neural regulation of smooth muscle, including peristalsis, and penile erection. NO is also responsible for endothelium-derived relaxing factor (EDRF) activity regulating blood pressure. In macrophages, NO mediates tumoricidal and bactericidal actions, as indicated by the fact that inhibitors of NO synthase (NOS, NITRIC OXIDE SYNTHASE 2A, NOS2A, NITRIC OXIDE SYNTHASE, INDUCIBLE; INOS, gene map locus 17cen-q11.2) block these effects. Neuronal NOS and macrophage NOS are distinct isoforms. Both the neuronal and the macrophage forms are unusual among oxidative enzymes in requiring several electron donors: FAD, FMN, NADPH, and tetrahydrobiopterin [233] NOS has been reported to be upregulated in OSCC. [234] More specifically, in the leukocytes of patients with stage II and III SCC, the p38 MAPK pathway performs an essential role in the induction of iNOSexpression, and the process of lipid peroxidation is not dependent on NO. In contrast, in patients with advanced-stage SCC, NOS expression did not seem to be linked with the p38 MAPK pathway, and NO directly influenced the process of lipid peroxidation.[234] The RNA interference technique was used to silence iNOS gene expression by transfecting an expression vector containing short hairpin RNA (shRNA) for NOS into Tca8113 tongue squamous cancer cells using cationic liposomes. NOS mRNA expression was significantly downregulated 24 and 36 h after transfection, and NOS protein expression was significantly downregulated at 36 and 48 h ($P<0.05$ versus control), showing that effective silencing could be achieved. [231] NOS shows correlation with cervical lymph node metastasis and tumor staging (TNM) of the patients and with angiogenesis.[230]

COX-2

COX (cyclooxygenase) is a key enzyme in the conversion of arachidonic acid to prostaglandins (PGs). COX-1 is constitutively expressed for the maintenance of homeostatic function in most of the cells, whereas COX-2 is induced during pathologic conditions such as inflammation and cancers. COX-2 levels have been found to be elevated in head and neck, esophageal, gastric, pancreatic, hepatocellular, colorectal, breast, and lung cancers, relative to the normal epithelia from which these tumors develop. [10, 235] COX-2 activation has been found to be an early event during carcinogenesis, and its increased expression has been associated with the development of genomic instability. [10] COX-2 plays an important role in tumor growth and spread of tumors by affecting mitogenesis, cellular adhesion, immune surveillance, apoptosis, and angiogenesis. In addition, inhibition of COX-2 increases radiation sensitivity without influencing normal tissue response to radiation.[140] There is an increasing amount of evidence revealing that a combined administration of non-selective COX1/COX-2 inhibitor and EGFR inhibitor prevents tumor progression in preclinical models. [140] COX-2 correlates with cervical lymph node metastasis. To summarize, high expression of iNOS, VEGF and COX-2 exists in OSCC.[230]

PPAR

The peroxisome proliferator-activated receptors (PPARs) are members of the nuclear hormone receptor subfamily of transcription factors. PPARs form heterodimers with retinoid X receptors (RXRs) and these heterodimers regulate transcription of various genes. There are 3 known subtypes of PPARs, PPAR-alpha, PPAR-delta, and PPAR-gamma. PPAR-gamma (PEROXISOME PROLIF-ERATOR-ACTIVATED RECEPTOR-GAMMA; PPARG, gene map locus 3p25) is believed to as a regulator of lipid metabolism and adipocyte differentiation and exists in 2 isoforms produced by the alternative splicing at the 50 end of the gene. [140] In OSCC, PPARg mRNA was detected in 17 of 28 cases using RT-PCR. [235] The function of PPARg in human OSCC cells was also investigated using the synthetic thiazolidine-dione derivative, TRO. Although the synthetic TRO, significantly suppressed the growth of OSCC cells, it did not induce transcriptional activity of PPARg even in human OSCC cells expressing PPARg mRNA. [235] Loss of PPARg expression and function may be associated with OSCC progression. [140]

6. Invade and Proliferate

NEDD9

NEDD9(NEURAL PRECURSOR CELL EXPRESSED, DEVELOPMENTALLY DOWNREG-ULATED 9;HUMAN ENHANCER OF FILAMENTATION 1;HEF1;gene map locus 6p25-p24) enhanced invasion *in vitro* and metastasis *in vivo* of both normal and malignant melanocytes, functionally interacted with focal adhesion kinase and modulated focal contact formation, and exhibited frequent robust overexpression in human metastatic melanoma when compared to primary melanoma. Roberg at al reported genetic changes in multiple cancer-associated genes not previously considered for OSCC, among them NEDD9.[236]

SLUG

SLUG(SNAIL, DROSOPHILA, HOMOLOG OF, 2;SNAI2;gene map locus 8q11) belongs to the Snail-family of zinc-finger transcription factors that share an evolutionarily conserved role in mesoderm formation in invertebrates and vertebrates. SLUG triggers epithelial-mesenchymal transitions and plays an important role in developmental processes.[237] Members of Snail family of transcription factors play an important role in oral cancer progression by inducing epithelial-mesenchymal transition, by promoting invasion and by increasing matrix metalloproteinase (MMP) expression. To further examine the role of Slug in OSCC progression, Joseph and colleagues generated UMSCC1 cells with inducible expression of Slug protein. Induction of Slug in UMSCC1 cells did not repress E-cadherin levels or regulate individual movement of UMSCC1 cells. Instead, Slug enhanced cohort migration and Matrigel invasion by UMSCC1 cells. Slug increased MMP-9 levels and MMP-9-specific siRNA blocked Slug-induced Matrigel invasion. Interestingly, Slug-specific siRNA attenuated TGF-beta1-induced MMP-9 expression and Matrigel invasion. These data demonstrate that TGF-beta1 increases Slug via ERK1/2 signaling, and thereby contributes to OSCC progression. [238]

S-allylcysteine (SAC) significantly inhibited the activation of MAPK/ERK signaling pathway. These findings were associated with the down-regulation of the SLUG repressor protein. [124]

SMN1

The SMN gene (SURVIVAL OF MOTOR NEURON 1, gene map locus 5q12.2-q13.3) is mutated or deleted in over 98% of patients with spinal muscular atrophy). SMN has been localized to a nuclear compartment called gems (gemini of coiled bodies). Liu et al. [239] identified a novel protein, SIP1 or SMN1 (SMN interacting protein-1, GEMIN2, gene map locus 14q13-q21). SIP1 is expressed as a 1.3-kb transcript that encodes a 279-amino acid protein with a calculated molecular mass of 32 kD.

Among a number of tumorrepressors including SNAIL, SLUG, SIP1, E12 and E47, SIP1 was inversely correlated to E-cadherin. [240] Chromatin immunoprecipitation showed that SIP1 specifically bound to the E-cadherin promoter region. SIP1 expression was immuno-histochemically detected in 27.7% of 47 oral carcinomas, and SIP1-positive carcinomas did not express E-cadherin. Thirteen patients with SIP1 staining showed a lower disease-specific survival rate. Multivariate risk factor analysis demonstrated that SIP1 expression was an independent prognostic value for disease-specific overall survival. These results suggest that SIP1 contributes to the loss of E-cadherin expression and that detection of SIP1 expression is a predictive and prognostic tool in clinical management of oral carcinomas.[240]

E-cadherin

ECAD(CADHERIN 1; E-CADHERIN; gene map locus 16q22.1) is a specific calcium ion-dependent cell adhesion molecule. In mice it expresses its adhesive function during the preimplantation stage of development in epithelial cells, where it is concentrated in the intermediate junctions. Activation of SLUG expression plays an important role in down-regulation of E-cadherin and tumorigenesis. [124, 238, 240]

E-cadherin immunoreactivity was found to inversely correlate with the loss of cell differentiation in a clinical study. The expression of E-cadherin decreased significantly in advanced cases of OSCC. However, increase in E-cadherin immunoreactivity was noted in early lesions. Furthermore, E-cadherin was negative in majority of metastatic lymph nodes. Down regulation of , E-cadherin expression is associated with de-differentiation and metastasis in OSCC.[241] Cruz et al reported no significant differences in the expression of E-cadherin and CD44v6 were recorded between SCCs of the lower lip and tongue. The expression of these adhesion molecules revealed association only with tumor histological grading of malignancy[.242]

Oral squamous cell carcinomas displayed overexpression of DPAGT1 DOLICHYL - PHOSPHATEN - ACETYLGLUCOSAMINE PHOSPHOTRANSFERASE; DPAGT1, GlcNAc-1-P TRANS-FERASE, gene map locus 11q23.3) that correlated with diminished localization of E-cadherin and alpha-catenin at the sites of adherens junctions. Studies that DPAGT1 is an upstream regulator of E-cadherin N-glycosylation status and adherens junction composition and suggest that dysregulation of DPAGT1 causes disturbances in intercellular adhesion in oral cancer.[243] In the head and neck squamous cell carcinoma, the correlation between the p16 and ECAD methylation profile in tumor and paired saliva is reported to be excellent ; thus methylation analysis in saliva is a very promising approach for early cancer detection in high risk patients or for the post treatment follow up and rapid diagnosis of relapse.[244] E-cadherin expression at the invasive tumor front is lower than that in center/superficial part for most of OSCCs. E-cadherin at the invasive tumor front is reported to be statistically associated with tumor thickness and poor survival of OSCC patients. [245]

S-allylcysteine (SAC) dose dependently inhibited the growth of human oral squamous cancer cells. SAC induced the expression of E-cadherin adhesion molecule. Immunocyto-chemical staining result also revealed that SAC could restore the distribution of E-cadherin molecule on cell membrane. SAC stabilized the adherent junction complex of E-cadherin/beta-catenin in oral cancer cells. Treatment with the MAPK/MEK specific inhibitor, PD098059, could up-regulate the expression of E-cadherin molecule. SAC effectively inhibited the proliferation, up-regulated the expression of E-cadherin molecule and stabilized the E-cadherin/beta-catenin adherent junction complex in human oral squamous cancer cells. The mechanism of action was in part through the suppression of MAPK/ERK signaling pathway and down-regulation of the SLUG repressorprotein.[124]

Overexpression of N-cadherin and beta-catenin were associated with progression of SCC of the tongue, whereas, E-cadherin showed a reverse result. In addition, N-cadherin and beta-catenin expression was associated with lymph node metastasis in SCC of the tongue. N-cadherin and beta-catenin silencing RNAs (siRNA)swhen transfected into Tca8113, a tongue SCC cell line, showed an obviously decreased invasion compared to that of control and control siRNA, but after co-transfection with both N-cadherin and beta-catenin siRNAs, a more profoundly decreased invasion was observed. Down-regulation of N-cadherin and beta-catenin in Tca8113 cells following transfection with N-cadherin and beta-catenin siRNAs, gave rise to inhibition of invasion and metastasis of Tca8113 cells in vitro, probably associated with down-regulation of MMP-2 and MMP-9 proteins and up-regulation of the cell cycle inhibitor p21. Further, transfection of N-cadherin and beta-catenin siRNAs gave rise to proliferation suppression of the cells, accompanied with a cell cycle inhibition at the G0/G1 phase and cell apoptosis. These findings suggest that N-cadherin and beta-catenin are of vital importance in the invasion and metastasis of SCC of the tongue.[170]

Analyzing the signalling mechanism behind it, Bauer and colleagues found glycogen-synthase-kinase-3beta (GSK-3beta) to be bound to Snail in all cell clones. Furthermore, P-cadherin-over-expressing cell lines showed activated GSK-3beta that phosphorylated Snail leading to its cytoplasmic translocation. In summary, P-cadherin appears to be a major component in reconfiguring mesenchymal cells with epithelial features by triggering GSK-3beta-mediated inactivation and cytoplasmatic translocation of Snail in OSCC.[246]

MMP

Type IV collagenase, 72-kD, is officially designated matrix metalloproteinase-2 (MATRIX METALLOPROTEINASE 2, MMP2, COLLAGENASE TYPE IV, 72-KD, GELATINASE, gene map locus 16q13). Type IV collagenase is a metalloproteinase that specifically cleaves type IV collagen, the major structural component of basement membranes. The metastatic potential of tumor cells has been found to correlate with the activity of this enzyme. The 72- and 92-kD (MATRIX METALLOPROTEINASE 9; MMP9, COLLAGENASE TYPE IV, 92-KD, GELATINASE B; GELB, gene map locus 20q11.2-q13.1) type IV collagenases are members of a group of secreted zinc metalloproteases which, in mammals, degrade the collagens of the extracellular matrix. The oral cavity is exposed to chronic or recurrent, physical and chemical trauma that could lead to mucosal reactions (e.g. hyperplasia, dysplasia and tumors). These reactions involvechanges in the expression of the two matrix metalloproteinases MMP-2 and MMP-9 in normal and pathological human oral mucosa samples.[247] In hyperplasia samples MMPs expression is reported to be limited to epithelial layers but the immunoreactivity is more intense than in the control. In dysplasia and carcinoma samples the two matrix metalloproteases are reported to be expressed not only in epithelium but also in some cells of the connective tissue and in the vessel walls. Qualitative RT-PCR and image analysis confirmed these immunohistochemical data. The authors suggested the existence of a possible relationship between the entity of morphological disorganization of the oral mucosa in different pathologies and the increase of MMP-2 and MMP-9 expression.[247]

History of radio- or radiochemotherapy was the only factor significantly predicting free flap complications. Radiochemotherapy resulted in a significant increase in TGF-beta(1)- and Tissue Inhibitor of Matrix-Metallo-Proteinase(TISSUE INHIBITOR OF METALL-OPROTEINASE 1; TIMP1, gene map locus Xp11.3-p11.23)-1-expression, while MMP-1-expression was not significantly altered. Radiotherapy alone significantly increased TIMP-1-expression without detectable effects on TGF-beta(1) and MMP-1.[248]

Germani and colleagues studied MM1 (MATRIX METALLOPROTEINASE 1; MMP1, gene map locus 11q22-q23) expression in OSCC patients who underwent sentinel lymph node biopsy. Twenty one percent of evaluable specimens stained positively in the sentinel lymph node biopsy negative group and 67 percent stained positively in the sentinel lymph node biopsy positive group. No statistically significant association was recorded between any marker's staining pattern and sentinel lymph node biopsy status alone. When MMP1 staining was evaluated in tumors with positive sentinel lymph node biopsy or perineural invasion present on histopathology, 67% stained positively for MMP1, vs 9% in specimens lacking either negative prognosticator. Preliminary results suggest that MMP1 positivity in primary tumor specimens may identify aggressive tumor types, evidenced by the presence of micrometastasis or perineural invasion. [249]

MMP1 and also MMP10(MATRIX METALLOPROTEINASE 10; MMP10, STROMELYSIN II; STMY2 gene map locus 11q22.3-q23) were reported as suitable biomarkers for cancer detection with gingiva and margin as control tissues. Using neck tissue as the control, only MMP10 was suitable for cancer detection.[250]

Epithelial to Mesenchymal Transition

Metastasis remains the most poorly understood aspect of oral cancer, which continues to have an extremely poor prognosis (5-year survival rate, 50%). [251] Recently., a clinical study in cervical squamous cell carcinoma shed new light in EMT transition. Along the process of acquiring metastatic capacities, polarized epithelial cancer cells are converted into motile mesenchymal cells that invade the basement membrane beneath and enter blood vessels to disseminate to secondary organs. The initiation of these processes is associated with morphogenetic changes referred to as the epithelial to mesenchymal transition (EMT) which has long been suggested to be an important process in many types of epithelial cancer. [252] The molecular basis of the EMT process involves changes in the expression, distribution and function of a number of proteins that play a role in extracellular matrix (ECM) remodeling or in cell–cell adhesion, such as matrix metalloproteinases (MMPs), E-cadherin, and integrins.[251] Loss of epithelial cell polarity and acquisition of the motile phenotype requires loss of cell to cell adhesion, reorganization of the cytoskeleton, and alterations in gene expression profiles [253]. E-cadherin has been reported above to bea key “read-out molecule” in the EMT that mediates cell–cell adhesion between adjacent epithelial cells and helps maintain epithelial integrity. E-cadherin expression and its subcellular localization might be altered during tumor progression, as cells change shape and become more like mesenchymal cells. Cell-surface receptors, like integrins, bind to ECM components and have a major role in modifying the cell attachment required for cell motility and invasion; they could also serve as transducers of cell survival signals. An invasive carcinoma cell must acquire the ability to interrelate with distinct interstitial matrices following its transgression of the basement membrane. Unexpectedly little is known with reference to how integrin expression and function are regulated during the EMT. The upregulation of ECM molecules for instance tenascin C (TENASCIN C; TNC, gene map locus 9q33) is repeatedly seen in epithelial tumors of the head and neck, thereby conveying a mesenchymal property to these tumor cells [254] The integrin $\alpha v\beta 6$ is an epithelial specific integrin and has been shown to be a receptor for Arg–Gly–Asp sites in fibronectin, TNC and vitronectin. Activation of TGFβ1 (TRANSFORMING GROWTH FACTOR, BETA-1; TGFB1, TGFB, gene map locus 19q13.1) occurs through the binding of $\alpha v\beta 6$ to a latency-associated peptide [255] When the full length β6 integrin was expressed in poorly invasive squamous cell carcinoma OSCC cells, the resulting OSCC β6 positive cells acquired a fibroblast-like morphology, increased expression of the mesenchymal marker vimentin and reduced expression of the epithelial markers keratin and E-cadherin. In contrast OSCC β6D1 cells, a subgroup of cells which express a truncated form of β6 subunit lacking the C-terminal 11 amino acids, retained their epithelial morphology and did not alter vimentin or E-cadherin expression. [251] Taken together these evidence suggest that there is an interplay of molecules with cadherins, integrins andMMPs holding the main acts, that when elucidated might help towards prediction or even involution of OSCC metastatic potential.

EPILOGUE

To endure in time, a literature review in a book chapter, should not provide just a re-hash of the literature. Rather, the author of the chapter needs to shape the literature of a field into a story in order to enlist the support ofreaderstocontinuethatstory. [256] In this chapter, we have tried our best to select froma wide list of researchpapers, put themside by side and create a story that combines them, a theatre play with actors and events but still without an ending. We hope that this way the current chapter attracts the reader into the deeper understanding or oral cancer biology and the implications for novel biomarkers. Ideally, by reaching this point, the reader should be able to understand the complex mechanisms involved in oral carcinogenesis in a straightforward manner and also foresee what can be done in the future. The aim of this chapter was not to merely provide information on what is currently known and acceptedwith regard to oral carcinogenesis but also to allow the reconstruction of oral carcinogenesis knowledge.[256]

Table 2. Current clinical Implications of Molecular Alterations in oral cancer

Biomarker	Clinical Significance	Citation
HPV 16	Positive tumors better prognosis, especially those with wild type p53	[108]
Ki67	p53 and Ki67 expression associated with tumor volume Ki67 value in distant mucosa for overall survival	[136] [137]
EGFR	EGFR inhibition plus radiotherapy or chemotherapy for overall survival	[141, 142]
CDKN2A (P16INKA)	Biomarker to detect HPV infection with greater sensitivity Detect cases of epithelial dysplasia with increased risk for malignant advancement	[114 161]
P53	Predict response to chemotherapy	[176]
hTERT	Increased risk for recurrence if nuclear labeling score >100%	[214]
Aneuploidy	Presence of Aneuploidy and tetraploidy in epithelial dysplasia denote high risk cancer progression	[220]
VEGF	Prognostic factor for disease-specific survival	[226]
MMP1	Adjunct to sentinel lymph node biopsy for prognostication	[249]

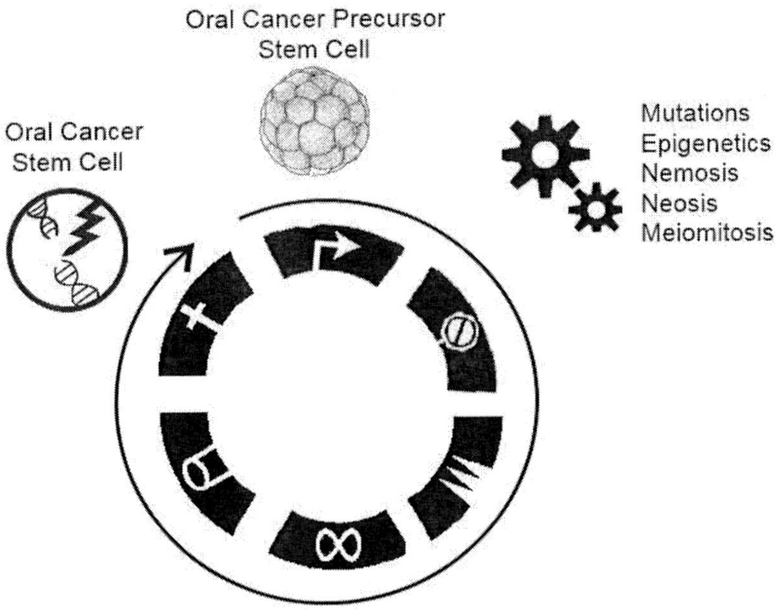

Figure 4. Oral carcinogenesis at a glance. Precursor cancer cells need to advance through the hallmarks of cancer. This is only feasible for cancer precursor stem cells that live long enough to acquire the hallmarks. The machinery that moves precursor stem cells round the hallmarks of cancer is multifarious. Key roles are assigned to mutations, epigenetic changes, nemosis, neosis and meiomitosis among other phenomena (like irradiated fibroblast bystander effect and/or epithelial to mesenchymal transition-see text for details). When cancer precursor stem cells circle round the six hallmarks of cancer, they become oral cancer stem cells.

It is evident that oral cancer will eventually end being a "black box" for researchers. Cancer precursor cells -stem cells more likely- undergo several genome changes. These changes could be either mutations or epigenetic. These changes provide the stem cells with the ability to self-invoke growth signals, the ability to suppress anti-growth signals, to avoid apoptosis, to replicate without limit, to invade, proliferate and sustain blood supply. Stem cells are able to collect progressively these changes in their genome. Mutations, epigenetic changes, nemosis, neosis and meiomitosis all have roles in the machinery that moves precursor stem cells round the hallmarks of cancer (Figure 4).

Contemporary use of biomarkers although limited, is a reality. Table 2 summarizes selected biomarkers reported in this chapter, which are supported by adequate evidence to justify their clinical use, with HPV tumor discrimination, EGFR targeted therapy and aneuploidy being the most well documented.

Future Pespectives for Researchers and Clinicians

Considerable effort is currently focused on patient-selection on the basis of molecular profiling and on combination of drugs targeting cancer-specific aberrations in signaling and apoptotic pathways to over come the many resistance mechanisms in cancer cells. Pharmacogenomics deal with the influence of genetic variations on drug response in patients by correlating gene expression or single nucleotide polymorphisms with a drug's efficacy or toxicity. Pharmacogenomics aim to develop rational means to optimize drug therapy, with respect to the patients' genotype, thus to ensure maximum efficacy with minimal adverse effects.[70] Pharmacogenomics constitute a promising field with regard to OSCC patients. We reviewed a number of treatment approaches that can form the basis of pharmacogenomic profiling.

Development of novel monoclonal antibodies is also another important field in future OSCC patient care. With growing knowledge of the aetiopathogenesis of the disease, we investigate ways to block more molecular signals and impair more cellular metabolic paths. Erbitux® is a licensed example of such treatment while other antibodies, like anti-VEGF (trastuzumab, Avastin®) may soon find their way in routine oncology practice of OSCC patients.

EGFR inhibitors (gefitinib, erlotinib, and cetuximab), COX-2 inhibitors (celecoxib), synthetic PPARg ligands, and hormonal therapy have been demonstrated to be promising molecular targeting agents against oral malignant neoplasms. [140] Combined therapies using these molecules may improve the outcome of these patients. However, more translational research, and subsequently, randomized clinical trials are needed before the broad introduction of such therapies in the clinical practice.

References

[1] La Vecchia C, Tavani A, Franceschi S, Levi F, Corrao G, Negri E. Epidemiology and prevention of oral cancer. *Oral Oncology* 1997;33(5):302-312.

[2] Society. AC. Cancer Facts and Figures 2009. Atlanta: American Cancer Society; 2009.

[3] Kyrgidis A, Nokolaou A, Rachvitsas D, Antoniades A, Vital V. Demographic clinical and histopathological characteristics of oral cavity cancer: Survival analysis in a single center retrospective study. *Hellenic Otorhinolaryngology, Head and Neck Surgery* 2008;33:8-18.

[4] Sudbo J, Reith A. The evolution of predictive oncology and molecular-based therapy for oral cancer prevention. *Int. J. Cancer* 2005;115(3):339-45.

[5] Lee JJ, Hong WK, Hittelman WN, et al. Predicting cancer development in oral leukoplakia: ten years of translational research. *Clin. Cancer Res.* 2000;6(5):1702-10.

[6] Boyle P, Macfarlane GJ, Scully C. Oral cancer: necessity for prevention strategies. *Lancet* 1993;342(8880):1129.

[7] Joseph BK. Oral cancer: prevention and detection. Med Princ Pract 2002;11 Suppl. 1:32-5.

[8] Kim J, Shin DM, El-Naggar A, et al. Chromosome polysomy and histological characteristics in oral premalignant lesions. *Cancer Epidemiol. Biomarkers Prev.*2001;10(4):319-25.

[9] Chimenos-Kustner E, Font-Costa I, Lopez-Lopez J. Oral cancer risk and molecular markers. *Med. Oral Patol. Oral Cir. Bucal.* 2004;9(5):381-4; 377-80.

[10] Kyrgidis A, Kountouras J, Zavos C, Chatzopoulos D. New molecular concepts of Barrett's esophagus: clinical implications and biomarkers. *J. Surg. Res* 2005; 125(2): 189-212.

[11] Kyrgidis A, Tzellos TG, Triaridis S. Melanoma: Stem cells, sun exposure and hallmarks for carcinogenesis, molecular concepts and future clinical implications. *Journal of Carcinogenesis* 2010;9(3).

[12] Hanahan D, Weinberg RA. The hallmarks of cancer. *Cell* 2000;100(1):57-70.

[13] Neville BW, Day TA. Oral cancer and precancerous lesions. *CA Cancer J. Clin.* 2002;52(4):195-215.

[14] Eckardt A, Barth EL, Kokemueller H, Wegener G. Recurrent carcinoma of the head and neck: treatment strategies and survival analysis in a 20-year period. *Oral Oncology* 2004;40(4):427-432.

[15] Jong RJBd, Hermans J, Molenaar J, Briaire JJ, Cessie Sl. Prediction of survival in patients with head and neck cancer. *Head and Neck* 2001;23(9):718-724.

[16] Hombach-Klonisch S, Paranjothy T, Wiechec E, et al. Cancer stem cells as targets for cancer therapy: selected cancers as examples. *Arch. Immunol. Ther. Exp.* (Warsz) 2008;56(3):165-80.

[17] Bouquot JE, Gorlin RJ. Leukoplakia, lichen planus, and other oral keratoses in 23,616 white Americans over the age of 35 years. *Oral Surg. Oral Med. Oral Pathol.* 1986;61(4):373-81.

[18] Suarez P, Batsakis JG, el-Naggar AK. Leukoplakia: still a gallimaufry or is progress being made?--A review. *Adv. Anat. Pathol.* 1998;5(3):137-55.

[19] Lumerman H, Freedman P, Kerpel S. Oral epithelial dysplasia and the development of invasive squamous cell carcinoma. *Oral Surg. Oral Med. Oral Pathol. Oral Radiol. Endod.* 1995;79(3):321-9.

[20] Watanabe S, Sato K, Okazaki Y, Tonogi M, Tanaka Y, Yamane G-y. Activation of PI3K-AKT Pathway in Oral Epithelial Dysplasia and Early Cancer of Tongue. *The Bulletin of Tokyo Dental College* 2009;50(3):125-133.

[21] van der Waal I, Axell T. Oral leukoplakia: a proposal for uniform reporting. *Oral Oncol.* 2002;38(6):521-6.

[22] Reichart PA, Way TH. Oral cancer and pre-cancer in Myanmar: a short review. *J. Oral Pathol. Med.* 2006;35(4):193-6.

[23] Karabulut A, Reibel J, Therkildsen MH, Praetorius F, Nielsen HW, Dabelsteen E. Observer variability in the histologic assessment of oral premalignant lesions. *J. Oral Pathol. Med.* 1995;24(5):198-200.

[24] Mao L, El-Naggar AK, Fan YH, et al. Telomerase activity in head and neck squamous cell carcinoma and adjacent tissues. *Cancer Res.* 1996;56(24):5600-4.

[25] Rosin MP, Cheng X, Poh C, et al. Use of allelic loss to predict malignant risk for low-grade oral epithelial dysplasia. *Clin. Cancer Res.* 2000;6(2):357-62.

[26] Gogas H, Eggermont AM, Hauschild A, et al. Biomarkers in melanoma. *Ann. Oncol.* 2009;20 Suppl 6:vi8-13.

[27] Cruz GD, Ostroff JS, Kumar JV, Gajendra S. Preventing and detecting oral cancer. Oral health care providers' readiness to provide health behavior counseling and oral cancer examinations. *J. Am. Dent. Assoc.* 2005;136(5):594-601; quiz 681-2.

[28] Kujan O, Glenny AM, Duxbury J, Thakker N, Sloan P. Evaluation of screening strategies for improving oral cancer mortality: a Cochrane systematic review. *J. Dent. Educ.* 2005;69(2):255-65.

[29] Chang CJ, Wilder-Smith P. Topical application of photofrin for photodynamic diagnosis of oral neoplasms. *Plast. Reconstr. Surg.* 2005;115(7):1877-86.

[30] Skala MC, Squirrell JM, Vrotsos KM, et al. Multiphoton microscopy of endogenous fluorescence differentiates normal, precancerous, and cancerous squamous epithelial tissues. *Cancer Res*. 2005;65(4):1180-6.

[31] Zhang L, Williams M, Poh CF, et al. Toluidine blue staining identifies high-risk primary oral premalignant lesions with poor outcome. *Cancer Res.* 2005;65(17):8017-21.

[32] Onofre MA, Sposto MR, Navarro CM. Reliability of toluidine blue application in the detection of oral epithelial dysplasia and in situ and invasive squamous cell carcinomas. *Oral Surg. Oral Med. Oral Pathol. Oral Radiol. Endod.* 2001;91(5):535-40.

[33] Piazza C, Cocco D, Bon FD, et al. Narrow band imaging and high definition television in evaluation of oral and oropharyngeal squamous cell cancer: A prospective study. *Oral Oncology* 2010;46(4):307-310.

[34] Maruvada P, Wang W, Wagner PD, Srivastava S. Biomarkers in molecular medicine: cancer detection and diagnosis. *Biotechniques* 2005;Suppl:9-15.

[35] Proia NK, Paszkiewicz GM, Sullivan Nasca MA, Franke GE, Pauly JL. Smoking and Smokeless Tobacco-Associated Human Buccal Cell Mutations and Their Association with Oral Cancer—A Review. *Cancer Epidemiology Biomarkers and Prevention* 2006;15(6):1061-1077.

[36] Ried T, Heselmeyer-Haddad K, Blegen H, Schrock E, Auer G. Genomic changes defining the genesis, progression, and malignancy potential in solid human tumors: a phenotype/genotype correlation. *Genes Chromosomes Cancer* 1999;25(3):195-204.

[37] Lengauer C, Kinzler KW, Vogelstein B. Genetic instabilities in human cancers. *Nature* 1998;396(6712):643-9.

[38] Bardelli A, Cahill DP, Lederer G, et al. Carcinogen-specific induction of genetic instability. *Proc. Natl. Acad. Sci. USA* 2001;98(10):5770-5.

[39] Sen S. Aneuploidy and cancer. Curr Opin Oncol 2000;12(1):82-8.

[40] Brandizzi D, Lanfranchi HE, Cabrini RL. Ploidy study in oral carcinomas: use of improved methodology to assess its clinical prognostic value. *Oral Surg. Oral Med. Oral Pathol. Oral Radiol. Endod.* 2009;108(3):406-12.

[41] Tsui IF, Garnis C, Poh CF. A dynamic oral cancer field: unraveling the underlying biology and its clinical implication. *Am. J. Surg. Pathol.* 2009;33(11):1732-8.

[42] Thornberry NA, Lazebnik Y. Caspases: Enemies Within. *Science* 1998;281(5381): 1312-1316.

[43] Hocker TL, Singh MK, Tsao H. Melanoma Genetics and Therapeutic Approaches in the 21st Century: Moving from the Benchside to the Bedside. *J. Invest. Dermatol.* 2008;128(11):2575-2595.

[44] Shaw R. The epigenetics of oral cancer. *Int. J. Oral Maxillofac. Surg.* 2006;35(2):101-8.

[45] Ha PK, Califano JA. Promoter methylation and inactivation of tumour-suppressor genes in oral squamous-cell carcinoma. *Lancet Oncol.* 2006;7(1):77-82.

[46] Perez-Sayans M, Somoza-Martin JM, Barros-Angueira F, Reboiras-Lopez MD, Gandara Rey JM, Garcia-Garcia A. Genetic and molecular alterations associated with oral squamous cell cancer (Review). *Oncol. Rep.* 2009;22(6):1277-82.

[47] Rajaraman R, Guernsey DL, Rajaraman MM, Rajaraman SR. Stem cells, senescence, neosis and self-renewal in cancer. *Cancer Cell Int.* 2006;6:25.

[48] Räsänen K, Virtanen I, Salmenperä P, Grenman R, Vaheri A. Differences in the Nemosis Response of Normal and Cancer-Associated Fibroblasts from Patients with Oral Squamous Cell Carcinoma. *PLoS ONE* 2009;4(9):e6879.

[49] Aswini Y. The genomics of oral cancer and wound healing; 2009. 2-5 p.

[50] Sundaram M, Guernsey DL, Rajaraman MM, Rajaraman R. Neosis: a novel type of cell division in cancer. *Cancer Biol. Ther.* 2004;3(2):207-18.

[51] Erenpreisa J, Cragg MS. Cancer: a matter of life cycle? Cell Biol. Int. 2007;31(12):1507-10.

[52] Grichnik JM. Melanoma, Nevogenesis, and Stem Cell Biology. *J. Invest. Dermatol.* 2008;128(10):2365-2380.

[53] Reya T, Morrison SJ, Clarke MF, Weissman IL. Stem cells, cancer, and cancer stem cells. *Nature* 2001;414(6859):105-111.

[54] Oback B, Wells DN. Donor cell differentiation, reprogramming, and cloning efficiency: Elusive or illusive correlation? *Molecular Reproduction and Development* 2007;74(5):646-654.

[55] Chere RL, Linda LS, John CM, Sarah AM, Russell PH, James MG. Early melanoma detection: Nonuniform dermoscopic features and growth. *Journal of the American Academy of Dermatology* 2003;48(5):663-671.

[56] Zhou ZT, Jiang WW. Cancer stem cell model in oral squamous cell carcinoma. *Curr. Stem. Cell Res. Ther.* 2008;3(1):17-20.

[57] Costea DE, Tsinkalovsky O, Vintermyr OK, Johannessen AC, Mackenzie IC. Cancer stem cells - new and potentially important targets for the therapy of oral squamous cell carcinoma. *Oral Dis.* 2006;12(5):443-54.

[58] Harper LJ, Piper K, Common J, Fortune F, Mackenzie IC. Stem cell patterns in cell lines derived from head and neck squamous cell carcinoma. *Journal of Oral Pathology and Medicine* 2007;36(10):594-603.

[59] Wallace-Brodeur RR, Lowe SW. Clinical implications of p53 mutations. *Cell Mol. Life Sci.* 1999;55(1):64-75.

[60] Boyle JO, Hakim J, Koch W, et al. The incidence of p53 mutations increases with progression of head and neck cancer. *Cancer Res.* 1993;53(19):4477-80.

[61] Chen Q, Samaranayake LP, Zhen X, Luo G, Nie M, Li B. Up-regulation of Fas ligand and down-regulation of Fas expression in oral carcinogenesis. *Oral Oncol.* 1999;35(6):548-53.

[62] Gastman BR, Atarshi Y, Reichert TE, et al. Fas ligand is expressed on human squamous cell carcinomas of the head and neck, and it promotes apoptosis of T lymphocytes. *Cancer Res.* 1999;59(20):5356-64.

[63] Imai Y, Sasaki T, Shinagawa Y, Akimoto K, Fujibayashi T. Expression of metastasis suppressor gene (KAI1/CD82) in oral squamous cell carcinoma and its clinico-pathological significance. *Oral Oncol.* 2002;38(6):557-61.

[64] Moles JP, Watt FM. The epidermal stem cell compartment: variation in expression levels of E-cadherin and catenins within the basal layer of human epidermis. J. Histochem. Cytochem. 1997;45(6):867-74.

[65] Yokoyama K, Kamata N, Hayashi E, et al. Reverse correlation of E-cadherin and snail expression in oral squamous cell carcinoma cells in vitro. *Oral Oncol.* 2001;37(1):65-71.

[66] Lowell S, Jones P, Le Roux I, Dunne J, Watt FM. Stimulation of human epidermal differentiation by Delta Notch signalling at the boundaries of stem-cell clusters. 2000;10(9):491-500.

[67] Fuchs E. Epidermal differentiation: the bare essentials. *The Journal of Cell Biology* 1990;111(6):2807-2814.

[68] Ryuhei O, Hachiro T, Setsuya A. Notch signaling: Its role in epidermal homeostasis and in the pathogenesis of skin diseases. *Journal of dermatological science* 2008;49(3):187-194.

[69] Kyrgidis A, Tzellos TG, Vahtsevanos K, Triaridis S. New Concepts for Basal Cell Carcinoma. Demographic, Clinical, Histological Risk Factors, and Biomarkers. A Systematic Review of Evidence Regarding Risk for Tumor Development, Susceptibility for Second Primary and Recurrence. *J. Surg. Res.* 2010;159(1):545-556.

[70] Kyrgidis A. Risk Factors for Non-Melanoma Skin Cancer. In: Maibach H, Gorouchi F, editors. Evidence Based Dermatology: PMH Publishers USA; 2010. p. in press.

[71] Aust G, Eichler W, Laue S, et al. CD97: a dedifferentiation marker in human thyroid carcinomas. *Cancer Res.* 1997;57(9):1798-806.

[72] Liu Y, Chen L, Peng SY, Chen ZX, Hoang-Vu C. Role of CD97(stalk) and CD55 as molecular markers for prognosis and therapy of gastric carcinoma patients. *J. Zhejiang. Univ. Sci.* B 2005;6(9):913-8.

[73] Mustafa T, Eckert A, Klonisch T, et al. Expression of the epidermal growth factor seven-transmembrane member CD97 correlates with grading and staging in human oral squamous cell carcinomas. *Cancer Epidemiol. Biomarkers Prev.* 2005;14(1):108-19.

[74] Zhang P, Zuo H, Ozaki T, Nakagomi N, Kakudo K. Cancer stem cell hypothesis in thyroid cancer. *Pathol. Int.* 2006;56(9):485-9.

[75] Irié T, Aida T, Tachikawa T. Gene expression profiling of oral squamous cell carcinoma using laser microdissection and cDNA microarray. *Medical Electron. Microscopy* 2004;37(2):89-96.

[76] Taybos G. Oral changes associated with tobacco use. *Am. J. Med. Sci.* 2003; 326(4):179-82.

[77] Parkin DM, Bray F, Ferlay J, Pisani P. Global cancer statistics, 2002. *CACancer J. Clin.* 2005;55(2):74-108.

[78] Taybos G. Oral Changes Associated with Tobacco Use. *The American Journal of the Medical Sciences* 2003;326(4):179-182.

[79] Joseph AM, Hecht SS, Murphy SE, et al. Relationships between cigarette consumption and biomarkers of tobacco toxin exposure. *Cancer Epidemiol. Biomarkers Prev.* 2005;14(12):2963-8.

[80] Xing S, Khanavkar B, Nakhosteen JA, Atay Z, Jockel KH, Marek W. Predictive value of image cytometry for diagnosis of lung cancer in heavy smokers. *Eu.r Respir. J.* 2005;25(6):956-63.

[81] Hecht SS, Murphy SE, Carmella SG, et al. Similar uptake of lung carcinogens by smokers of regular, light, and ultralight cigarettes. *Cancer Epidemiol. Biomarkers Prev.* 2005;14(3):693-8.

[82] Hecht SS, Carmella SG, Murphy SE, et al. Similar exposure to a tobacco-specific carcinogen in smokeless tobacco users and cigarette smokers. *Cancer Epidemiol. Biomarkers Prev.* 2007;16(8):1567-72.

[83] Bonassi S, Ugolini D, Kirsch-Volders M, Stromberg U, Vermeulen R, Tucker JD. Human population studies with cytogenetic biomarkers: review of the literature and future prospectives. *Environ. Mol. Mutagen.* 2005;45(2-3):258-70.
[84] Scaros O, Fisler R. Biomarker technology roundup: from discovery to clinical applications, a broad set of tools is required to translate from the lab to the clinic. *Biotechniques* 2005;Suppl:30-2.
[85] Shulman JD, Beach MM, Rivera-Hidalgo F. The prevalence of oral mucosal lesions in U.S. adults: data from the Third National Health and Nutrition Examination Survey, 1988-1994. *J. Am. Dent. Assoc.* 2004;135(9):1279-86.
[86] Bloching M, Hofmann A, Lautenschlager C, Berghaus A, Grummt T. Exfoliative cytology of normal buccal mucosa to predict the relative risk of cancer in the upper aerodigestive tract using the MN-assay. *Oral Oncol.* 2000;36(6):550-5.
[87] Bonassi S, Neri M, Lando C, et al. Effect of smoking habit on the frequency of micronuclei in human lymphocytes: results from the Human MicroNucleus project. *Mutat. Res.* 2003;543(2):155-66.
[88] Bonassi S, Znaor A, Ceppi M, et al. An increased micronucleus frequency in peripheral blood lymphocytes predicts the risk of cancer in humans. *Carcinogenesis* 2007;28(3):625-31.
[89] Majer BJ, Laky B, Knasmuller S, Kassie F. Use of the micronucleus assay with exfoliated epithelial cells as a biomarker for monitoring individuals at elevated risk of genetic damage and in chemoprevention trials. *Mutat. Res.* 2001;489(2-3):147-72.
[90] Castellsague X, Quintana MJ, Martinez MC, et al. The role of type of tobacco and type of alcoholic beverage in oral carcinogenesis. *Int. J. Cancer* 2004;108(5):741-9.
[91] Squier CA, Cox P, Hall BK. Enhanced penetration of nitrosonornicotine across oral mucosa in the presence of ethanol. *J. Oral Pathol.* 1986;15(5):276-9.
[92] Petti S, Scully C. Oral cancer: the association between nation-based alcohol-drinking profiles and oral cancer mortality. *Oral Oncol.* 2005;41(8):828-34.
[93] McCullough MJ, Farah CS. The role of alcohol in oral carcinogenesis with particular reference to alcohol-containing mouthwashes. *Aust. Dent. J.* 2008;53(4):302-5.
[94] Maserejian NN, Joshipura KJ, Rosner BA, Giovannucci E, Zavras AI. Prospective study of alcohol consumption and risk of oral premalignant lesions in men. *Cancer Epidemiol. Biomarkers Prev.* 2006;15(4):774-81.
[95] Howie NM, Trigkas TK, Cruchley AT, Wertz PW, Squier CA, Williams DM. Short-term exposure to alcohol increases the permeability of human oral mucosa. *Oral Dis.* 2001;7(6):349-54.
[96] Mascres C, Ming-Wen F, Joly JG. Morphologic changes of the esophageal mucosa in the rat after chronic alcohol ingestion. *Exp. Pathol.* 1984;25(3):147-53.
[97] Muller P, Hepke B, Meldau U, Raabe G. Tissue damage in the rabbit oral mucosa by acute and chronic direct toxic action of different alcohol concentrations. *Exp. Pathol.* 1983;24(2-3):171-81.
[98] Maier H, Weidauer H, Zoller J, et al. Effect of chronic alcohol consumption on the morphology of the oral mucosa. *Alcohol Clin. Exp. Res.* 1994;18(2):387-91.
[99] Hsu TC, Furlong C, Spitz MR. Ethyl alcohol as a cocarcinogen with special reference to the aerodigestive tract: a cytogenetic study. *Anticancer Res.* 1991;11(3):1097-101.

[100] Dong YJ, Peng TK, Yin SJ. Expression and activities of class IV alcohol dehydrogenase and class III aldehyde dehydrogenase in human mouth. *Alcohol* 1996;13(3):257-62.

[101] Seitz HK, Matsuzaki S, Yokoyama A, Homann N, Vakevainen S, Wang XD. Alcohol and cancer. *Alcohol Clin. Exp. Res.* 2001;25(5 Suppl ISBRA):137S-143S.

[102] Kurkivuori J, Salaspuro V, Kaihovaara P, et al. Acetaldehyde production from ethanol by oral streptococci. *Oral Oncol.* 2007;43(2):181-6.

[103] Velly AM, Franco EL, Schlecht N, et al. Relationship between dental factors and risk of upper aerodigestive tract cancer. *Oral Oncology* 1998;34(4):284-291.

[104] Warnakulasuriya S, Parkkila S, Nagao T, et al. Demonstration of ethanol-induced protein adducts in oral leukoplakia (pre-cancer) and cancer. *J. Oral Pathol. Med.* 2008;37(3):157-65.

[105] Ritchie JM, Smith EM, Summersgill KF, et al. Human papillomavirus infection as a prognostic factor in carcinomas of the oral cavity and oropharynx. *Int. J. Cancer* 2003;104(3):336-44.

[106] Smith EM, Ritchie JM, Summersgill KF, et al. Human papillomavirus in oral exfoliated cells and risk of head and neck cancer. *J. Natl. Cancer Inst.* 2004;96(6):449-55.

[107] Wiest T, Schwarz E, Enders C, Flechtenmacher C, Bosch FX. Involvement of intact HPV16 E6/E7 gene expression in head and neck cancers with unaltered p53 status and perturbed pRb cell cycle control. *Oncogene* 2002;21(10):1510-7.

[108] van Houten VM, Snijders PJ, van den Brekel MW, et al. Biological evidence that human papillomaviruses are etiologically involved in a subgroup of head and neck squamous cell carcinomas. *Int. J. Cancer* 2001;93(2):232-5.

[109] Wong M, Pagano JS, Schiller JT, Tevethia SS, Raab-Traub N, Gruber J. New associations of human papillomavirus, Simian virus 40, and Epstein-Barr virus with human cancer. *J. Natl. Cancer Inst.* 2002;94(24):1832-6.

[110] Katiyar S, Thelma BK, Murthy NS, et al. Polymorphism of the p53 codon 72 Arg/Pro and the risk of HPV type 16/18-associated cervical and oral cancer in India. *Mol. Cell Biochem.* 2003;252(1-2):117-24.

[111] Xian-Lu Z, Qi L, Yan Z, et al. Study on TP53 Codon 72 Polymorphisms with Oral Carcinoma Susceptibility. Archives of medical research 2009;40(7):625-634.

[112] Salem A. Dismissing links between HPV and aggressive tongue cancer in young patients. *Annals of Oncology* 2010;21(1):13-17.

[113] Yang S-W, Lee Y-S, Chen T-A, Wu C-J, Tsai C-N. Human papillomavirus in oral leukoplakia is no prognostic indicator of malignant transformation. Cancer *Epidemiology* 2009;33(2):118-122.

[114] Jung AC, Briolat J, Millon R, et al. Biological and clinical relevance of transcriptionally active human papillomavirus (HPV) infection in oropharynx squamous cell carcinoma. *International Journal of Cancer* 2010;126(8):1882-1894.

[115] SahebJamee M, Boorghani M, Ghaffari SR, AtarbashiMoghadam F, Keyhani A. Human papillomavirus in saliva of patients with oral squamous cell carcinoma. *Med. Oral Patol. Oral Cir. Bucal.* 2009;14(10):e525-8.

[116] Szarka K, Tar I, Fehér E, et al. Progressive increase of human papillomavirus carriage rates in potentially malignant and malignant oral disorders with increasing malignant potential. *Oral Microbiology and Immunology* 2009;24(4):314-318.

[117] Melle C, Ernst G, Winkler R, et al. Proteomic analysis of human papillomavirus-related oral squamous cell carcinoma: Identification of thioredoxin and epidermal-fatty acid binding protein as upregulated protein markers in microdissected tumor tissue. *PROTEOMICS* 2009;9(8):2193-2201.

[118] Marshall CJ, Hall A, Weiss RA. A transforming gene present in human sarcoma cell lines. *Nature* 1982;299(5879):171-3.

[119] Hall A, Marshall CJ, Spurr NK, Weiss RA. Identification of transforming gene in two human sarcoma cell lines as a new member of the ras gene family located on chromosome 1. *Nature* 1983;303(5916):396-400.

[120] Hauser-Urfer IH, Stauffer J. Comparative chromosome analysis of nine squamous cell carcinoma lines from tumors of the head and neck. *Cytogenet Cell Genet.* 1985;39 (1):35-9.

[121] Adjei AA, Cohen RB, Franklin W, et al. Phase I pharmacokinetic and pharma codynamic study of the oral, small-molecule mitogen-activated protein kinase kinase 1/2 inhibitor AZD6244 (ARRY-142886) in patients with advanced cancers. *J. Clin. Oncol.* 2008;26(13):2139-46.

[122] Houben R, Becker JC, Rapp UR. Absence of mutations in the coding sequence of the potential tumor suppressor 3pK in metastatic melanoma. *J. Carcinog.* 2005;4:23.

[123] Mishima K, Inoue K, Hayashi Y. Overexpression of extracellular-signal regulated kinases on oral squamous cell carcinoma. *Oral Oncol.* 2002;38(5):468-74.

[124] Feng-Yao T, En-Pei Isabel C, Jing-Gung C, Hong-Zin L, Chia-Yun H. S-Allylcysteine modulates the expression of E-cadherin and inhibits the malignant progression of human oral cancer. *The Journal of nutritional biochemistry* 2009;20(12):1013-1020.

[125] Ding H, Han C, Guo D, Wang D, Chen C-S, D'Ambrosio SM. OSU03012 activates Erk1/2 and Cdks leading to the accumulation of cells in the S-phase and apoptosis. *International Journal of Cancer* 2008;123(12):2923-2930.

[126] VAIRAKTARIS E, LOUKERI S, VASSILIOU S, et al. EGFR and c-Jun Exhibit the Same Pattern of Expression and Increase Gradually During the Progress of Oral Oncogenesis. *In Vivo* 2007;21(5):791-796.

[127] Yang L-C, Yang S-H, Tai K-W, Chou M-Y, Yang J-J. MEK inhibition enhances bleomycin A5-induced apoptosis in an oral cancer cell line: signaling mechanisms and therapeutic opportun-ities. *Journal of Oral Pathology and Medicine* 2004;33(1):37-45.

[128] Wioletta R-W, Ewa J, Magdalena M, Zyta G, Leszek P. Role of p38 MAPK Pathway in Induction of iNOS Expression in Neutrophils and Peripheral Blood Mononuclear Cells in Patients With Squamous Cell Carcinoma of the Oral Cavity. *Journal of oral and maxillofacial surgery : official journal of the American Association of Oral and Maxillofacial Surgeons* 2009;67(11):2354-2363.

[129] Hong K-O, Kim J-H, Hong J-S, et al. Inhibition of Akt activity induces the mesenchymal-to-epithelial reverting transition with restoring E-cadherin expression in KB and KOSCC-25B oral squamous cell carcinoma cells. *Journal of Experimental and Clinical Cancer Research* 2009;28(1):28.

[130] Yao J-e, Yan M, Guan Z, et al. Aurora-A down-regulates IkappaBalpha via Akt activation and interacts with insulin-like growth factor-1 induced phosphatidylinositol 3-kinase pathway for cancer cell survival. *Molecular Cancer* 2009;8(1):95.

[131] Husvik C, Bryne M, Halstensen TS. Epidermal growth factor-induced cyclooxygenase-2 expression in oral squamous cell carcinoma cell lines is mediated through

extracellular signal-regulated kinase 1/2 and p38 but is Src and nuclear factor-kappa B independent. *European Journal of Oral Sciences* 2009;117(5):528-535.

[132] Huang K-H, Huang S-F, Chen I-H, Liao C-T, Wang H-M, Hsieh L-L. Methylation of RASSF1A, RASSF2A, and HIN-1 Is Associated with Poor Outcome after Radiotherapy, but not Surgery, in Oral Squamous Cell Carcinoma. *Clinical Cancer Research* 2009;15(12):4174-4180.

[133] Rothschild G, Sottas CM, Kissel H, et al. A role for kit receptor signaling in Leydig cell steroidogenesis. *Biol. Reprod.* 2003;69(3):925-32.

[134] Ettl T, Schwarz S, Kleinsasser N, Hartmann A, Reichert TE, Driemel O. Overexpression of EGFR and absence of C-KIT expression correlate with poor prognosis in salivary gland carcinomas. *Histopathology* 2008;53(5):567-577.

[135] Traut W, Scholzen T, Winking H, Kubbutat MHG, Gerdes J. Assignment 1 of the murine Ki-67 gene (Mki67) to chromosome band 7F3–F5 by in situ hybridization. *Cytogenetic and Genome Research* 1998;83(1-2):12-13.

[136] Motta RDR, Zettler CG, Cambruzzi E, Jotz GP, Berni RB. Ki-67 and p53 correlation prognostic value in squamous cell carcinomas of the oral cavity and tongue. *Brazilian Journal of Otorhinolaryngology (Impresso)* 2009;75:544-549.

[137] Montebugnoli L, Badiali G, Marchetti C, Cervellati F, Farnedi A, Foschini MP. Prognostic value of Ki67 from clinically and histologically 'normal' distant mucosa in patients surgically treated for oral squamous cell carcinoma: a prospective study. *International journal of oral and maxillofacial surgery* 2009;38(11):1165-1172.

[138] Shpitzer T, Hamzany Y, Bahar G, et al. Salivary analysis of oral cancer biomarkers. *Br. J. Cancer* 2009;101(7):1194-1198.

[139] Torres-Rendon A, Roy S, Craig GT, Speight PM. Expression of Mcm2, geminin and Ki67 in normal oral mucosa, oral epithelial dysplasias and their corresponding squamous-cell carcinomas. *Br. J. Cancer* 2009;100(7):1128-1134.

[140] Hamakawa H, Nakashiro K-i, Sumida T, et al. Basic evidence of molecular targeted therapy for oral cancer and salivary gland cancer. *Head and Neck* 2008;30(6):800-809.

[141] Bonner JA, Harari PM, Giralt J, et al. Radiotherapy plus cetuximab for locoregionally advanced head and neck cancer: 5-year survival data from a phase 3 randomised trial, and relation between cetuximab-induced rash and survival. *Lancet. Oncol.* 2010;11(1):21-8.

[142] Vermorken JB, Mesia R, Rivera F, et al. Platinum-Based Chemotherapy plus Cetuximab in Head and Neck Cancer. *N. Engl. J. Med.* 2008;359(11):1116-1127.

[143] Specenier P, Vermorken JB. Advances in the systemic treatment of head and neck cancers. *Curr. Opin. Oncol.* 2010.

[144] Michael R, Darawalee W, Kerstin H-H, et al. EGFR protein overexpression and gene copy number increases in oral tongue squamous cell carcinoma. *European journal of cancer* (Oxford, England : 1990) 2009;45(9):1700-1708.

[145] Huang S-F, Chuang W-Y, Chen I-H, Liao C-T, Wang H-M, Hsieh L-L. EGFR protein overexpression and mutation in areca quid-associated oral cavity squamous cell carcinoma in Taiwan. *Head and Neck* 2009;31(8):1068-1077.

[146] Sheu JJ-C, Hua C-H, Wan L, et al. Functional Genomic Analysis Identified Epidermal Growth Factor Receptor Activation as the Most Common Genetic Event in Oral Squamous Cell Carcinoma. *Cancer Res.* 2009;69(6):2568-2576.

[147] Dang D, Sadler S, Ramos DM. Modulation of EGFR by oral squamous cell carcinoma cell lines. *J. Calif. Dent. Assoc.* 2009;37(12):869-74.

[148] Williams M. Integration of Biomarkers Including Molecular Targeted Therapies in Head and Neck Cancer. *Head and Neck Pathology* 2010;4(1):62-69.

[149] Chen JY, Hung CC, Huang KL, et al. Src family kinases mediate betel quid-induced oral cancer cell motility and could be a biomarker for early invasion in oral squamous cell carcinoma. *Neoplasia* 2008;10(12):1393-401.

[150] Hamada N, Matsumoto H, Hara T, Kobayashi Y. Intercellular and Intracellular Signaling Pathways Mediating Ionizing Radiation-Induced Bystander Effects. *Journal of Radiation Research* 2007;48(2):87-95.

[151] Kamochi N, Nakashima M, Aoki S, et al. Irradiated fibroblast-induced bystander effects on invasive growth of squamous cell carcinoma under cancerand#x2013;stromal cell interaction. *Cancer Science* 2008;99(12):2417-2427.

[152] Shah NG, Trivedi TI, Tankshali RA, et al. Prognostic significance of molecular markers in oral squamous cell carcinoma: A multivariate analysis. *Head and Neck* 2009;31(12):1544-1556.

[153] Jayasurya R, Sathyan KM, Lakshminarayanan K, et al. Phenotypic alterations in Rb pathway have more prognostic influence than p53 pathway proteins in oral carcinoma. *Mod. Pathol.* 2005;18(8):1056-1066.

[154] RIBEIRO DA, FRACALOSSI ACC, UATARI SA, OSHIMA CTF, SALVADORI DMF. Imbalance of Tumor Suppression Genes Expression Following Rat Tongue Carcinogenesis Induced by 4-Nitroquinoline 1-Oxide. *In Vivo* 2009;23(6):937-942.

[155] Fu M, Wang C, Li Z, Sakamaki T, Pestell RG. Minireview: Cyclin D1: Normal and Abnormal Functions. *Endocrinology* 2004;145(12):5439-5447.

[156] Filmus J, Robles AI, Shi W, Wong MJ, Colombo LL, Conti CJ. Induction of cyclin D1 overexpression by activated ras. *Oncogene* 1994;9(12):3627-33.

[157] Zhou X, Zhang Z, Yang X, Chen W, Zhang P. Inhibition of cyclin D1 expression by cyclin D1 shRNAs in human oral squamous cell carcinoma cells is associated with increased cisplatin chemosensitivity. *International Journal of Cancer* 2009;124(2):483-489.

[158] Robertson KD, Jones PA. Tissue-specific alternative splicing in the human INK4a/ARF cell cycle regulatory locus. *Oncogene* 1999;18(26):3810-20.

[159] Buajeeb W, Poomsawat S, Punyasingh J, Sanguansin S. Expression of p16 in oral cancer and premalignant lesions. *Journal of Oral Pathology and Medicine* 2009;38(1):104-108.

[160] Tang X-H, Albert M, Scognamiglio T, Gudas LJ. A DNA Methyltransferase Inhibitor and All-trans Retinoic Acid Reduce Oral Cavity Carcinogenesis Induced by the Carcinogen 4-Nitroquinoline 1-Oxide. *Cancer Prevention Research* 2009;2(12):1100-1110.

[161] Cao J, Zhou J, Gao Y, et al. Methylation of p16 CpG Island Associated with Malignant Progression of Oral Epithelial Dysplasia: A Prospective Cohort Study. *Clinical Cancer Research* 2009;15(16):5178-5183.

[162] Sinha P, Bahadur S, Thakar A, et al. Significance of promoter hypermethylation of <I>p16</I> gene for margin assessment in carcinoma tongue. *Head and Neck* 2009;31(11):1423-1430.

[163] Li J, Yen C, Liaw D, et al. PTEN, a Putative Protein Tyrosine Phosphatase Gene Mutated in Human Brain, Breast, and Prostate Cancer. *Science* 1997;275(5308):1943-1947.
[164] Kurasawa Y, Shiiba M, Nakamura M, et al. PTEN expression and methylation status in oral squamous cell carcinoma. Oncol Rep 2008;19(6):1429-34.
[165] Eiwa I, Mitsutoshi N, Miwa I, et al. Promotor hypermethylation of p14ARF is a key alteration for progression of oral squamous cell carcinoma. *Oral Oncology* 2005;41(6):614-622.
[166] Chakraborty S, Mohiyuddin SA, Gopinath K, Kumar A. Involvement of TSC genes and differential expression of other members of the mTOR signaling pathway in oral squamous cell carcinoma. *BMC Cancer* 2008;8(1):163.
[167] Xie SM, Shen LJ, Yin C, Ruan P, Yao X. [Expression of tumor suppressor gene PTEN, PIP3 and cyclin D1 in oral squamous cell carcinoma and their correlations]. *Zhonghua Kou Qiang Yi Xue Za Zhi* 2006;41(7):407-10.
[168] Xavier FCA, Rodini CO, Ramalho LMP, Mantesso A, Nunes FD. WNT-5A, but not matrix metalloproteinase 3 or and#x03B2;-catenin protein, expression is related to early stages of lip carcinogenesis. *Journal of Oral Pathology and Medicine* 2009;38(9):708-715.
[169] Fracalossi ACC, Silva MdS, Oshima CTF, Ribeiro DA. Wnt/[beta]-catenin signalling pathway following rat tongue carcinogenesis induced by 4-nitroquinoline 1-oxide. *Experimental and Molecular Pathology* 2010;88(1):176-183.
[170] Li S, Jiao J, Lu Z, Zhang M. An essential role for N-cadherin and beta-catenin for progression in tongue squamous cell carcinoma and their effect on invasion and metastasis of Tca8113 tongue cancer cells. *Oncol. Rep.* 2009;21(5):1223-33.
[171] Lo Muzio L. A Possible Role for the Wnt~1 Pathway in Oral Carcinogenesis. *Critical Reviews in Oral Biology and Medicine* 2001;12(2):152-165.
[172] Fernanda Ferreira L, Márcia Cristina da Costa M, Antônio Luiz Amaral P, et al. Changes in immunoexpression of E-cadherin and β-catenin in oral squamous cell carcinoma with and without nodal metastasis. *Annals of diagnostic pathology* 2009;13(1):22-29.
[173] Bidaud P, Chasle J, Sichel F, et al. Expression of p53 family members and CD44 in oral squamous cell carcinoma (OSCC) in relation to tumorigenesis. *Histol. Histopathol.* 2010;25(3):331-9.
[174] Fernando Augusto Cervantes Garcia de S, Thaís Cachuté P, Yasmin Rodarte C, Luiz Eduardo Blumer R. Comparative analysis of the expression of proliferating cell nuclear antigen, p53, bax, and bcl-2 in oral lichen planus and oral squamous cell carcinoma. *Annals of diagnostic pathology* 2009;13(5):308-312.
[175] Li Y, Li L-J, Zhang S-T, et al. In vitro and Clinical Studies of Gene Therapy with Recombinant Human Adenovirus-p53 Injection for Oral Leukoplakia. *Clinical Cancer Research* 2009;15(21):6724-6731.
[176] Perrone F, Bossi P, Cortelazzi B, et al. TP53 Mutations and Pathologic Complete Response to Neoadjuvant Cisplatin and Fluorouracil Chemotherapy in Resected Oral Cavity Squamous Cell Carcinoma. *J. Clin. Oncol.* 2010;28(5):761-766.
[177] Mroz EA, Rocco JW. Functional p53 Status As a Biomarker for Chemotherapy Response in Oral-Cavity Cancer. *J. Clin. Oncol.* 2010;28(5):715-717.

[178] Poeta ML, Manola J, Goldwasser MA, et al. TP53 Mutations and Survival in Squamous-Cell Carcinoma of the Head and Neck. *N. Engl. J. Med.* 2007;357(25):2552-2561.

[179] Bao Q, Lu W, Rabinowitz JD, Shi Y. Calcium Blocks Formation of Apoptosome by Preventing Nucleotide Exchange in Apaf-1. 2007;25(2):181-192.

[180] Lo Muzio L, Santarelli A, Emanuelli M, et al. Genetic analysis of oral squamous cell carcinoma by cDNA microarrays focused apoptotic pathway. *Int. J. Immunopathol. Pharmacol.* 2006;19(3):675-82.

[181] Hayashi K, Yokozaki H, Naka K, Yasui W, Lotan R, Tahara E. Overexpression of retinoic acid receptor beta induces growth arrest and apoptosis in oral cancer cell lines. *Jpn. J. Cancer Res.* 2001;92(1):42-50.

[182] Azuma M, Tamatani T, Ashida Y, Takashima R, Harada K, Sato M. Cisplatin induces apoptosis in oral squamous carcinoma cells by the mitochondria-mediated but not the NF-κB-suppressed pathway. Oral Oncology 2003;39(3):282-289.

[183] Soengas MS, Lowe SW. Apoptosis and melanoma chemoresistance. *Oncogene* 2003; 22(20):3138-3151.

[184] Danial NN, Korsmeyer SJ. Cell Death: *Critical Control Points*. 2004;116(2):205-219.

[185] Pegoraro L, Palumbo A, Erikson J, et al. A 14;18 and an 8;14 chromosome translocation in a cell line derived from an acute B-cell leukemia. *Proc. Natl. Acad. Sci. USA* 1984;81(22):7166-70.

[186] Bakhshi A, Jensen JP, Goldman P, et al. Cloning the chromosomal breakpoint of t(14;18) human lymphomas: clustering around JH on chromosome 14 and near a transcriptional unit on 18. Cell 1985;41(3):899-906.

[187] Tsujimoto Y, Finger L, Yunis J, Nowell P, Croce C. Cloning of the chromosome breakpoint of neoplastic B cells with the t(14;18) chromosome translocation. *Science* 1984;226(4678):1097-1099.

[188] Sousa FACGd, Paradella T, iacute, s C, Carvalho YR, Rosa LEB. Immuno-histochemical expression of PCNA, p53, bax and bcl-2 in oral lichen planus and epithelial dysplasia. *Journal of Oral Science* 2009;51(1):117-121.

[189] Sohrabi M, Kalati FA, Vatansever S, et al. Effect of dietary and topical Celecoxib on expression of bcl-2, bax, c-erb-B2 and Ki67 in carcinogen-induced tongue carcinoma in rat. *Pak. J. Biol. Sci.* 2009;12(10):750-7.

[190] CHIU T-H, LAI W-W, HSIA T-C, et al. Aloe-emodin Induces Cell Death through S-Phase Arrest and Caspase-dependent Pathways in Human Tongue Squamous Cancer SCC-4 Cells. *Anticancer Research* 2009;29(11):4503-4511.

[191] Boise LH, Gonzalez-Garcia M, Postema CE, et al. bcl-x, a bcl-2-related gene that functions as a dominant regulator of apoptotic cell death. *Cell* 1993;74(4):597-608.

[192] Han Z, Chatterjee D, Early J, Pantazis P, Hendrickson EA, Wyche JH. Isolation and Characterization of an Apoptosis-resistant Variant of Human Leukemia HL-60 Cells That Has Switched Expression from Bcl-2 to Bcl-XL. *Cancer Res.* 1996;56(7):1621-1628.

[193] Arriola EL, Rodriguez-Lopez AM, Hickman JA, Chresta CM. Bcl-2 overexpression results in reciprocal downregulation of Bcl-X(L) and sensitizes human testicular germ cell tumours to chemotherapy-induced apoptosis. *Oncogene* 1999;18(7):1457-64.

[194] Noda T, Iwai S, Hamada M, Fujita Y, Yura Y. Induction of apoptosis of detached oral squamous cell carcinoma cells by safingol. Possible role of Bim, focal adhesion kinase and endonuclease G. *Apoptosis* 2009;14(3):287-297.
[195] Kajihara A, Takahashi A, Ohnishi K, et al. Protein microarray analysis of apoptosis-related protein expression following heat shock in human tongue squamous cell carcinomas containing different p53 phenotypes. *International Journal of Hyperthermia* 2008;24(8):605-612.
[196] Li D, Ueta E, Kimura T, Yamamoto T, Osaki T. Reactive oxygen species (ROS) control the expression of Bcl-2 family proteins by regulating their phosphorylation and ubiquitination. *Cancer Science* 2004;95(8):644-650.
[197] Mott JL, Kobayashi S, Bronk SF, Gores GJ. mir-29 regulates Mcl-1 protein expression and apoptosis. *Oncogene* 2007;26(42):6133-6140.
[198] Nikiforov MA, Riblett M, Tang W-H, et al. Tumor cell-selective regulation of NOXA by c-MYC in response to proteasome inhibition. *Proceedings of the National Academy of Sciences* 2007;104(49):19488-19493.
[199] Zhai D, Jin C, Huang Z, Satterthwait AC, Reed JC. Differential Regulation of Bax and Bak by Anti-apoptotic Bcl-2 Family Proteins Bcl-B and Mcl-1. *Journal of Biological Chemistry* 2008;283(15):9580-9586.
[200] Willis SN, Chen L, Dewson G, et al. Proapoptotic Bak is sequestered by Mcl-1 and Bcl-xL, but not Bcl-2, until displaced by BH3-only proteins. *Genes. Dev.* 2005; 19(11):1294-305.
[201] Nagata M, Wada K, Nakajima A, et al. Role of Myeloid Cell Leukemia-1 in Cell Growth of Squamous Cell Carcinoma. *Journal of Pharmacological Sciences* 2009;110(3):344-353.
[202] Jabłońska E, Garley M, Jabłoński J. The expressions of intrinsic and extrinsic apoptotic pathway proteins in neutrophils of oral cavity cancer patients: a preliminary study. *Archivum Immunologiae et Therapiae Experimentalis* 2009;57(3):229-234.
[203] Mallick S, Patil R, Gyanchandani R, et al. Human oral cancers have altered expression of Bcl-2 family members and increased expression of the anti-apoptotic splice variant of <I>Mcl-1</I>. *The Journal of Pathology* 2009;217(3):398-407.
[204] Kiefer MC, Brauer MJ, Powers VC, et al. Modulation of apoptosis by the widely distributed Bcl-2 homologue Bak. *Nature* 1995;374(6524):736-739.
[205] Chittenden T, Harrington EA, O'Connor R, et al. Induction of apoptosis by the Bcl-2 homologue Bak. *Nature* 1995;374(6524):733-736.
[206] Baltaziak M, Koda M, Barwijuk-Machala M, et al. The role of Bak expression in apoptosis of the oral squamous cell carcinoma (OSCC) and metastases to lymph nodes (LNMs). *Rocz. Akad. Med. Bialymst.* 2004;49 Suppl 1:14-5.
[207] Xie X, Clausen OP, Boysen M. Prognostic value of Bak expression in oral tongue squamous cell carcinomas. *Oncol. Rep.* 2003;10(2):369-74.
[208] Oltvai ZN, Milliman CL, Korsmeyer SJ. Bcl-2 heterodimerizes in vivo with a conserved homolog, Bax, that accelerates programmed cell death. *Cell* 1993;74(4):609-19.
[209] HO Y-T, LU C-C, YANG J-S, et al. Berberine Induced Apoptosis via Promoting the Expression of Caspase-8, -9 and -3, Apoptosis-inducing Factor and Endonuclease G in SCC-4 Human Tongue Squamous Carcinoma Cancer Cells. *Anticancer Research* 2009;29(10):4063-4070.

[210] Kipling D. Telomerase: immortality enzyme or oncogene? *Nat. Genet.* 1995;9(2):104-6.
[211] Morin GB. The human telomere terminal transferase enzyme is a ribonucleoprotein that synthesizes TTAGGG repeats. *Cell* 1989;59(3):521-9.
[212] Kang X, Chen W, Kim RH, Kang MK, Park NH. Regulation of the hTERT promoter activity by MSH2, the hnRNPs K and D, and GRHL2 in human oral squamous cell carcinoma cells. *Oncogene* 2008;28(4):565-574.
[213] Freier K, Pungs S, Flechtenmacher C, et al. Frequent high telomerase reverse transcriptase expression in primary oral squamous cell carcinoma. *Journal of Oral Pathology and Medicine* 2007;36(5):267-272.
[214] Huang-Hsu C, Chuan-Hang Y, Jeng-Tzung W, et al. Expression of human telomerase reverse transcriptase (hTERT) protein is significantly associated with the progression, recurrence and prognosis of oral squamous cell carcinoma in Taiwan. *Oral Oncology* 2007;43(2):122-129.
[215] Wu KJ, Grandori C, Amacker M, et al. Direct activation of TERT transcription by c-MYC. *Nat. Genet.* 1999;21(2):220-4.
[216] BEKTAŞ-KAYHAN K, ÜNÜR M, YAYLIM-ERALTAN İ, et al. Role of L-MYC Polymorphism in Oral Squamous Cell Carcinoma in Turkey. *Anticancer Research* 2009;29(7):2519-2524.
[217] Koehn J, Krapfenbauer K, Huber S, et al. Potential Involvement of MYC- and p53-Related Pathways in Tumorigenesis in Human Oral Squamous Cell Carcinoma Revealed by Proteomic Analysis. *Journal of Proteome Research* 2008;7(9):3818-3829.
[218] Hayry V, Makinen LK, Atula T, et al. Bmi-1 expression predicts prognosis in squamous cell carcinoma of the tongue. *Br. J. Cancer* 2010;102(5):892-897.
[219] Klanrit P, Sperandio M, Brown AL, et al. DNA ploidy in proliferative verrucous leukoplakia. *Oral Oncology* 2007;43(3):310-316.
[220] Sudbo J. Human papillomavirus infection as a risk factor for squamous-cell carcinoma of the head and neck. *N. Engl. J. Med.* 2001;345(5):376-7.
[221] Couzin J. CANCER RESEARCH: Fake Data, but Could the Idea Still Be Right? *Science* 2006;313(5784):154-.
[222] Schliephake H. Prognostic relevance of molecular markers of oral cancer--A review. *International journal of oral and maxillofacial surgery* 2003;32(3):233-245.
[223] Kim J, Shin DM, El-Naggar A, et al. Chromosome Polysomy and Histological Characteristics in Oral Premalignant Lesions. *Cancer EpidemiologyBiomarkers and Prevention* 2001;10(4):319-325.
[224] Matsuura M, Onimaru M, Yonemitsu Y, et al. Autocrine Loop between Vascular Endothelial Growth Factor (VEGF)-C and VEGF Receptor-3 Positively Regulates Tumor-Associated Lymphangiogenesis in Oral Squamoid Cancer Cells. *Am. J. Pathol.* 2009;175(4):1709-1721.
[225] Bin X, Jiu-Ming L, Na T, et al. VEGFA + 936C>T polymorphism and cancer risk: a meta-analysis. *Cancer genetics and cytogenetics* 2010;198(1):7-14.
[226] Young-Hoon J, Chan-Kwon J, Min-Sik K, Dong-Il S. Relationship between vascular endothelial growth factor and Notch1 expression and lymphatic metastasis in tongue cancer Otolaryngology - *Head and Neck Surgery* 2009;140(4):512-518.
[227] Sugiura T, Inoue Y, Matsuki R, et al. VEGF-C and VEGF-D expression is correlated with lymphatic vessel density and lymph node metastasis in oral squamous cell

carcinoma: Implications for use as a prognostic marker. *Int. J. Oncol.* 2009 34(3):673-80.
[228] Shane J, Richard ML. The role of vascular endothelial growth factor (VEGF) in oral dysplasia and oral squamous cell carcinoma. *Oral Oncology* 2006;42(4):337-342.
[229] Li C, Shintani S, Terakado N, et al. Microvessel density and expression of vascular endothelial growth factor, basic fibroblast growth factor, and platelet-derived endothelial growth factor in oral squamous cell carcinomas. *International journal of oral and maxillofacial surgery* 2005;34(5):559-565.
[230] Sappayatosok K, Maneerat Y, Swasdison S, et al. Expression of pro-inflammatory protein, iNOS, VEGF and COX-2 in oral squamous cell carcinoma (OSCC), relationship with angiogenesis and their clinico-pathological correlation. *Med. Oral Patol. Oral Cir. Bucal.* 2009;14(7):E319-24.
[231] Lan Y, Wei-liang C, Shu-guang Z, Yong-jie W, Zhi-bao B. Inhibition of VEGF expression in tongue squamous cancer cells via RNA interference silencing of iNOS gene. *International journal of oral and maxillofacial surgery* 2009;38(4):369-373.
[232] Ali MA. Lymphatic Microvessel Density and the Expression of Lymphangiogenic Factors in Oral Squamous Cell Carcinoma. *Medical Principles and Practice* 2008;17(6):486-492.
[233] Lowenstein CJ, Glatt CS, Bredt DS, Snyder SH. Cloned and expressed macrophage nitric oxide synthase contrasts with the brain enzyme. *Proc. Natl. Acad. Sci. USA* 1992;89(15):6711-5.
[234] Ratajczak-Wrona W, Jablonska E, Marcinczyk M, Grabowska Z, Piotrowski L. Role of p38 MAPK pathway in induction of iNOS expression in neutrophils and peripheral blood mononuclear cells in patients with squamous cell carcinoma of the oral cavity. *J. Oral Maxillofac. Surg.* 2009;67(11):2354-63.
[235] Nakashiro K, Begum NM, Uchida D, et al. Thiazolidinediones inhibit cell growth of human oral squamous cell carcinoma in vitro independent of peroxisome proliferator-activated receptor gamma. *Oral Oncol.* 2003;39(8):855-61.
[236] Roberg K, Ceder R, Farnebo L, Norberg-Spaak L, Grafstrom RC. Multiple genotypic aberrances associate to terminal differentiation-deficiency of an oral squamous cell carcinoma in serum-free culture. *Differentiation* 2008;76(8):868-80.
[237] Perez-Mancera PA, Bermejo-Rodriguez C, Gonzalez-Herrero I, et al. Adipose tissue mass is modulated by SLUG (SNAI2). *Hum. Mol. Genet.* 2007;16(23):2972-2986.
[238] Joseph MJ, Dangi-Garimella S, Shields MA, et al. Slug is a downstream mediator of transforming growth factor-beta1-induced matrix metalloproteinase-9 expression and invasion of oral cancer cells. *Journal of Cellular Biochemistry* 2009;108(3):726-736.
[239] Liu LK, Jiang XY, Zhou XX, Wang DM, Song XL, Jiang HB. Upregulation of vimentin and aberrant expression of E-cadherin/beta-catenin complex in oral squamous cell carcinomas: correlation with the clinicopathological features and patient outcome. *Mod. Pathol.* 2010;23(2):213-24.
[240] Maeda G, Chiba T, Okazaki M, et al. Expression of SIP1 in oral squamous cell carcinomas: implications for E-cadherin expression and tumor progression. *Int. J. Oncol.* 2005;27(6):1535-41.
[241] Kaur G, Carnelio S, Rao N, Rao L. Expression of E-cadherin in primary oral squamous cell carcinoma and metastatic lymph nodes: *An immunohistochemical study*; 2009. 71-76 p.

[242] Cruz MC, Pereira AL, Lopes FF, et al. Immunohistochemical expression of E-cadherin and CD44v6 in squamous cell carcinomas of the lower lip and tongue. *Braz. Dent. J.* 2009;20(1):64-9.

[243] Nita-Lazar M, Noonan V, Rebustini I, Walker J, Menko AS, Kukuruzinska MA. Overexpression of DPAGT1 Leads to Aberrant N-Glycosylation of E-Cadherin and Cellular Discohesion in Oral Cancer. *Cancer Res.* 2009;69(14):5673-5680.

[244] Righini CA, de Fraipont F, Reyt E, Favrot MC. [Aberrant methylation of tumor suppressor genes in head and neck squamous cell carcinoma: is it clinically relevant?]. *Bull. Cancer* 2007;94(2):191-7.

[245] Xinhong W, Jiali Z, Mingwen F, et al. The expression of E-cadherin at the invasive tumor front of oral squamous cell carcinoma: immunohistochemical and RT-PCR analysis with clinicopathological correlation. *Oral surgery, oral medicine, oral pathology, oral radiology, and endodontics* 2009;107(4):547-554.

[246] Bauer K, Dowejko A, Bosserhoff A-K, Reichert TE, Josef Bauer R. P-cadherin induces an epithelial-like phenotype in oral squamous cell carcinoma by GSK-3beta-mediated Snail phosphorylation. *Carcinogenesis* 2009;30(10):1781-1788.

[247] Lipari L, Mauro A, Tortorici S, et al. Immunohistochemical and transcriptional expression of the matrix metalloproteinases MMP-2 and MMP-9 in normal and pathological human oral mucosa. *J. Biol. Regul. Homeost. Agents* 2009;23(4):259-67.

[248] Mueller CK, Schultze-Mosgau S. Radiation-induced microenvironments--the molecular basis for free flap complications in the pre-irradiated field? *Radiother. Oncol.* 2009;93(3):581-5.

[249] Germani RM, Civantos FJ, Elgart G, Roberts B, Franzmann EJ. Molecular markers of micrometastasis in oral cavity carcinomas. *Otolaryngol Head Neck Surg.* 2009;141(1):52-8.

[250] Yen CY, Chen CH, Chang CH, et al. Matrix metalloproteinases (MMP) 1 and MMP10 but not MMP12 are potential oral cancer markers. *Biomarkers* 2009;14(4):244-9.

[251] RAMOS DM, DANG D, SADLER S. The Role of the Integrin αvβ6 in Regulating the Epithelial to Mesenchymal Transition in Oral Cancer. *Anticancer Research* 2009;29(1):125-130.

[252] Lee M-Y, Chou C-Y, Tang M-J, Shen M-R. Epithelial-Mesenchymal Transition in Cervical Cancer: Correlation with Tumor Progression, Epidermal Growth Factor Receptor Overexpr-ession, and Snail Up-Regulation. *Clinical Cancer Research* 2008;14(15):4743-4750.

[253] Christofori G. New signals from the invasive front. *Nature* 2006;441(7092):444-450.

[254] Ramos DM, Chen BL, Boylen K, et al. Stromal fibroblasts influence oral squamous-cell carcinoma cell interactions with tenascin-C. *International Journal of Cancer* 1997;72(2):369-376.

[255] Munger JS, Huang X, Kawakatsu H, et al. A Mechanism for Regulating Pulmonary Inflammation and Fibrosis: The Integrin ±v²6 Binds and Activates *Latent* TGF ²1. 1999;96(3):319-328.

[256] Ketcham CM, Crawford JM. The impact of review articles. *Lab. Invest.* 2007; 87(12):1174-85.

In: Stem Cell Research: New Developments
Editors: Hiroshi Tanaka and Michael C. F. Chang
ISBN: 978-1-61942-081-6

Chapter 7

WNT SIGNALING IN COLON CANCER STEM CELLS

Tianxin Yu, Xi Chen and Chunming Liu*
University of Kentucky, Lexington, US

ABSTRACT

Colorectal cancer is the second leading cause of cancer-related death in the United States. Among many gene mutations associated with colorectal cancer, mutation of APC (adenomatous polyposis coli) or β-catenin, which activates Wnt signaling, represents the initiation step of colon tumorigenesis. Wnt signaling is known to play multiple roles in early development and formation of human cancers. In addition, Wnt signaling also regulates the self-renewal and differentiation of adult stem cells. Recently, cancer stem cells have emerged as an exciting new concept in cancer research. However, many challenging questions have also arisen. What is the definition of a cancer stem cell? Where do such cells originate and what are the markers for these cells? What's the genetic and epigenetic machinery that regulate the homeostasis of this cell population? What is the mechanism underlying the process of cancer stem cell-involved tumorigenesis? In this review, we will discuss the development and trends in the field of cancer stem cell research, with emphasis on colon cancer stem cells. Since Wnt signaling is involved in both intestinal stem cells and colon cancers, we will first discuss the mechanisms of the Wnt signal transduction pathway, and then discuss the roles of Wnt signaling in normal intestine and in colon cancer. Finally, we will discuss the challenges and opportunities in colon cancer stem cell research.

WNT SIGNALING PATHWAY

The Wnt gene was first identified as a preferential insertion site for the Murine Mammary Tumor Virus, resulting in overexpression of the Wnt-1 protein and the formation of mammary tumors [1]. Wnts are secreted glycoproteins. In human and mouse genomes, nineteen Wnt

* Correspondence concerning this article should be addressed to: Chunming Liu, Markey Cancer Center and the Department of Molecular and Cellular Biochemistry, University of Kentucky, Lexington, KY 40506. E-mail: chunming.liu@uky.edu.

genes have been found. Each individual Wnt protein may have similar or drastically different functions. Some activate the canonical Wnt pathway, whereas others activate the non-canonical pathway, including the PCP pathway, and/or the Ca^{2+} pathway [2,3]. Wnt signaling is one of the major signaling pathways that controls cell proliferation and differentiation, and it also regulates the homeostasis of many tissues [4-6]. Deregulation of Wnt signaling plays a vital role in tumorigenesis [7,8].

The canonical pathway is also called the Wnt/β-catenin pathway. The central task of canonical Wnt signaling is to regulate β-catenin. β-catenin is a multifunctional protein depending on cellular localization. When on the cell membrane, it binds E-cadherin and regulates cell adhesion, whereas when in the nucleus, it binds TCF/LEF and regulates gene transcription. The level of cytoplasmic β-catenin is tightly controlled by the Axin degradation complex (Figure 1A). Axin is a scaffold protein; it interacts with APC, GSK-3, Casein Kinase Iα (CKIα) and β-catenin through different domains. In the absence of Wnt, β-catenin is sequentially phosphorylated by CKIα and GSK-3 within the Axin complex [9,10]. Phosphorylated β-catenin is recognized by β-Trcp, a component of E3 ubiquitin ligase complex, for ubiquitination [11-15]. Poly-ubiquitinated β-catenin is then degraded by the proteasome (Figure 1A). β-catenin phosphorylation is also regulated by Protein phosphatase 2A (PP2A). The specificity of PP2A-mediated β-catenin dephosphorylation is regulated by PR55α, a regulatory subunit of PP2A [16]. Whether β-catenin ubiquitination is regulated by a deubiquitinase is currently unknown.

In the presence of Wnt, Wnt binds to the receptor Frizzled (Fz) [17,18] and co-receptor Lrp5/6 (low-density-lipoprotein receptor-related proteins 5 and 6) [19-21] (Figure 1B). Fz receptors are seven trans-membrane repeat proteins that contain an extra-cellular N-terminal cysteine-rich domain (CRD) and an intra-cellular tail domain [22,23]. Binding of Wnt induces structural changes in the receptor that result in recruitment of Dvl to the cytoplasmic tail of Fz through its intra-cellular domain [24-27]. Fz can also activate signaling through heterotrimeric G proteins [28,29]. Lrp5/6 are single transmembrane proteins; binding of Wnt induces phosphorylation of Lrp5/6, creating a docking site for Axin [30], which is an inhibitory downstream component of the Wnt pathway. Recruitment of Axin to the co-receptor inhibits its function, and leads to stabilization of β-catenin by releasing it from the destruction complex [31] (Figure 1B).

Stabilized β-catenin translocates into the nucleus. In the nucleus, β-catenin interacts with the TCF family of transcription factors, which includes TCF-1, lymphoid enhancer factor-1 (LEF-1), TCF-3, and TCF-4 [32,33]. In the absence of β-catenin, TCF/LEF family members bind co-repressors such as CtBP [34], HDAC1 [35,36], and Groucho/TLE [37-39] and repress transcription (Figure 1A). When Wnt signaling is activated, β-catenin binds TCF/LEF and recruits co-activators through its N- and C-terminal transactivation domains, and subsequently activates downstream genes (Figure 1B). The C-terminus of β-catenin contains a strong transactivation domain [32,40,41]. This transactivation domain recruits p300/CBP which is required for Wnt signaling [40,42]. p300 and CBP are paralogous transcriptional co-activators; they acetylate nearby histones, thereby loosening chromatin in order to facilitate binding of other transcription factors [43,44]. The N-terminal transactivation domain of β-catenin directly associates with BCL9/Legless, which in turn recruits the transcriptional co-activator Pygopus [45-48] (Figure 1B). Pygopus contains a plant homeodomain (PHD). The PHD domain of ING (inhibitor of growth) can interact with tri-methylated histone H3, and is thought to regulate epigenetic modifications on target genes [49].

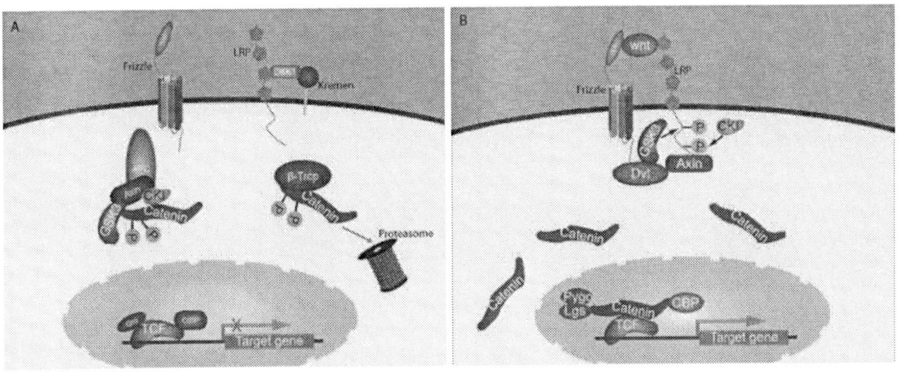

Figure 1. Wnt Signaling Pathway. (A) In the absence of Wnt, β-catenin is phosphorylated by the Axin destruction complex consisting of Axin, APC, GSK3 and CKIα. Phosphorylated β-catenin is recognized by β-Trcp for ubiquitination and proteasome degradation. In the nucleus, TCF recruits co-repressors such as CtBP and Groucho (Gro) to inhibit transcription. (B) Wnt binds to its receptor Frizzled and co-receptor LRP5/6. Wnt stimulates LRP5/6 phosphorylation and recruitment of Axin to LRP5/6, leading to release of β-catenin from the destruction complex. Stablized β-catenin enters the nucleus, binds to TCF, and recruits co-activators such as Pygopus (Pygo), Legless (Lgs) and P300/CBP to activate target gene expression.

WNT SIGNALING IN THE INTESTINE

The intestine is a tube-like organ. The luminal surface of the gut is covered by a continuous sheet of epithelial cells (Figure 2A). In the epithelium of the small intestine, this sheet folds into finger-like protrusions that extend into the lumen, called villi. In between each villus, the epithelial sheet additionally invaginates inward to form the crypts of Lieberkühn [50]. The colonic epithelium has no villi, but consists entirely of crypts. Intestinal stem cells are located at the bottom of the crypts. Crypt stem cells produce transit-amplifying cells that ultimately differentiate into enterocytes, goblet cells, and enteroendocrine cells (Figure 2B). In the small intestine, transit-amplifying cells additionally differentiate into Paneth cells [50,51]. Enterocytes are the most abundant cell type of the intestine, and perform the primary absorptive function of the intestine. Goblet cells secrete mucins that protect the luminal surface. Enteroendocrine cells are located throughout the crypt-villus axis and secrete intestinal hormones. Paneth cells are found at the bottom of crypts and release lysozyme as well as other anti-microbial molecules. With the exception of Paneth cells, terminally differentiated cells migrate along the crypt-villi axis and are shed into lumen after 3-5 days [51].

Wnt signaling is the major player in regulating cell fate along the crypt-villus axis [52-54]. Since TCF4-deficient mice lack proliferating cells in the intestinal crypts [54], Wnt signaling is known to be essential for self-renewal of intestine stem cells, and the bottom of the crypt is thought to be a stem cell niche in which Wnt plays a vital role controlling the differentiation, migration and proliferation of the epithelial stem cells [55]. Overexpression of Dkk1, a Wnt inhibitor, in the intestine causes loss of crypt and secretory cell lineages [56]. APC is a negative regulator of β-catenin and the major tumor suppressor in colorectal cancer. Deletion of APC in the mouse intestine activates Wnt signaling and results in expansion of the crypts [57]. As a well-established target of Wnt, MYC deletion in the intestine rescues the defects in proliferation and migration in APC$^{-/-}$ mice [58]. In addition, expression of the Wnt agonist R-spondin1 in mice induces crypt cell proliferation [59]. These data further suggest that Wnt signaling plays essential roles in maintaining the stem cell compartment and regulating cell proliferation and differentiation in the intestine.

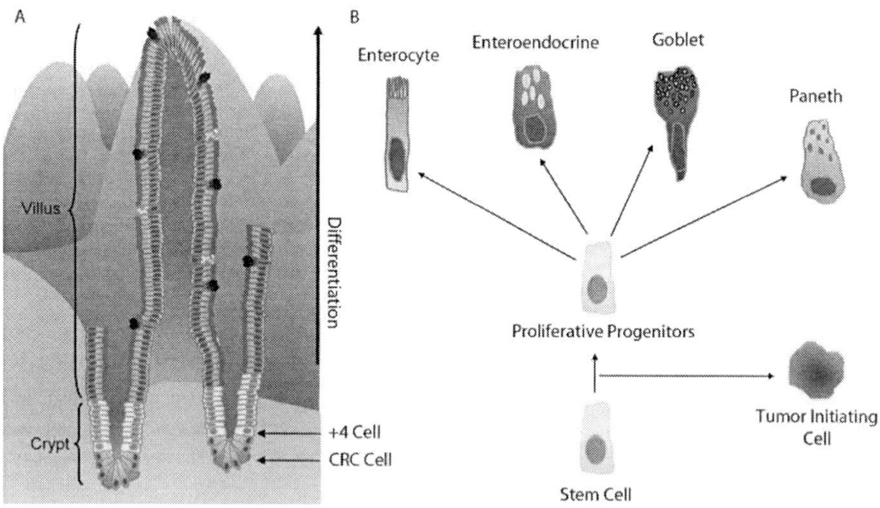

Figure 2. Wnt signaling in the intestine. (A) Structure of the intestine. The epithelium of the small intestine is composed of the crypt and villus. Stem cells (+4 and CBCs) are located at the bottom of crypts. Self-renewal and differentiation of the stem cells are regulated by Wnt signaling. (B) Lineage of intestinal stem cells. Intestinal stem cells produce transit-amplifying cells, which ultimately differentiate into enterocytes, goblet cells, enteroendocrine cells and Paneth cells. Tumor initiating cells likely originate from stem cells or transit-amplifying cells containing APC or β-catenin mutations.

Wnt Signaling in Colon Cancer

Aberrant Wnt signaling was first linked to colon cancer by the observation that FAP patients had a mutation in the *APC* gene [60-63]. In addition, APC mutations have been found in more than 80% of sporadic colon cancer. These APC mutants contain C-terminal truncations. Since the Axin-binding domain and part of the β-catenin-binding domains are missing, these APC mutants are unable to regulate β-catenin phosphorylation, ubiquitination or degradation [64]. This allows β-catenin to accumulate and results in constitutively active Wnt signaling [65,66]. The APC$^{min/+}$ mouse model provided clear evidence showing the role of mutant APC in initiation of formation of tumors in the intestine [67,68]. Moreover, conditional deletion of the *APC* gene in the adult mouse intestine results in a "crypt progenitor-like" phenotype with altered patterns of proliferation and differentiation [57,69], which eventually leads to the formation of tumors [70].

In sporadic colorectal tumors that retain wild-type *APC*, mutations are frequently found in the β-catenin (*CTNNB1*) [66,71] or Axin2 gene [72]. Mutations of the β-catenin gene prevent β-catenin phosphorylation by CKIα or GSK-3, and prevent β-Trcp-mediated ubiquitination/degradation [9]. These mutations result in chronic activation of Wnt signaling that ultimately lead to colon cancer. As an example, targeted deletion of the N-terminus of β-catenin in the intestinal epithelium of mice produces thousands of adenomatous polyps within weeks [73]. Moreover, in a mouse model of colitis-associated colorectal carcinoma, using 1,2-dimethylhydrazine and dextran sulfate sodium, mice develop dysplastic lesions and invasive colorectal cancer that strongly stains for β-catenin in the nuclei [74].

Although, APC and β-catenin mutations are the initiating step of colonic tumorigenesis [8], down-regulation of other tumor suppressor genes may also contribute to the development of colon cancer. For example, Krüppel like factor 4 (KLF4), interacts with β-catenin to repress Wnt signaling and inhibit tumor growth [75]. $KLF^{+/-}/APC^{Min/+}$ mice developed, on average, 59% more intestinal adenomas than $Apc^{Min/+}$ mice [76]. In addition, it is important to further analyze the cross-talk between Wnt signaling and other signaling pathways, such as PTEN/Akt, Notch, BMP and Hedgehog in the tumorigenesis of colon cancer as well as other cancers.

Intestinal Stem Cells

Intestinal stem cells are located in the bottom of crypts (Figure 2A). Hierarchies of stem cell models suggest that there are 4 to 6 stem cells per crypt, which decide the ultimate pattern of the entire crypt [77]. Due to the lack of specific markers, the exact position of these cells within the crypts is still unclear. Currently, there are two models for intestinal stem cells: the +4 label-retaining cells (LRC) model and the crypt columnar base cells (CBC) model [77,78].

Since the relative "quiescent" status is thought to be one of the characters of stem cells [79], DNA label retention is used as a marker for "stemness" [80]. The +4 LRC model is based on the results of DNA label retention experiments. Long-term BrdU and ^{3}H-thymidine label-retaining cells are located at the +4 position, just above the crypt base columnar and Paneth cells at the base of the crypt [51]. These cells have the quiescent or slow cycling character [51,81]. Additional evidence suggests that these +4 cells indeed have stem cell activity [82]. The neural RNA-binding protein Musashi-1, which has been proposed as a stem cell marker of human colon epithelium, is expressed in the +4 cells as well as CBC cells [83,84]. Several other stem cell markers such as Sox4 [85], phosphorylated PTEN, phosphorylated AKT and AKT-phosphorylated β-catenin (S552) [86], are also localized in the +4 cells. S552-phosphorylated β-catenin is associated with its nuclear localization. These observations support the notion that the +4 cells are potential intestinal stem cells. However, the label retention property of the stem cells does not address the functional characteristics of these cells. Thus, functional evidence is lacking to fully support the +4 LRC model. In addition, there are about 16 cells around the +4 position; the exact position of +4 LRCs in the intestine is not well defined [77,78].

By analyzing Wnt target genes, Lgr5 (or Grp49) was identified as a novel intestinal stem cell marker. Lgr5 (leucine-rich-repeat-containing G-protein-coupled receptor 5) encodes an orphan G-protein-coupled receptor with a leucine-rich extracellular domain [87]. Lgr5 was identified as a Wnt target gene in a micro-array study [88]. *In situ* hybridization and Lrg5-EGFP knock-in studies suggest that Lgr5 is expressed the crypt columnar base cells (CBC) which are intermingled with the Paneth cells [89]. Lineage-tracing experiments with an inducible Cre knock-in allele and the Rosa26-lacZ reporter strain demonstrated that these CBC cells are cable of maintaining epithelial self-renewal over long periods of time and generate all of the major differentiated cell types, thus strongly suggesting that the CBCs are intestinal stem cells and the Lgr5 is a marker for these cells [89,90]. When Lrg5$^+$ cells were isolated from the crypt and sorted with the GFP marker, a single Lgr5$^+$ cell was shown to generate a crypt-villus structure [91]. These data further support that Lgr5 is a specific marker for intestinal stem cells. The current barrier to use Lgr5 as a stem cell marker is the lack of a specific antibody that recognizes the extracellular domain of Lrg5.

Following the discovery of Lgr5, the stem cell transcription profile was analyzed using sorted Lrg5 stem cells. Among the genes tested by in situ hybridization, olfactomedin-4 (Olfm4) and achaete scute-like-2 (Ascl2) have been identified as novel stem cell markers that are expressed in Lrg5 stem cells [92,93]. Olfm4 is a secreted protein with unknown function. An Olfm4 family member, ONT1, acts as a BMP antagonist in Xenopus [94]. Ascl2 is a basic helix-loop-helix transcription factor. Expression of Ascl2 induces ectopic crypts on the villi; deletion of Ascl2 gene in the small intestine results in loss of Lgr5 stem cells, suggesting that Ascl2 plays a key role in regulating intestinal stem cells [93]. As Lgr5, Ascl2 is a Wnt target gene, while Olfm4 is not, implying that these cells are regulated by multiple signaling pathways [92,93].

Using similar lineage-tracing methods described above [89,90], Bmi1 was identified as another intestinal stem cell marker [95]. Bmi1 belongs to the polycomb group (PcG) gene family, which functions in gene silencing through chromatin modifications. Bmi1 was initially identified as an oncogene that regulates cell proliferation and transformation [96,97]. Later it was found to play an important role in hematopoiesis and development of the nervous systems [98]. Bmi1 is also crucial for self-renewal of stem cells and cancer initiation [99-101]. The role of Bmi1 in controlling cell proliferation and self-renewal might be through its function as a polycomb group (PcG) protein , which facilitates histone modification and regulates gene silencing [102-104]. Although it was originally reported that Bmi1 is expressed in the +4 cells in the intestine, Van de Flier et al. reported that Bmi1 expression is enriched in Lgr5 cells, suggesting that these two stem cell markers may be express in overlapping cells in the intestine [92]. Again, the exact position of +4 LRCs requires further refinement.

Prominin1 (Prom1 or CD133) is a five-transmembrane-domain-containing glycoprotein. It has been proposed as a marker for cancer stem cells, including colon cancer stem cells [105,106]. To determine if Prom1 is a marker for normal intestinal stem cells, lineage-tracing experiments were performed by two groups [107,108]. Zhu et al. reported that expression of Prom1 overlaps with Lgr5 expression in the small intestine; YFP-labeled Prom1 cells remained present at 60 days and gave rise to four differentiated cell types [108]. However, Snippert et al. demonstrated that Prom1 expression is not restricted to the CBCs, but rather is also detected in transit-amplifying progenitor cells [107]. Snippert et al. further demonstrated the stem cell tracing should be analyzed quantitatively. Most of the Prom1-YFP tracing is initiated in the transit-amplifying cells, which can only last for a few days, whereas about 10% of tracing is initiated in the stem cells, which can last 60 days [107]. In contrast, the frequency of long-term tracing in Lgr5 cells is much higher [89]. This also raises a concern of the stem cell tracing technique: it can only determine if a gene is expressed in the stem cells but it cannot give a definitive answer as to whether this gene is a stem cell-specific gene.

Recently, doublecortin and Ca^{2+}/calmodulin-dependent kinase-like-1 (DCAMKL-1) was identified as a putative intestinal stem cell marker, which specifically marks the quiescent cells in the lower two-thirds of the intestinal crypt epithelium and occasionally marks CBCs [109]. DCAMKL-1 is a microtubule-associated kinase expressed in post-mitotic neurons

[110]. Using Gene Ontology (GO) term enrichment analysis, DCAMKL-1 was found to be expressed in comparison with gastric epithelial progenitor and whole stomach libraries [111]. It was later found to be expressed in gastric stem cells [112]. Most frequently, DCAMKL-1 was found at or near position +4; much less frequently, it was localized in CBC cells [109]. Using conjugated anti-DCAMKL-1 antibody, which targets the extracellular C-terminal epitope, epithelial stem cells from mouse small intestine were labeled and isolated by FACS. Sorted cells were grown in suspension culture for further analysis. It was demonstrated that the resulting spheroids in suspension culture have proliferation capacity and are positive for stem cell markers and progenitor cell markers [109]. It has been proposed that DCAMKL-1 marks the quiescent stem cells and Lgr5 marks the cycling stem cells in the intestine. However, another group demonstrated only 21% of the DCAMKL-1 cells were localized in the crypts, while about 50% were localized on villi and 29% were localized in the crypt-villus junction. This group found that these cells also express Cox-1 and Cox-2, markers for tuft cells. Thus, DCAMKL-1 cells are probably tuft cells rather than stem cells [113]. Tuft cells are also called brush cells; the function of these cells is currently not known. It will be interesting to investigate the lineage of tuft cells in the intestine. Despite the interesting properties of DCAMKL-1 cells in *in vitro* cultures, the role of DCAMKL-1 in stem cells has yet to be determined.

Colon Cancer Stem Cells

Since Wnt signaling plays essential roles in both normal intestinal stem cells and colon cancers, it was hypothesized that colon cancer is initiated from intestinal stem cells or progenitor cells [88] (Figure 2B). Lgr5 is a Wnt target gene as well as a stem cell marker; deletion of APC genes in Lgr5 cells leads to rapid transformation of these cells [114]. In contrast, deletion of APC in non-stem cells fails to induce transformation [114]. In these Wnt signaling-induced adenomas, the expression of Lgr5-EGFP was restricted to a small population of cells, suggesting that stem cells or progenitor cells are maintained in these tumors, thus strongly supporting the cancer stem cell concept [114].

Like many other types of stem cells, cancer stem cells are basically defined by the ability to self-renew and the capability of generating differentiated cells. In addition, two other characteristics of cancer stem cells differ from other stem cells: 1) the potential of transformation toward adenomas, i.e., the ability to give rise to heterogeneous progeny of cells, and to maintain diverse and specialized progression [115], and 2) the ability to 'escape' from normal cell cycle regulation and enter into the tumorigenic status, which is parallel to the difference in property between embryonic carcinoma and normal embryonic stem cells [116]. In the small intestine, transformed cells are originally and mainly located at the bottom of the crypt, which is also considered to be the main location of cells that give rise to intestinal cancer [114].

The major challenge in the field of colon cancer stem cells is one characterized by the lack of a widely accepted specific cancer stem cell marker. Two groups independently reported the identification of a colorectal cancer stem cell based on the surface marker CD133 (Prom1) [105-106]. Purified $CD133^{+}$ cells grew exponentially *in vitro* for long periods of time as undifferentiated tumor spheres. Limiting dilution analysis suggested that the tumor initiating cells enriched more than 200-fold in $CD133^+$ cells [105,106]. However, as discussed above, CD133 (Prom1) is not likely a specific marker for normal intestinal stem cells, and whether it is a specific marker for colon cancer stem cell is also questionable [117]. Shmelkov et al. demonstrated that $CD133^-$ and $CD133^+$ cells were equally capable of tumor initiation, butthe metastatic $CD133^-$ cells form more aggressive tumors in the xenograft model [117]. Clearly, other markers for colon cancer stem cells need to be identified and characterized.

Markers such as epithelial cell adhesion molecule (EpCAM) and CD44 have been used to isolate human colorectal cancer stem cells in a reproducible and consistent way. The isolated population was studied and demonstrated to have a certain gene expression profile, though variable, indicating correlation among expression of other stem cell markers such as CD44, CD133 and CD166 [107,108,118,119]. The normal intestinal stem cell markers, such as Lgr5, Bmi1 and DCAMKL-1, are also potential markers for colon cancer stem cells. In addition to its expression in intestinal stem cells and adenomas, Lrg5 is also expressed in the ovarian and hepatocellular carcinomas [120,121]. Further analysis of Lgr5 as a marker for cancer stem cells, particularly stem cells from human colon cancer, requires a specific antibody for immunohistochemistry and flow cytometry.

SUMMARY

Constitutive activation of Wnt/β-catenin signaling is a hallmark of colorectal cancer. Moreover, this signal transduction event also governs intestinal stem cell identity and tissue homeostasis. The concept of cancer stem cells implies that stem cells are the culprit of cancer origin and progression. The findings that Lgr5 is a stem cell marker and a Wnt target gene substantiate the importance of Wnt signaling in stem cell biology. Lgr5, together with other intestinal stem cell markers, provides surrogate index to track the role of the Wnt pathway in intestinal stem cells and in tumorigenesis. Stem cells usually reside in a specialized niche. Communication between the niche and stem cell, such as through Wnt signaling, plays a critical role in stem cell self-renewal and differentiation. It is of great interest to investigate how cancer stem cells abduct the normal stroma for cancer growth. *In vitro* culture of a single Lgr5+ cell is able to recapitulate the basic organization of intestine epithelia. The requirement of Wnt and Notch signaling highlights the importance of these two pathways in regulating intestinal stem cells. This *in vitro* model will greatly facilitate research on intestinal stem cell biology and extend our understanding of the role of stem cells in colon cancer initiation and progression.

Because of its roles in colon cancer and stem cells, Wnt signaling becomes a very attractive target for colon cancer prevention and therapeutics. It is expected that inhibiting Wnt signaling would inhibit colon cancer stem cells. From high throughput screenings, several small molecular inhibitors targeting the Wnt pathway have been identified. For example, CPG049090 inhibits the β-catenin/TCF interaction; IGC-001 inhibits the interaction of β-catenin/CBP [122,123]; XAV939 and IWRs stabilize Axin [124,125]. Wnt signaling is required for both tumorigenesis and stem cell self-renewal; how to inhibit cancer stem cells but not normal intestinal stem cells will be an exciting but challenging question.

ACKNOWLEDGMENTS

We thank Drs. B. Mark Evers and Nathan Vanderford for critically reading this manuscript and Donna A. Gilbreath for helping with the figures. C.L. is supported by R01 DK071976 from the NIH.

REFERENCES

[1] Nusse R, Varmus HE. Many tumors induced by the mouse mammary tumor virus contain a provirus integrated in the same region of the host genome. *Cell* 1982; 31 (1):99-109.

[2] Clevers H. Wnt/beta-catenin signaling in development and disease. *Cell* 2006; 127 (3):469-480.

[3] Logan CY, Nusse R. The Wnt signaling pathway in development and disease. *Annu Rev Cell Dev Biol* 2004; 20:781-810.

[4] Czyz J, Wobus A. Embryonic stem cell differentiation: the role of extracellular factors. *Differentiation* 2001; 68 (4-5):167-174.

[5] Malhotra S, Kincade PW. Wnt-related molecules and signaling pathway equilibrium in hematopoiesis. *Cell Stem Cell* 2009; 4 (1):27-36.

[6] Wodarz A, Nusse R. Mechanisms of Wnt signaling in development. *Annu Rev Cell Dev Biol* 1998; 14:59-88.

[7] Giles RH, van Es JH, Clevers H. Caught up in a Wnt storm: Wnt signaling in cancer. *Biochim Biophys Acta* 2003; 1653 (1):1-24.

[8] Kinzler KW, Vogelstein B. Lessons from hereditary colorectal cancer. *Cell* 1996; 87 (2):159-170.

[9] Liu C, Li Y, Semenov M *et al.* Control of beta-catenin phosphorylation/degradation by a dual-kinase mechanism. *Cell* 2002; 108 (6):837-847.

[10] Amit S, Hatzubai A, Birman Y *et al.* Axin-mediated CKI phosphorylation of beta-catenin at Ser 45: a molecular switch for the Wnt pathway. *Genes Dev* 2002; 16 (9):1066-1076.

[11] Hart M, Concordet JP, Lassot I *et al.* The F-box protein beta-TrCP associates with phosphorylated beta catenin and regulates its activity in the cell. *Curr Biol* 1999; 9 (4):207-210.

[12] Jiang J, Struhl G. Regulation of the Hedgehog and Wingless signalling pathways by the F-box/WD40-repeat protein Slimb. *Nature* 1998; 391 (6666):493-496.

[13] Liu C, Kato Y, Zhang Z *et al.* beta-Trcp couples beta-catenin phosphorylation-degradation and regulates Xenopus axis formation. *Proc Natl Acad Sci USA* 1999; 96 (11):6273-6278.

[14] Spencer E, Jiang J, Chen ZJ. Signal-induced ubiquitination of IkappaBalpha by the F-box protein Slimb/beta-TrCP. *Genes Dev* 1999; 13 (3):284-294.

[15] Winston JT, Strack P, Beer-Romero P *et al.* The SCFbeta-TRCP-ubiquitin ligase complex associates specifically with phosphorylated destruction motifs in IkappaBalpha and beta-catenin and stimulates IkappaBalpha ubiquitination in vitro. *Genes Dev* 1999; 13 (3):270-283.

[16] Zhang W, Yang J, Liu Y *et al.* PR55 alpha, a regulatory subunit of PP2A, specifically regulates PP2A-mediated beta-catenin dephosphorylation. *J Biol Chem* 2009; 284 (34):22649-22656.
[17] Bhanot P, Brink M, Samos CH *et al.* A new member of the frizzled family from Drosophila functions as a Wingless receptor. *Nature* 1996; 382 (6588):225-230.
[18] Yang-Snyder J, Miller JR, Brown JD, Lai CJ, Moon RT. A frizzled homolog functions in a vertebrate Wnt signaling pathway. *Curr Biol* 1996; 6 (10):1302-1306.
[19] Pinson KI, Brennan J, Monkley S, Avery BJ, Skarnes WC. An LDL-receptor-related protein mediates Wnt signalling in mice. *Nature* 2000; 407 (6803):535-538.
[20] Tamai K, Semenov M, Kato Y *et al.* LDL-receptor-related proteins in Wnt signal transduction. *Nature* 2000; 407 (6803):530-535.
[21] Wehrli M, Dougan ST, Caldwell K *et al.* arrow encodes an LDL-receptor-related protein essential for Wingless signalling. *Nature* 2000; 407 (6803):527-530.
[22] Dann CE, Hsieh JC, Rattner A *et al.* Insights into Wnt binding and signalling from the structures of two Frizzled cysteine-rich domains. *Nature* 2001; 412 (6842):86-90.
[23] Hsieh JC, Rattner A, Smallwood PM, Nathans J. Biochemical characterization of Wnt-frizzled interactions using a soluble, biologically active vertebrate Wnt protein. *Proc Natl Acad Sci USA* 1999; 96 (7):3546-3551.
[24] Umbhauer M, Djiane A, Goisset C *et al.* The C-terminal cytoplasmic Lys-thr-X-X-X-Trp motif in frizzled receptors mediates Wnt/beta-catenin signalling. *Embo J* 2000; 19 (18):4944-4954.
[25] Wong HC, Bourdelas A, Krauss A *et al.* Direct binding of the PDZ domain of Dishevelled to a conserved internal sequence in the C-terminal region of Frizzled. *Mol Cell* 2003; 12 (5):1251-1260.
[26] Rothbacher U, Laurent MN, Deardorff MA *et al.* Dishevelled phosphorylation, subcellular localization and multimerization regulate its role in early embryogenesis. *Embo J* 2000; 19 (5):1010-1022.
[27] Axelrod JD, Miller JR, Shulman JM, Moon RT, Perrimon N. Differential recruitment of Dishevelled provides signaling specificity in the planar cell polarity and Wingless signaling pathways. *Genes Dev* 1998; 12 (16):2610-2622.
[28] Katanaev VL, Ponzielli R, Semeriva M, Tomlinson A. Trimeric G protein-dependent frizzled signaling in Drosophila. *Cell* 2005; 120 (1):111-122.
[29] Liu X, Rubin JS, Kimmel AR. Rapid, Wnt-induced changes in GSK3beta associations that regulate beta-catenin stabilization are mediated by Galpha proteins. *Curr Biol* 2005; 15 (22):1989-1997.
[30] Mao J, Wang J, Liu B *et al.* Low-density lipoprotein receptor-related protein-5 binds to Axin and regulates the canonical Wnt signaling pathway. *Mol Cell* 2001; 7 (4):801-809.
[31] Tamai K, Zeng X, Liu C *et al.* A mechanism for Wnt coreceptor activation. *Mol Cell* 2004; 13 (1):149-156.
[32] van de Wetering M, Cavallo R, Dooijes D *et al.* Armadillo coactivates transcription driven by the product of the Drosophila segment polarity gene dTCF. *Cell* 1997; 88 (6):789-799.
[33] Brunner E, Peter O, Schweizer L, Basler K. pangolin encodes a Lef-1 homologue that acts downstream of Armadillo to transduce the Wingless signal in Drosophila. *Nature* 1997; 385 (6619):829-833.

[34] Brannon M, Brown JD, Bates R, Kimelman D, Moon RT. XCtBP is a XTcf-3 co-repressor with roles throughout Xenopus development. *Development* 1999; 126 (14):3159-3170.

[35] Billin AN, Thirlwell H, Ayer DE. Beta-catenin-histone deacetylase interactions regulate the transition of LEF1 from a transcriptional repressor to an activator. *Mol Cell Biol* 2000; 20 (18):6882-6890.

[36] Kioussi C, Briata P, Baek SH *et al.* Identification of a Wnt/Dvl/beta-Catenin --> Pitx2 pathway mediating cell-type-specific proliferation during development. *Cell* 2002; 111 (5):673-685.

[37] Cavallo RA, Cox RT, Moline MM *et al.* Drosophila Tcf and Groucho interact to repress Wingless signalling activity. *Nature* 1998; 395 (6702):604-608.

[38] Roose J, Molenaar M, Peterson J *et al.* The Xenopus Wnt effector XTcf-3 interacts with Groucho-related transcriptional repressors. *Nature* 1998; 395 (6702):608-612.

[39] Levanon D, Goldstein RE, Bernstein Y *et al.* Transcriptional repression by AML1 and LEF-1 is mediated by the TLE/Groucho corepressors. *Proc Natl Acad Sci USA* 1998; 95 (20):11590-11595.

[40] Hecht A, Vleminckx K, Stemmler MP, van Roy F, Kemler R. The p300/CBP acetyltransferases function as transcriptional coactivators of beta-catenin in vertebrates. *Embo J* 2000; 19 (8):1839-1850.

[41] Cox RT, Pai LM, Kirkpatrick C, Stein J, Peifer M. Roles of the C terminus of Armadillo in Wingless signaling in Drosophila. *Genetics* 1999; 153 (1):319-332.

[42] Takemaru KI, Moon RT. The transcriptional coactivator CBP interacts with beta-catenin to activate gene expression. *J Cell Biol* 2000; 149 (2):249-254.

[43] Ogryzko VV, Schiltz RL, Russanova V, Howard BH, Nakatani Y. The transcriptional coactivators p300 and CBP are histone acetyltransferases. *Cell* 1996; 87 (5):953-959.

[44] Goldman PS, Tran VK, Goodman RH. The multifunctional role of the co-activator CBP in transcriptional regulation. *Recent Prog Horm Res* 1997; 52:103-119; discussion 119-120.

[45] Belenkaya TY, Han C, Standley HJ *et al.* pygopus Encodes a nuclear protein essential for wingless/Wnt signaling. *Development* 2002; 129 (17):4089-4101.

[46] Kramps T, Peter O, Brunner E *et al.* Wnt/wingless signaling requires BCL9/legless-mediated recruitment of pygopus to the nuclear beta-catenin-TCF complex. *Cell* 2002; 109 (1):47-60.

[47] Parker DS, Jemison J, Cadigan KM. Pygopus, a nuclear PHD-finger protein required for Wingless signaling in Drosophila. *Development* 2002; 129 (11):2565-2576.

[48] Thompson B, Townsley F, Rosin-Arbesfeld R, Musisi H, Bienz M. A new nuclear component of the Wnt signalling pathway. *Nat Cell Biol* 2002; 4 (5):367-373.

[49] Soliman MA, Riabowol K. After a decade of study-ING, a PHD for a versatile family of proteins. *Trends Biochem Sci* 2007; 32 (11):509-519.

[50] Crosnier C, Stamataki D, Lewis J. Organizing cell renewal in the intestine: stem cells, signals and combinatorial control. *Nat Rev Genet* 2006; 7 (5):349-359.

[51] Marshman E, Booth C, Potten CS. The intestinal epithelial stem cell. *Bioessays* 2002; 24 (1):91-98.

[52] Reya T, Clevers H. Wnt signalling in stem cells and cancer. *Nature* 2005; 434 (7035):843-850.

[53] Batlle E, Henderson JT, Beghtel H *et al.* Beta-catenin and TCF mediate cell positioning in the intestinal epithelium by controlling the expression of EphB/ephrinB. *Cell* 2002; 111 (2):251-263.
[54] Korinek V, Barker N, Moerer P *et al.* Depletion of epithelial stem-cell compartments in the small intestine of mice lacking Tcf-4. *Nat Genet* 1998; 19 (4):379-383.
[55] Pardal R, Clarke MF, Morrison SJ. Applying the principles of stem-cell biology to cancer. *Nat Rev Cancer* 2003; 3 (12):895-902.
[56] Pinto D, Gregorieff A, Begthel H, Clevers H. Canonical Wnt signals are essential for homeostasis of the intestinal epithelium. *Genes Dev* 2003; 17 (14):1709-1713.
[57] Sansom OJ, Reed KR, Hayes AJ *et al.* Loss of Apc in vivo immediately perturbs Wnt signaling, differentiation, and migration. *Genes Dev* 2004; 18 (12):1385-1390.
[58] Sansom OJ, Meniel VS, Muncan V *et al.* Myc deletion rescues Apc deficiency in the small intestine. *Nature* 2007; 446 (7136):676-679.
[59] Kim KA, Kakitani M, Zhao J *et al.* Mitogenic influence of human R-spondin1 on the intestinal epithelium. *Science* 2005; 309 (5738):1256-1259.
[60] Groden J, Thliveris A, Samowitz W *et al.* Identification and characterization of the familial adenomatous polyposis coli gene. *Cell* 1991; 66 (3):589-600.
[61] Kinzler KW, Nilbert MC, Su LK *et al.* Identification of FAP locus genes from chromosome 5q21. *Science* 1991; 253 (5020):661-665.
[62] Nishisho I, Nakamura Y, Miyoshi Y *et al.* Mutations of chromosome 5q21 genes in FAP and colorectal cancer patients. *Science* 1991; 253 (5020):665-669.
[63] Powell SM, Zilz N, Beazer-Barclay Y *et al.* APC mutations occur early during colorectal tumorigenesis. *Nature* 1992; 359 (6392):235-237.
[64] Yang J, Zhang W, Evans PM *et al.* Adenomatous polyposis coli (APC) differentially regulates beta-catenin phosphorylation and ubiquitination in colon cancer cells. *J Biol Chem* 2006; 281 (26):17751-17757.
[65] Korinek V, Barker N, Morin PJ *et al.* Constitutive transcriptional activation by a beta-catenin-Tcf complex in APC-/- colon carcinoma. *Science* 1997; 275 (5307):1784-1787.
[66] Morin PJ, Sparks AB, Korinek V *et al.* Activation of beta-catenin-Tcf signaling in colon cancer by mutations in beta-catenin or APC. *Science* 1997; 275 (5307):1787-1790.
[67] Moser AR, Pitot HC, Dove WF. A dominant mutation that predisposes to multiple intestinal neoplasia in the mouse. *Science* 1990; 247 (4940):322-324.
[68] Su LK, Kinzler KW, Vogelstein B *et al.* Multiple intestinal neoplasia caused by a mutation in the murine homolog of the APC gene. *Science* 1992; 256 (5057):668-670.
[69] Andreu P, Colnot S, Godard C *et al.* Crypt-restricted proliferation and commitment to the Paneth cell lineage following Apc loss in the mouse intestine. *Development* 2005; 132 (6):1443-1451.
[70] Shibata H, Toyama K, Shioya H *et al.* Rapid colorectal adenoma formation initiated by conditional targeting of the Apc gene. *Science* 1997; 278 (5335):120-123.
[71] Munemitsu S, Albert I, Rubinfeld B, Polakis P. Deletion of an amino-terminal sequence beta-catenin in vivo and promotes hyperphosporylation of the adenomatous polyposis coli tumor suppressor protein. *Mol Cell Biol* 1996; 16 (8):4088-4094.
[72] Liu W, Dong X, Mai M *et al.* Mutations in AXIN2 cause colorectal cancer with defective mismatch repair by activating beta-catenin/TCF signalling. *Nat Genet* 2000; 26 (2):146-147.

[73] Harada N, Tamai Y, Ishikawa T *et al.* Intestinal polyposis in mice with a dominant stable mutation of the beta-catenin gene. *Embo J* 1999; 18 (21):5931-5942.

[74] Wang JG, Wang DF, Lv BJ, Si JM. A novel mouse model for colitis-associated colon carcinogenesis induced by 1,2-dimethylhydrazine and dextran sulfate sodium. *World J Gastroenterol* 2004; 10 (20):2958-2962.

[75] Zhang W, Chen X, Kato Y *et al.* Novel cross talk of Kruppel-like factor 4 and beta-catenin regulates normal intestinal homeostasis and tumor repression. *Mol Cell Biol* 2006; 26 (6):2055-2064.

[76] Ghaleb AM, McConnell BB, Nandan MO *et al.* Haploinsufficiency of Kruppel-like factor 4 promotes adenomatous polyposis coli dependent intestinal tumorigenesis. *Cancer Res* 2007; 67 (15):7147-7154.

[77] van der Flier LG, Clevers H. Stem cells, self-renewal, and differentiation in the intestinal epithelium. *Annu Rev Physiol* 2009; 71:241-260.

[78] Scoville DH, Sato T, He XC, Li L. Current view: intestinal stem cells and signaling. *Gastroenterology* 2008; 134 (3):849-864.

[79] Tumbar T, Guasch G, Greco V *et al.* Defining the epithelial stem cell niche in skin. *Science* 2004; 303 (5656):359-363.

[80] Kiel MJ, He S, Ashkenazi R *et al.* Haematopoietic stem cells do not asymmetrically segregate chromosomes or retain BrdU. *Nature* 2007; 449 (7159):238-242.

[81] Potten CS, Owen G, Booth D. Intestinal stem cells protect their genome by selective segregation of template DNA strands. *J Cell Sci* 2002; 115 (Pt 11):2381-2388.

[82] Bjerknes M, Cheng H. The stem-cell zone of the small intestinal epithelium. III. Evidence from columnar, enteroendocrine, and mucous cells in the adult mouse. *Am J Anat* 1981; 160 (1):77-91.

[83] Nishimura S, Wakabayashi N, Toyoda K, Kashima K, Mitsufuji S. Expression of Musashi-1 in human normal colon crypt cells: a possible stem cell marker of human colon epithelium. *Dig Dis Sci* 2003; 48 (8):1523-1529.

[84] Imai T, Tokunaga A, Yoshida T *et al.* The neural RNA-binding protein Musashi1 translationally regulates mammalian numb gene expression by interacting with its mRNA. *Mol Cell Biol* 2001; 21 (12):3888-3900.

[85] Van der Flier LG, Sabates-Bellver J, Oving I *et al.* The Intestinal Wnt/TCF Signature. *Gastroenterology* 2007; 132 (2):628-632.

[86] He XC, Zhang J, Tong WG *et al.* BMP signaling inhibits intestinal stem cell self-renewal through suppression of Wnt-beta-catenin signaling. *Nat Genet* 2004; 36 (10):1117-1121.

[87] Hsu SY, Liang SG, Hsueh AJ. Characterization of two LGR genes homologous to gonadotropin and thyrotropin receptors with extracellular leucine-rich repeats and a G protein-coupled, seven-transmembrane region. *Mol Endocrinol* 1998; 12 (12):1830-1845.

[88] van de Wetering M, Sancho E, Verweij C *et al.* The beta-catenin/TCF-4 complex imposes a crypt progenitor phenotype on colorectal cancer cells. *Cell* 2002; 111 (2):241-250.

[89] Barker N, van Es JH, Kuipers J *et al.* Identification of stem cells in small intestine and colon by marker gene Lgr5. *Nature* 2007; 449 (7165):1003-1007.

[90] Barker N, van de Wetering M, Clevers H. The intestinal stem cell. *Genes Dev* 2008; 22 (14):1856-1864.

[91] Sato T, Vries RG, Snippert HJ *et al.* Single Lgr5 stem cells build crypt-villus structures in vitro without a mesenchymal niche. *Nature* 2009; 459 (7244):262-265.

[92] van der Flier LG, Haegebarth A, Stange DE, van de Wetering M, Clevers H. OLFM4 is a robust marker for stem cells in human intestine and marks a subset of colorectal cancer cells. *Gastroenterology* 2009; 137 (1):15-17.

[93] van der Flier LG, van Gijn ME, Hatzis P *et al.* Transcription factor achaete scute-like 2 controls intestinal stem cell fate. *Cell* 2009; 136 (5):903-912.

[94] Inomata H, Haraguchi T, Sasai Y. Robust stability of the embryonic axial pattern requires a secreted scaffold for chordin degradation. *Cell* 2008; 134 (5):854-865.

[95] Sangiorgi E, Capecchi MR. Bmi1 is expressed in vivo in intestinal stem cells. *Nat Genet* 2008; 40 (7):915-920.

[96] Haupt Y, Alexander WS, Barri G, Klinken SP, Adams JM. Novel zinc finger gene implicated as myc collaborator by retrovirally accelerated lymphomagenesis in E mu-myc transgenic mice. *Cell* 1991; 65 (5):753-763.

[97] Jacobs JJ, Scheijen B, Voncken JW *et al.* Bmi-1 collaborates with c-Myc in tumorigenesis by inhibiting c-Myc-induced apoptosis via INK4a/ARF. *Genes Dev* 1999; 13 (20):2678-2690.

[98] van der Lugt NM, Domen J, Linders K *et al.* Posterior transformation, neurological abnormalities, and severe hematopoietic defects in mice with a targeted deletion of the bmi-1 proto-oncogene. *Genes Dev* 1994; 8 (7):757-769.

[99] Valk-Lingbeek ME, Bruggeman SW, van Lohuizen M. Stem cells and cancer; the polycomb connection. *Cell* 2004; 118 (4):409-418.

[100] Lessard J, Sauvageau G. Bmi-1 determines the proliferative capacity of normal and leukaemic stem cells. *Nature* 2003; 423 (6937):255-260.

[101] Kang MK, Kim RH, Kim SJ *et al.* Elevated Bmi-1 expression is associated with dysplastic cell transformation during oral carcinogenesis and is required for cancer cell replication and survival. *Br J Cancer* 2007; 96 (1):126-133.

[102] Wei J, Zhai L, Xu J, Wang H. Role of Bmi1 in H2A ubiquitylation and Hox gene silencing. *J Biol Chem* 2006; 281 (32):22537-22544.

[103] Wang H, Wang L, Erdjument-Bromage H *et al.* Role of histone H2A ubiquitination in Polycomb silencing. *Nature* 2004; 431 (7010):873-878.

[104] Rajasekhar VK, Begemann M. Concise review: roles of polycomb group proteins in development and disease: a stem cell perspective. *Stem Cells* 2007; 25 (10):2498-2510.

[105] O'Brien CA, Pollett A, Gallinger S, Dick JE. A human colon cancer cell capable of initiating tumour growth in immunodeficient mice. *Nature* 2007; 445 (7123):106-110.

[106] Ricci-Vitiani L, Lombardi DG, Pilozzi E *et al.* Identification and expansion of human colon-cancer-initiating cells. *Nature* 2007; 445 (7123):111-115.

[107] Snippert HJ, van Es JH, van den Born M *et al.* Prominin-1/CD133 marks stem cells and early progenitors in mouse small intestine. *Gastroenterology* 2009; 136 (7):2187-2194 e2181.

[108] Zhu L, Gibson P, Currle DS *et al.* Prominin 1 marks intestinal stem cells that are susceptible to neoplastic transformation. *Nature* 2009; 457 (7229):603-607.

[109] May R, Sureban SM, Hoang N *et al.* Doublecortin and CaM Kinase-like-1 and Leucine-Rich-Repeat-Containing G-Protein-Coupled Receptor Mark Quiescent and Cycling Intestinal Stem Cells, Respectively. *Stem Cells* 2009; 27 (10):2571-2579.

[110] Lin PT, Gleeson JG, Corbo JC, Flanagan L, Walsh CA. DCAMKL1 encodes a protein kinase with homology to doublecortin that regulates microtubule polymerization. *J Neurosci* 2000; 20 (24):9152-9161.

[111] Giannakis M, Stappenbeck TS, Mills JC *et al.* Molecular properties of adult mouse gastric and intestinal epithelial progenitors in their niches. *J Biol Chem* 2006; 281 (16):11292-11300.

[112] Giannakis M, Chen SL, Karam SM, Engstrand L, Gordon JI. Helicobacter pylori evolution during progression from chronic atrophic gastritis to gastric cancer and its impact on gastric stem cells. *Proc Natl Acad Sci USA* 2008; 105 (11):4358-4363.

[113] Gerbe F, Brulin B, Makrini L, Legraverend C, Jay P. DCAMKL-1 expression identifies Tuft cells rather than stem cells in the adult mouse intestinal epithelium. *Gastroenterology* 2009; 137 (6):2179-2180; author reply 2180-2171.

[114] Barker N, Ridgway RA, van Es JH *et al.* Crypt stem cells as the cells-of-origin of intestinal cancer. *Nature* 2009; 457 (7229):608-611.

[115] Dalerba P, Cho RW, Clarke MF. Cancer stem cells: models and concepts. *Annu Rev Med* 2007; 58:267-284.

[116] Chambers I, Smith A. Self-renewal of teratocarcinoma and embryonic stem cells. *Oncogene* 2004; 23 (43):7150-7160.

[117] Shmelkov SV, Butler JM, Hooper AT *et al.* CD133 expression is not restricted to stem cells, and both CD133+ and CD133- metastatic colon cancer cells initiate tumors. *J Clin Invest* 2008; 118 (6):2111-2120.

[118] Dalerba P, Dylla SJ, Park IK *et al.* Phenotypic characterization of human colorectal cancer stem cells. *Proc Natl Acad Sci USA 2007*; 104 (24):10158-10163.

[119] Takaishi S, Okumura T, Tu S *et al.* Identification of gastric cancer stem cells using the cell surface marker CD44. *Stem Cells* 2009; 27 (5):1006-1020.

[120] McClanahan T, Koseoglu S, Smith K *et al.* Identification of overexpression of orphan G protein-coupled receptor GPR49 in human colon and ovarian primary tumors. *Cancer Biol Ther* 2006; 5 (4):419-426.

[121] Yamamoto Y, Sakamoto M, Fujii G *et al.* Overexpression of orphan G-protein-coupled receptor, Gpr49, in human hepatocellular carcinomas with beta-catenin mutations. *Hepatology* 2003; 37 (3):528-533.

[122] Emami KH, Nguyen C, Ma H *et al.* A small molecule inhibitor of beta-catenin/CREB-binding protein transcription [corrected]. *Proc Natl Acad Sci USA* 2004; 101 (34):12682-12687.

[123] Lepourcelet M, Chen YN, France DS *et al.* Small-molecule antagonists of the oncogenic Tcf/beta-catenin protein complex. *Cancer Cell* 2004; 5 (1):91-102.

[124] Chen B, Dodge ME, Tang W *et al.* Small molecule-mediated disruption of Wnt-dependent signaling in tissue regeneration and cancer. *Nat Chem Biol* 2009; 5 (2):100-107.

[125] Huang SM, Mishina YM, Liu S *et al.* Tankyrase inhibition stabilizes axin and antagonizes Wnt signalling. *Nature* 2009; 461 (7264):614-620.

In: Stem Cell Research: New Developments
Editors: Hiroshi Tanaka and Michael C. F. Chang
ISBN: 978-1-61942-081-6

Chapter 8

CANCER STEM CELLS IN LUNG CANCER: DISTINCT DIFFERENCES BETWEEN SMALL CELL LUNG CARCINOMA AND NON-SMALL CELL LUNG CARCINOMA

Koji Okudela[1], Noriyuki Nagahara[2], Akira Katayama[2] and Hitoshi Kitamura[1,*]
[1]Graduate School of Medicine, Yokohama City University, Yokohama, Japan
[2]Graduate School of Medicine, Nippon Medical School, Tokyo, Japan

ABSTRACT

Of the many markers for cancer stem cells (CSCs) in lung cancer reported to date, the cell surface antigen CD133, nuclear β-catenin accumulation, the side population phenotype, and high aldehyde dehydrogenase (ALDH) activity seem to be most reliable. In this chapter, we review the results of studies on lung CSCs and discuss the significance of these markers from a biological, pathological, and clinical viewpoint. In addition, we present our own data, focusing primarily upon ALDH1A1. Twenty-seven lung cancer cell lines (nine small cell lung carcinoma (SCLC) cell lines and eighteen non-small cell lung carcinoma (NSCLC) cell lines) were examined for mRNA and protein expression and fractions of cells with activity. ALDH1A1 mRNA was strongly expressed in five cell lines, of which three were SCLC cell lines and two were NSCLC cell lines. Two of the SCLC cell lines consistently expressed the protein and had a large fraction of cells with ALDH activity, but the third did not. Both the NSCLC cell lines expressed the protein, but only one had a large fraction of cells with strong ALDH activity. In brief, the level of ALDH1A1 mRNA did not always parallel that of the protein in SCLC cell lines, while the level of ALDH1A1 protein did not necessarily parallel that of ALDH activity in NSCLC cell lines. The ALDH1A1 protein level or ALDH activity level was well associated with the mRNA level of CD133, which is the most commonly used marker for

* Correspondence concerning this article should be addressed to: Dr. Hitoshi Kitamura, M.D., Ph.D. Department of Pathology, Graduate School of Medicine, Yokohama City University, 3-9 Fukuura, Kanazawa-ku, Yokohama 236-0004, Japan. (Tel: +81-45-787-2583; Fax: +81-45-789-0588; E-mail address: pathola@med.yokohama-cu.ac.jp.

CSCs, in SCLC cell lines, but not in NSCLC cell lines, suggesting an abundance of CSC populations in SCLC compared to in NSCLC. From the current findings, the mechanism and pathway that regulate the expression of ALDH1A1 mRNA and its protein, and its enzymatic activity as well differ greatly between SCLC and NSCLC cells. We speculate that ALDH (its expression and activity) is only one of the factors determining the stemness of CSCs in lung cancers. In conclusion, the CSCs in SCLC and NSCLC differ distinctly in terms not only of their abundance but also of the regulatory mechanism of ALDH1A1 expression and activity, as well as its role in the maintenance/activation of stemness. Exploring the mechanism of ALDH's activation and its role in the maintenance of the stemness not only of CSCs but also of normal stem cells would provide a novel paradigm for stem cell biology.

Keywords: Cancer stem cell; Small cell lung carcinoma; Non-small cell lung carcinoma; Aldehyde dehydrogenase

ABBREVIATIONS

SCLC: small cell lung carcinoma;
NSCLC: non-small cell lung carcinoma;
SQC: squamous cell carcinoma;
DC: adenocarcinoma;
LCC: large cell carcinoma;
RB: retinoblastoma;
TP53: tumor protein 53;
EGFR: epidermal growth factor receptor;
ASCL1: achaete-scute complex homolog 1;
TTF-1: thyroid transcription factor-1;
ALDH: aldehyde dehydrogenase;
CSC: cancer stem cell;
ABCG2, ATP binding cassette transporter superfamily member G2;
CIC: cancer initiating cell;
SP: side population;
FACS: fluorescence activating cell sorting;
UV: ultraviolet;
uPAR: urokinase plasminogen activator receptor;
uPA: urokinase plasminogen activator;
Shh: Sonic hedgehog;
BMP: bone morphogenetic protein;
Bmi1: B cell-specific Mo-MuLV integration site 1;
PODXL-1: podocalyxin-like protein 1;
RT-PCR: reverse transcription polymerase chain reaction;
mRNA, messenger ribonucleic acid: cDNA;
complementary deoxyribonucleic acid;
siRNA: small interfering RNA;
PI: propidium iodide.

INTRODUCTION

Lung cancer is one of the most common malignancies worldwide and a leading cause of cancer-related deaths. It is increasing year by year in almost all areas of the world, except for a slight decrease in certain countries [1]. Lung cancer consists of heterogeneous groups in terms of pathological features and is commonly classified into the following two major types, small cell lung carcinoma (SCLC) and non-small cell lung carcinoma (NSCLC). NSCLC also is a group of heterogeneous histological types, the majority of which are squamous cell carcinoma (SQC) and adenocarcinoma (ADC) with roughly similar frequencies (30-40% each), and large cell carcinoma (LCC) with a lower frequency (< 10%). SCLC comprises nearly 20% of lung cancer. ADC and LCC are further sub-classified into several categories, respectively. The classification of lung cancer is not only of academic interest but also of practical necessity, because the biological aggressiveness, responsiveness to therapeutic intervention and patients' prognosis are greatly different among the respective types [2].

Lung cancer originates from the airway epithelia of larger and smaller bronchi as well as of alveoli. While it is generally accepted that cancer cells are derived from progenitor or tissue stem cells, relatively little has been elucidated with regard to the identification of airway stem cells and the molecular mechanisms underlying their self-renewal and differentiation abilities [3-5], in contrast to other epithelial tissues such as the intestine, mammary gland, and skin [6].

The heterogeneity of lung cancer likely reflects differences in the site of origin (proximal versus peripheral), and, more importantly, in the type of cell of origin, i.e., progenitor (tissue stem) cells. The diversity of etiologic factors and target genes, the types of genetic insults, and the ensuing effects, activation or inactivation, on the genes involved, would also be responsible for the heterogeneity of lung cancer. In fact, tobacco smoke, containing more than 60 carcinogens, is generally accepted as the most important cause of almost all types of lung cancer, among which the genetic and molecular mechanisms of carcinogenesis differ considerably. The ensuing genetic alteration and epigenetic changes as well, could lead to dysfunction of molecular signal transduction pathways, which relate directly or indirectly to proliferation, differentiation, and death of the cell.

In our recent review article, we underscored that silencing alterations of both the *RB* and *TP53* genes are most likely to be important and early events in the development of SCLC, whereas alterations of the epidermal growth factor receptor (EGFR) signaling pathway play significant and important roles in NSCLC carcinogenesis [7]. We also emphasized that alterations of both the *RB* and *TP53* genes are central to the carcinogenesis of SCLC, while many other factors including achaete-scute complex homolog 1 (ASCL1) and thyroid transcription factor-1 (TTF-1) contribute to the development and biological behavior of SCLC [8].

The cancer stem cell (CSC) theory has proposed that a tumor cell subpopulation possessing self-renewal capacity which forms only a small fraction of tumor tissue is central in sustaining neoplastic lesions and is a potentially crucial target of cancer therapy [9-23]. The CSCs are possibly produced by either transformation of normal stem cells or multistep dedifferentiation of specialized progenitor cells through a progressive accumulation of genetic aberrations. Rapp, *et al.* [12] proposed a model of oncogene-induced plasticity for CSC origin by demonstrating reprogramming events triggered by a specific combination of oncogenes.

Li, *et al.* [16] suggested that genomic instability is a driving force for transforming normal stem cells into CSCs and, in CSCs, a potential mechanism for cancer cell heterogeneity. The origin of CSCs and this mechanism are discussed in more detail in other chapters [The publisher may modify this part].

The CSCs of lung cancers can be considered to originate from either airway stem cells, which have not been identified yet, or respective committed progenitor cells, such as bronchioloalveolar progenitor cells, basal/mucous secretory bronchial progenitor cells, and neuroendocrine progenitor cells (see the section Origin of CSCs in lung cancer).

The CSC theory is tremendously attractive to both researchers and physicians, because the CSC is central to cancer cell biology and cancer therapy. The discovery of specific markers of CSCs in the respective types of cancers is particularly important. Furthermore, it is necessary to clarify the function of these molecules, as the disruption of the signaling pathways and gene transcriptions that control the activity of CSCs is the final goal of CSC-targeting therapy. We emphasized that a knowledge of CSC signaling pathways may lead to new treatment that kill or induce differentiation of CSCs and could better contribute to cures [24]. These treatments could be designed to target CSCs in order to induce the differentiation of CSCs, or eliminate CSCs by inhibiting the maintenance of the stem-cell state. For instance, side population (SP) cells that are considered to represent CSCs (see below), of a human lung cancer cell line (A549) totally disappeared after treatment with the selective ATP-binding cassette transporter G2 (ABCG2) inhibitor fumitremorgin C [25]. As another example, a Hedgehog signaling inhibitor cyclopamine strikingly reduced the *in vitro* invasive capacity of pancreatic cancer cell lines and also profoundly inhibited metastatic spread in an orthotopic xenograft model [26].

In regard to lung cancer, we also stressed the extreme importance of identifying specific CSC markers for the respective subtypes of lung cancer, for instance SCLC and NSCLC (ADC, SQC, LCC, and others), since they are quite different not only in phenotype but also in pathogenesis and biological behavior. In particular, SCLC is highly metastatic, drug-resistant, and rapidly fatal. The aggressiveness of SCLC may be attributable to an abundance of CSCs, as CSCs are drug-resistant and play a crucial role in cancer recurrence and metastasis. Alternatively, it is also possible that the CSCs of SCLC are endowed with specific biological properties, for instance niche-independency or strong drug-resistance, or both. If SCLC-specific CSC markers were discovered, they would be extremely useful as targets of chemotherapy, for the establishment of therapeutic regimens, and for predictions of the prognosis (outcome) of patients.

In this chapter, we discuss the characteristics of normal airway stem/progenitor cells and CSCs in lung cancer by reviewing hitherto described study results. In addition, we demonstrate the potentially distinct differences in the mechanism of maintenance of CSCs between SCLC and NSCLC, primarily focusing upon aldehyde dehydrogenase (ALDH) based on our own experiments currently underway.

Stem Cells in Healthy and Injured Lungs

Although the airway stem cell in a strict sense has not been identified yet, several lines of evidence support the existence of regional progenitors cells, such as bronchioloalveolar progenitor cells, basal/mucous secretory bronchial progenitor cells, and neuroendocrine progenitor cells, which maintain normal homeostasis as well as play roles in repair [3-5]. These progenitor cells expand their populations in response to various insults including toxic substances, but do not become tumorigenic unless at least one genetic or epigenetic event occurs, for instance by tobacco smoke carcinogens [4,27].

Origin of CSCs in Lung Cancers

As in hematological malignancies and other solid cancers, the presence of subpopulations of cells endowed with CSC properties has been recognized in lung cancers. Like CSCs in other tissues, the CSCs of lung cancers can be considered to originate from either airway stem cells, which have not been identified yet, or respective committed progenitor cells, such as bronchioloalveolar progenitor cells, basal/mucous secretory bronchial progenitor cells, and neuroendocrine progenitor cells [3-5], resulting in the initiation of region-specific lung cancers [4].

Cell markers for CSCs in Lung Cancers

CSC markers for lung cancer are a matter of some controversy, probably reflecting the tremendous heterogeneity of lung cancers in terms of cell of origin, etiology, pathology, biology, and molecular/genetic pathogenesis [2,7]. We herein briefly discuss these markers, paying special attention to the differences between SCLC and NSCLC; representative lung CSC markers reported to date are listed in Table 1.

CD133

CD133 was first reported as a novel marker for human hematopoietic stem and progenitor cells [28], and later found in some types of leukemic cells [29]. Prominin-1, which was identified on neuroepithelial stem cells in mice in 1997, is a mouse homolog of the human CD133 antigen [30]. The expression of CD133 has been detected in human central nervous system stem cells [31], human trophoblasts [32], human lymphatic/vascular endothelial precursor cells [33], and human prostatic epithelial stem cells [34]. The CD133 antigen is a 120kDa five-transmembrane domain glycoprotein, and its chromosomal location (4p16.2-p12) and amino acid sequence have been clarified [35]. Although its function is still unknown, CD133 may have a role in stem cell activation/maintenance, as shown by its coexpression with β1-integrin in the epidermal basal cells [36], release of CD133-carrying membrane particles into the extracellular space from neural progenitors and some epithelial cells [37], and potential regulatory activity of cell-cell contacts [38].

Recent studies have demonstrated that CD133 is a specific marker of CSCs in a wide spectrum of malignant tumors including brain tumors, colorectal cancers, pancreatic cancers, breast cancers, prostate cancers, ovarian cancers [39-41], and some lung cancers [42]. In contrast to the general consensus that CD133 is a ubiquitous CSC marker, several studies demonstrated that CD133-negative cells in certain human tumors also possess tumorigenic activity upon xenotransplantation into immunocompromised rodents [43-45]. These results imply that the CD133-negative subpopulation also contains cells with cancer initiating cell (CIC) activity. Mizrak, *et al.* [46] pointed out that CD133 is actually detected by its glycosylated epitope, AC133, and it is likely that AC133, but not CD133, is a more reliable CSC marker. Bidlingmaier, *et al.* [47] also suggested that the use of CD133 expression as a marker for CSC should be critically evaluated. These reports may explain the discrepancy observed in the results from different studies.

Table 1. Cancer stem cell markers in small cell lung carcinoma and non-small cell lung carcinoma

Category	Molecule	SCLC	NSCLC
Cell surface marker	CD133	1. Eramo A, *et al.* [42] Cancer cells isolated from surgical specimens 2. Jiang T, *et al.* [52] H1688 cell line 3. Meng X, *et al.* [48] *H446 cell line	1. Eramo A, *et al.* [42] Cancer cells isolated from surgical specimens 2. Jiang T, *et al.* [52] H460, H125, H322, and H358 cell lines 3. Levina V, *et al.* [50] H460 cell line 4. Chen YC, *et al.* [51] Cancer cells isolated from surgical specimens 5. Meng X, *et al.* [48] *A549 cell line
	PODXL-1	Koch LK, *et al.* [69] Immunohistochemical analysis in surgical specimen tissue sections	
	uPAR	Gutova M, *et al.* [54] H1417, H69AR, H211, H1688, H1882, and H250 cell lines	
Transporter	SP	1. Meng X, *et al.* [48] *H446 cell line	1. Ho MM, *et al.* [48] A549, H23, H460, HTB-58, H2170, and H441 cell lines 2. Meng X, *et al.* [48] *A549 cell line
	ABCG2		Sung JM, *et al.* [25] A549 cell line
Enzymatic activity	ALDH	Jiang T, *et al.* [52] Aldefluor assay in H1618 cell line Moreb JS, *et al.* [93] RT-PCR, Western blotting, spectrophotometrical analysis and Aldefluor assay in SW210.5, H82, and SCLC-16HC cell lines	Ucar D, *et al.* [95] Spectrophotometrical analysis and Aldefluor assay in H522 cell line Patel M, *et al.* [96]. Immunohistochemical analysis in surgical specimen tissue sections Jiang F, *et al.* [49] Aldefluor assay in H460, H125, H322, and H358 cell lines Moreb JS, *et al.* [93] RT-PCR, Western blotting, spectrophotometrical analysis and Aldefluor assay in A549, H522, H322, H157, H125, H460, H1299, LCLC-103H and ADLC-5M2H lung cancer cell lines, as well as Beas-2B non-cancerous airway cell line

Category	Molecule	SCLC	NSCLC
Signaling pathway	Shh	Watkins DN, *et al.* [77] NCI-H1618, NCI-H60, NCI-H146, NCI-H209, NCI-H249, NCI-H82, and NCI-H417 cell lines Yagui-Beltrán A, *et al.* [78] Review Peacock CD, *et al.* [79] Review	Yagui-Beltrán A, *et al.* [78] Review Peacock CD, *et al.* [79] Review
	Wnt/β-catenin	Yagui-Beltrán A, *et al.* [78] Review Peacock CD, *et al.* [79] Review	Yagui-Beltrán A, *et al.* [78] Review Peacock CD, *et al.* [79] Review 3. Levina V, *et al.* [50] H460 cell line
Transcription factor	Bmi1	Koch LK, *et al.* [69] Immunohistochemical analysis in surgical specimen tissue sections	Dovey JS, *et al.* [85] Bronchioloalveolar carcinoma (mouse)
	Oct-4		1. Levina V, *et al.* [50] H460 cell line 2. Chen YC, *et al.* [51] Cancer cells isolated from surgical specimens

SCLC: small cell lung carcinoma; NSCLC: non-small cell lung carcinoma; PODXL-1: podocalyxin-like protein 1; uPAR: urokinase plasminogen activator receptor.

SP: side population; ABCG2: ATP binding cassette transporter superfamily member G2; ALDH: aldehyde dehydrogenase; Shh: Sonic hedgehog; Bmi1: B cell-specific Mo-MuLV integration site 1.

* These authors reported that both of CD133+ and CD133- cells and of SP cells and non-SP cells exhibited the cancer initiating activity.

The methods for analysis of ALDH activity and protein expression are specifically described, because the procedures employed may potentially lead to the differences in results.

In regard to lung cancers, Eramo, *et al.* [42] reported that CD133 is a useful CSC marker in both SCLC and NSCLC. In contrast, Meng, *et al.* [48] reported more than 45% of A549 (NSCLC) and H446 (SCLC) cells to be CICs regardless of CD133 expression based on the results of cloning and tumorigenic analyses. Jiang, *et al.* [49] reported that, in NSCLC, cancer cells with strong ALDH activity (see below), showed CSC features and CD133 expression. Levina, *et al.* [50] demonstrated that NSCLC cells (H460) propagated a CD133-positive CSC-like cell population, in association with the expression of Oct-4 and high nuclear β-catenin (see below), after an *in vitro* treatment with anti-cancer drugs. Chen, *et al.* [51] reported that CD133-positive NSCLC cell lines display self-renewal and chemo-radio-resistant properties. Intriguingly, in SCLC, Jiang, *et al.* [52] demonstrated that achaete-scute complex homolog 1 (ASCL1) directly regulates ALDH1A1 and CD133 and that the $CD133^{high}$-$ALDH1A1^{high}$-$ASCL1^{high}$ subpopulation exhibits the features of CSCs both *in vitro* and *in vivo*. ASCL1 is a specific marker of SCLC and thought to play important roles in its phenotypic expression and biological aggressiveness [8,53].

Side Population

Hoechst 33342 dye-efflux side population (SP) bone marrow cells were first discovered as hematopoietic stem cells in mice [54]. Since then, SP cells with stem-cell-like capabilities have been found in a variety of human hematologic and solid malignancies. These cells show the features of CSCs characterized by self-renewal activity, differentiated progeny production, tumorigenicity, as well as the expression of CSC markers and stem cell genes [55]. Thus, SP cells can be assumed to be CSCs. Importantly, SP cells are highly resistant to chemotherapeutic agents and crucial in therapy resistance and tumor recurrence [55-57]. Zhou, *et al.* [58] showed that expression of the *ATP binding cassette transporter superfamily member G2* (*ABCG2*) gene is an important determinant of the SP phenotype, and that it might serve as a marker for stem cells from various sources. SP cells are usually isolated and purified by fluorescence activating cell sorting (FACS) using an ultraviolet (UV) laser. Recently, a new technique using a Violet-excited cell-permeable DNA-binding dye has been reported [59]. This method is inexpensive and yields the same results as UV-excited FACS [59]. In contrast, Wu, *et al.* [55] pointed out the following problems in using the SP phenotype as a CSC marker: 1) cells resistant to the Hoechst dye's toxicity do not consist only of stem-like cells, 2) variables in staining times, dye concentrations, and cellular concentrations can greatly affect the SP phenotype, and 3) cytometric gating strategies used to isolate SP cells lack the consistency of gating strategies used when staining with markers. These problems potentially lead to cross contamination of the SP and the non-SP fractions ultimately resulting in the production of confounding data. They emphasized that more stringent gating strategies are necessary and that a combination of isolation methods are required to enhance the purity of CSCs.

In lung cancers, Ho, *et al.* [60] reported that the SP cells in NSCLC cell lines were an enriched source of tumor-initiating cells with stem cell properties. Sung, *et al.* [25] suggested that ABCG2 played an important role in the multidrug resistance phenotype of SP cells in a NSCLC cell line, A549. In contrast, Meng, *et al.* [48] reported more than 45% of A549 (NSCLC) and H446 (SCLC) cells to be CICs regardless of SP features based on the results of cloning and tumorigenic analyses.

Aldehyde Dehydrogenase

The ALDH superfamily represents a divergently related group of enzymes that metabolize a wide variety of endogenous and exogenous aldehydes. In the human genome, at least 19 functional genes and 3 pseudogenes have been identified [61]. ALDH also contributes to the oxidation of retinol to retinoic acid, a modulator of cell proliferation, which may also modulate stem cell proliferation [62]. Murine and human hematopoietic stem cells [63-64], murine neural stem cells [65], normal and malignant human mammary stem cells [66], and normal and malignant human colorectal stem cells [62,67] exhibit ALDH activity and express this enzyme, strongly suggesting that strong ALDH activity and/or antigen expression can be used as a marker for stem cells in a variety of cancers. ALDH activity has been measured as substrate-oxidizing activity in whole cell lysate, and the expression of the enzyme has been detected by immunoreactions with specific antibodies, such as Western blot and immunohistochemical analyses. Since the development of a new method using an

ALDH-activated fluorescent substrate as a marker for the isolation of human hematopoietic stem cells [68], the so-called Aldefluor assay has been widely applied to the measurement and isolation of normal and malignant stem-cell-like cells in a variety of tissues [49,64-67]. This method is useful for isolating and purifying viable cells with high levels of ALDH activity for assays of the CSC properties of these cell populations.

Other Lung CSC Markers

Koch, *et al.* [69] demonstrated that a majority of SCLC were immunohistochemically positive for the antibody against podocalyxin-like protein 1 (PODXL-1) and hypothesized that PODXL-1 is a potential CSC marker of SCLC. PODXL-1, belonging to a large family of cell surface sialomucins and being most closely related to CD34 and endoglycan [33,70,71], is expressed in primitive hematopoietic progenitors and thought to be a marker of embryonic and hematopoietic stem cells [72].

Gutova, *et al.* [73] found that SCLC cells positive for urokinase plasminogen activator receptor (uPAR) were resistant to traditional chemotherapies and speculated that they contain a putative CSC population. Urokinase plasminogen activator (uPA) and its receptor uPAR are instrumental in controlling membrane-associated extracellular proteolysis and transmembranous signaling, thus affecting cell migration and invasion [74]. uPAR is up-regulated by several oncogenic pathways including mutations of multiple oncogenes. Alfano, *et al.* [74] underlined the importance of uPAR signaling in the prevention of apoptosis.

Signaling Pathways in CSCs of Lung Cancers

Sonic Hedgehog

Sonic hedgehog (Shh) is expressed by the epithelial cells, and binds and signals to Patched1/2 receptors in the underlying mesenchyme [6,75,76].

Watkins, *et al.* [77] reported the significance of Hedgehog signaling in a subset of SCLCs. Yagui-Beltrán, *et al.* [78] and Peacock, *et al.* [79] reviewed the results of studies on CSC markers and signaling pathways in pulmonary carcinogenesis with special attention to the differences between SCLC and NSCLC. Both papers emphasized the potential importance of the Hedgehog and Wnt signaling pathways in SCLC and NSCLC (see below). Interestingly, human primary or immortalized bronchial epithelial cells exposed to cigarette smoke for only eight days in culture became tumorigenic in nude mice, in association with the activation of the Hedgehog and Wnt signaling pathways [80].

Wnt Signaling Pathway and Nuclear β-Catenin

For the maintenance and activation of normal stem cells, the Wnt/β-catenin signaling pathway is crucial, as distinctly demonstrated in the intestinal mucosa epithelia, epidermis, mammary gland [6], and other tissue [81]. The importance of Wnt signaling in cancer cells has been emphasized [82], and the Wnt/β-catenin signaling cascade is a critical regulator not only of normal stem cells but also of CSCs [83]. Disruption of this signaling pathway at any step potentially causes disorders of stem cell activity and plays a crucial role in the development of cancer. For instance, sustained Wnt signaling mediated by the membrane receptor Frizzled stimulates the release of β-catenin from a cytoplasmic degradation complex composed of APC, Axin, GSK3-β and Dsh, resulting in its movement into the nucleus and activation of Lef/Tcf transcription factors for c-Myc and cyclin D1 [82]. As another example, inactivation of APC due to a gene mutation also results in the release of β-catenin from the degradation complex, leading to the neoplastic transformation of colonic epithelial stem cells [11]. Thus, nuclear β-catenin is a hallmark for active Wnt signaling [75].

As described above, Yagui-Beltrán, *et al.* [87] and Peacock, *et al.* [79] emphasized the potential importance of the Wnt signaling pathway in SCLC and NSCLC in addition to the Hedgehog signaling pathway. Also as described above, human primary or immortalized bronchial epithelial cells exposed to cigarette smoke became tumorigenic in nude mice, being associated with the activation of not only the Hedgehog signaling pathway but also the Wnt signaling pathway [80].

Other Signaling Pathways and Transcription Factors in Lung CSCs

While the Wnt/β-catenin signaling pathway has been extensively investigated in many tissues including the lung, other signaling pathways are also important for controlling stem cell activity, including transmembranous Notch signaling and bone morphogenetic protein (BMP) signaling mediated by the cell membrane receptor Bmpr1a [8,75]. However, we are only beginning to understand the roles these pathways play in CSC populations of lung cancers.

B cell-specific Mo-MuLV integration site 1 (Bmi1) is a member of the Polycomb group family of proteins and a downstream effector of the extracellular signaling molecule Shh. Bmi1 is implicated in the self-renewal of multiple stem cells including hematopoietic and neural stem cells [84]. Dovey, *et al.* [85] suggested that Bmi1 is critical for both normal and tumor bronchioloalveolar stem cell expansion in mice. Koch, *et al.* [69] demonstrated that a majority of SCLCs were immunohistochemically positive for antibodies against Bmi1. From these results, they hypothesized that Bmi1 is a potential CSC marker of SCLC.

A couple of studies suggest that Oct-4 is a potential CSC marker for lung cancers. Levina, *et al.* [50] demonstrated that a human large cell cancer cell line (H460) propagated a CSC-like cell population that showed CD133, Oct-4, and high nuclear β-catenin expression after an *in vitro* treatment with anti-cancer drugs. Chen, *et al.* [51] reported that Oct-4 expression plays a crucial role in maintaining the self-renewing, CSC-like, and chemo-radio-resistant properties of CD133-positive NSCLC cell lines. Oct-4 is a member of the POU transcription factor family known to be expressed in pluripotent stem cells and to function as a transcriptional regulator of multiple genes related to stemness [86].

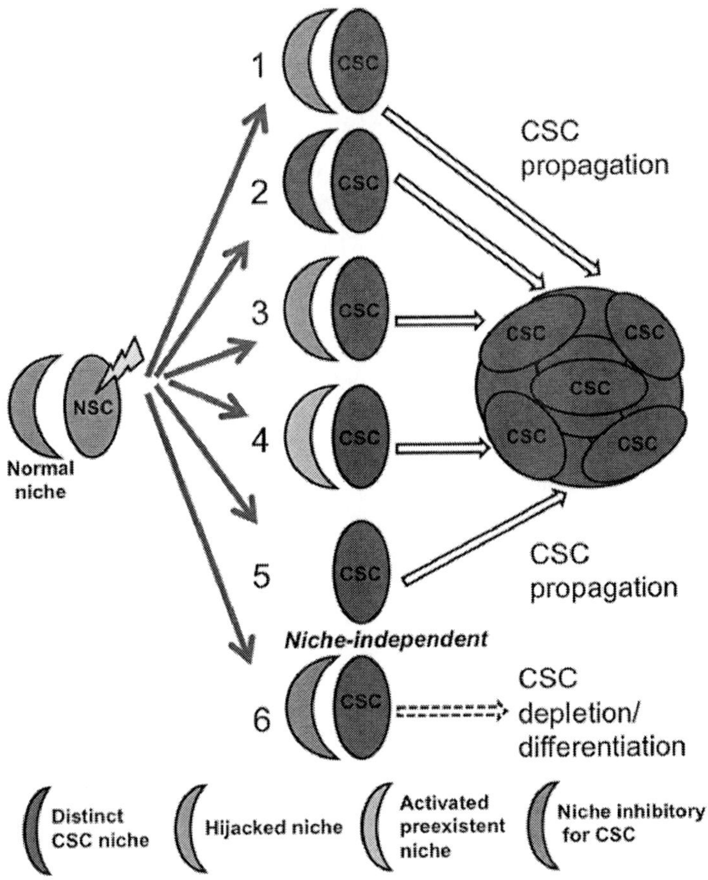

Figure 1. Hypothesis for the relationship between cancer stem cells (CSCs) and their niche. At least one genetic or epigenetic event (yellow arrow) is required to occur in a normal stem cell (NSC; or progenitor cell, not shown here) for a CSC initiation to develop (closed arrows). The CSCs may utilize the normal niche (1), require the distinct CSC niche (2), instruct an otherwise quiescent niche to become activated by providing signals ("hijacking the niche") (3), amplify an already existent activated niche (4), or become niche-independent (5). Furthermore, there may be a discrete niche that is inhibitory for CSC maintenance (6). (Modified from [24]).

In Vitro Assay

Several *in vitro* assays have been used to identify CSCs, including sphere-formation assays, serial colony-forming unit assays (re-plating assays), and label-retention assays [10,14]. Among them, sphere-formation assays are utilized in a wide range of tissue systems including lung cancers [42,87]. However, each of these methods has potential pitfalls that complicate interpretation of the results. For instance, difficulty in confirming clonality (single cell origin) has been pointed out [10]. In addition, the culture conditions used for these assays potentially exert selection pressures upon the cultured cells, resulting in the selection of only cell populations that are able to survive and proliferate under such specific conditions. The limitations of these *in vitro* assays should be kept in mind, and a combination of methods including *in vivo* assays is necessary for the identification and isolation of CSCs.

CSC Niche

The microenvironment surrounding normal and cancer stem cells, which provides the stem cell niche, plays multiple roles including as a mechanical anchorage for the stem cells and in cross-talk communication mediated by direct contact and/or indirect extracellular factors. For instance, Wnt ligands are produced and released from both stem cells and niche cells, BMP and Shh are released from niche cells and epithelial cells respectively, and Notch signaling is transmembranously transmitted between neighboring cells. The micro environment may also provide signaling via the cell receptor integrin as suggested by its expression in prostatic CSCs [88] and its co-expression with AC133 (CD133) in the epidermal basal cells [36], as well as through metalloprotease-mediated lysophopholipid signaling [89].

The concept of a CSC niche is a matter of debate [90]. Two fundamental questions need to be answered: 1) Does a specific CSC niche exist? 2) If it does, what are the differences between the normal stem cell niche and CSC niche? Sneddon, *et al.* [23] removed some of the confusion regarding the CSC niche by proposing several possible models (Figure 1): 1) CSCs are capable of surviving in the normal stem cell niche, 2) a distinct CSC niche is necessary for activation, 3) CSCs may be capable of providing signals that instruct an otherwise quiescent niche to become activated ("hijacking the niche"), 4) CSCs could amplify an already existent activated niche, 5) CSCs may be niche-independent, that is, they themselves acquire the ability to maintain activity, and 6) there may be a discrete niche that is inhibitory for CSC maintenance. Accumulating evidence suggests that no single model fits all the diverse types of cancer. Further study is required to establish a universally acceptable CSC niche theory.

While the niche may also play an important role in the maintenance of CSCs from lung cancers, little has been elucidated yet. Hilbe, *et al.* [91] demonstrated by immunohisto chemistry a significant increase in CD133-positive vascular endothelial cells in patients with NSCLC and suggested an involvement of endothelial progenitor cells in the tumor vasculature and tumor growth, as well as possibly the maintenance and activation of CSCs. More studies of the lung CSC niche are required not only to understand the biological relationship between lung CSCs and their niche but also for the development of therapeutic strategies for lung cancers.

Brief Summary of Lung CSC Markers and Potential Problems

While investigations into the CSC markers of lung cancer are insufficient at this time, as discussed above and summarized in Table 1, we tentatively summarize the findings to date as follows: 1) CD133 expression and the SP phenotype are common CSC markers for SCLC and NSCLC. 2) The Wnt/β-catenin signaling pathway is also important in the maintenance and activation of CSCs in SCLC and NSCLC. 3) PODXL-1 and uPAR are potential CSC markers for SCLC, but their expression has not been well examined in NSCLC. 4) In regard to ALDH, results reported to date appear to be complicated. Its enzymatic activity has been demonstrated in SCLC and NSCLC cells by the Aldefluor assay, as well as by a spectrophotometrical assay [92-97]. On the other hand, an immunohistochemical analysis using antibodies against ALDH1A1 and ALDH3A1 in tissue sections of surgical specimens of lung cancer demonstrated the expression of these ALDH isozymes in NSCLC cases, but not in SCLC cases, suggesting that the ALDH protein expression was limited to CSCs in NSCLC [96]. In contrast, Moreb, *et al.* [93] reported that in their studies using several SCLC and NSCLC cell lines there were good correlations between the results of a Western blot analysis, a spectrophotometrical analysis, and the Aldefluor assay, in spite of a few exceptions (see below). The discrepancy among these results may be attributable to the difference in the antibodies used, and the difference between the *in vitro* and *in vivo* conditions as well.

Though evidence is still poor, it is supposed that distinct differences in the mechanism of ALDH expression and activity, as well as the role of ALDH in the maintenance/activation of CSCs, exist between SCLC and NSCLC. Furthermore, the exact mechanism and role of ALDH in the maintenance of the stemness of normal stem cells and CSCs are still unknown. To try to resolve these issues, we have carried out investigations, which are described in the following section.

Recent Findings in ALDH and CSC of the Lung

As described above, ALDH activity and its protein expression have been reported to be useful normal stem cell and CSC markers in a wide range of tissues [66,92,96-98]. These ALDHs play pluripotent roles in endobiotic and xenobiotic metabolism through specific metabolic pathways. One important issue to be addressed is which ALDH isozymes are responsible for the ALDH activity used to identify stem cell progenitors. Several studies have demonstrated that ALDH activity is needed for the differentiation of primitive progenitors into mature cells, thus fulfilling one of the defining characteristics of multipotent stem cells, and some lines of evidence suggest that ALDH1A1 is an important marker of hematopoietic stem cell progenitors [92]. In fact, ALDH1A1 is one of the enzymes involved in the production of retinoic acid from retinol, and retinoic acid is considered significantly important in maintaining a balance between hematopoietic stem cell self-renewal and differentiation [92].

Moreb, *et al.* [93] systemically evaluated ALDH expression in several lung cancer cells lines (SCLC and NSCLC cell lines) utilizing the Aldefluor assay, a Western blotting, and a spectrophotometry and found a very good correlation between the results of all three. They concluded that the Aldefluor assay can be adapted successfully to measure ALDH activity in lung cancer cells, providing real time changes in ALDH activity in viable cells treated with chemotherapy or siRNA. They emphasized the importance of the use of mixed populations of cells with high ALDH levels and cells lacking ALDH activity when ALDH activity is measured by the Aldefluor assay in cells known to have high ALDH levels.

Importantly, they carried out double Aldefluor and propidium iodide (PI) staining to delineate dead cells. According to their results, while ALDH expression levels were heterogeneous among the cell lines examined, overall findings revealed low levels of ALDH activity in SCLC cell lines, while higher levels were detected in some, but not all, NSCLC cell lines. The results correlated very well with protein and enzymatic activity as measured by the Western blot analysis and the spectrophotometrical assay, respectively. Intriguingly, there was one exception: The SW210.5 (SCLC) cell line registered only a small amount of ALDH activity in the spectrophotometrical assay and expressed only small amounts of ALDH1A1 and ALDH3A1 proteins in the Western blot analysis, whereas the Aldefluor assay showed high levels of ALDH activity (50% of the cells). This SCLC cell line (SW210.5) was shown to express mRNA for ALDH1A1 and ALDH2, but not ALDH3A1, by the semi-quantitative reverse transcription polymerase chain reaction (RT-PCR) assay.

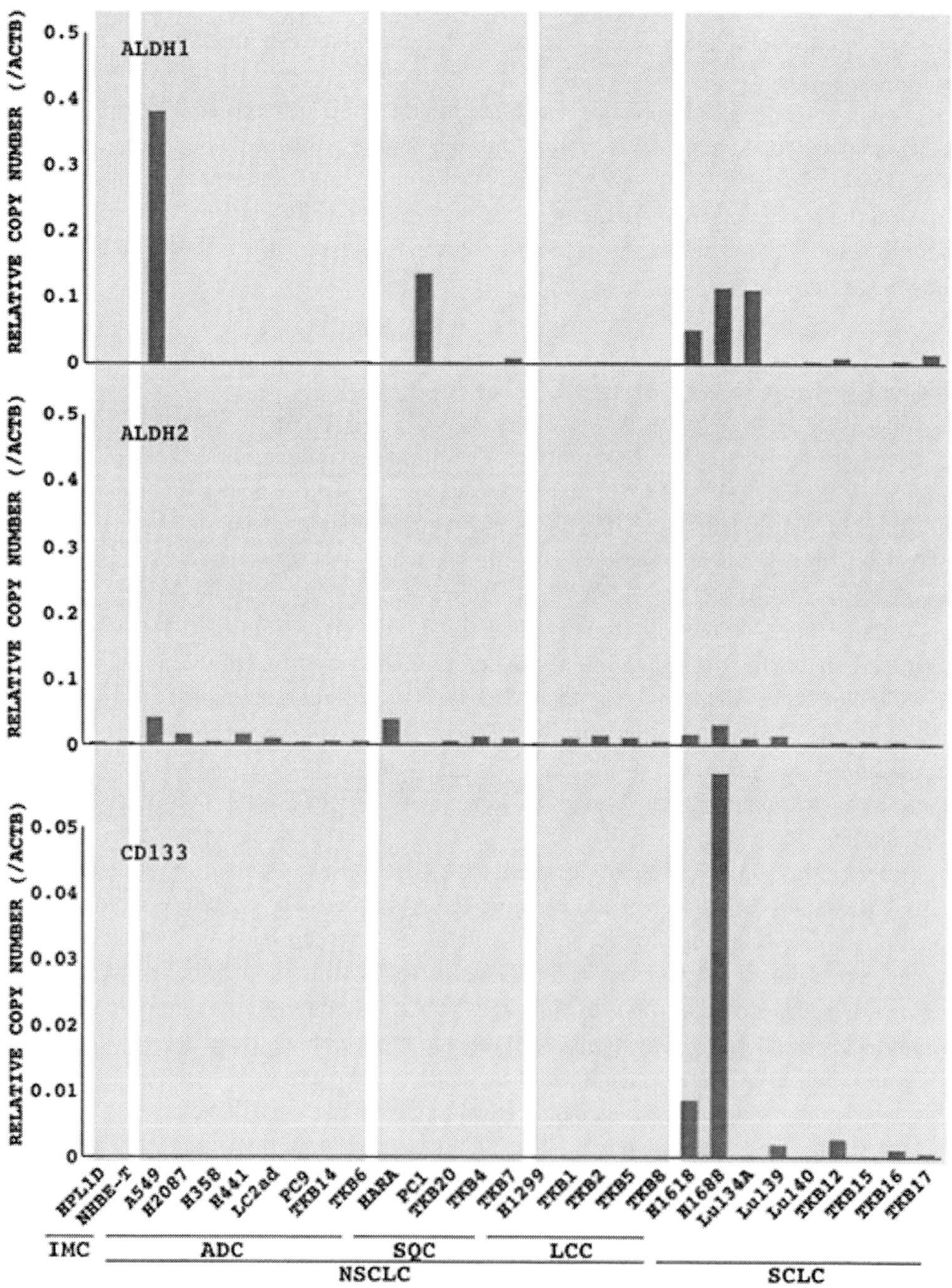

Figure 2. Expression of ALDH1, ALDH2 and CD133 mRNA in immortalized human airway cell and lung cancer cell lines. Levels of mRNA of ALDH1, ALDH2 and CD133 and β-actin (ACTB) were measured by quantitative RT-PCR. The mRNA levels of ALDH1 (upper panel), ALDH2 (second panel) and CD133 (lower panel) relative to that of ACTB in immortalized human airway cells and lung cancer

cells are presented. IMC, immortalized human airway cell lines; ADC, adenocarcinoma cell lines; SQC, squamous cell carcinoma cell lines; LCC, large cell carcinoma cell lines; NSCLC, non-small cell lung carcinoma cell lines; SCLC, small cell lung carcinoma cell lines. The experimental materials and methods are as follows. An immortalized human airway epithelial cell line (16HBE14o, Simian virus 40 (SV40)-transformed human bronchial epithelial cells) described by Cozens AL, *et al.* [102] was kindly provided by Gruenert DC (California Pacific Medical Center Research Institute, CA) via Kaneko T (Division of Respiratory Disease Center, Yokohama City Medical Center Hospital, Yokohama, Japan). A sub-clone of 16HBE14o cells, described as NHBE-T in this chapter, was used. An immortalized airway epithelial cell line (HPL1D, SV40-transformed human small airway epithelial cells) established by Masuda A, *et al.* [103], was provided by Takahashi T (Division of Molecular Carcinogenesis, Center for Neurological Disease and Cancer, Nagoya University Graduate School of Medicine, Nagoya, Japan). Human lung cancer cell lines (A549, H358, H2087, H1618, H1688 and H1299) were purchased from American Type Culture Collection (ATCC, Manassas, VA). Human lung cancer cell lines, LC2/ad, Lu134A and Lu140 were obtained form Riken Cell Bank (Tsukuba, Japan), and PC9, PC1 and HARA from Immuno-Biological Laboratories Co. (Gunma, Japan). Human lung cancer cell lines, TKB1, TKB2, TKB4, TKB5, TKB6, TKB7, TKB8, TKB12, TKB15, TKB16, TKB17 and TKB20, were kindly provided by Kamma H (Department of Pathology, Kyorin University School of Medicine, Tokyo, Japan) via Yazawa T (Department of Pathology, Yokohama City University School of Medicine, Yokohama Japan). The cells were cultured and grown in DEMEM (Sigma Aldrich, St. Louis, MO) (NHBE-T, HPL1D, A549, H358, H2087, PC9, PC1, HARA, LC2/ad, TKB1, TKB2, TKB4, TKB5, TKB6, TKB7, TKB8, TKB20 and H1299) or RPMI1640 medium (Sigma) (H1618, H1688, Lu130, Lu134A, Lu140, TKB12, TKB15, TKB16 and TKB17) supplemented with 10% heat-inactivated fetal bovine serum (FBS) (Sigma), 100 units/ml of penicillin (Sigma), and 100 μg/ml of streptomycin (Sigma). Total RNA was extracted from the cells with Isogen reagents (NIPPON GENE, Tokyo, Japan). First-strand cDNA was synthesized from total RNA using the SuperScript First-Strand Synthesis System according to the protocols of the manufacturer (Invitrogen, Carlsbad, CA). The cDNA generated was used as a template in real-time PCR with SYBR Premix EXTaq (Takara, Kyoto, Japan). The primer set used for ALDH1A1 was forward (F), 5'- agtgcccctttggtggattc; reverse (R), 5'-aagagcttctctccactcttg. That for ALDH2 was, F, 5'- ctacacacgccatgaacctg; R, 5'- caaccacgtttccagttg. That for CD133 was, F, 5'- ttgtggcaaatcaccaggta; R, 5'- gatgttgggtctcagtcggt. That for ACTB was, F, 5'-tggcacccagcacaatgaa; R, 5'- ctaagtcatagtccgcctagaagca. The mean of the copy number of ALDH1A1, ALDH2 or CD133 normalized to the value for ACTB mRNA was obtained from triplicate reactions.

Our preliminary experiments revealed very high levels of ALDH1A1 mRNA expression in some SCLC and NSCLC cell lines. We also observed considerable discrepancies between mRNA levels detected by the quantitative RT-PCR assay, protein levels analyzed by Western blotting, and the proportion of cells with enzymatic activity measured by the Aldefluor assay in several SCLC and NSCLC cell lines.

Aiming to elucidate the mechanism underlying the discrepancies observed in preliminary experiments and the previous study, we carried out the following experiments.

ALDH mRNA Expression - Its Correlation with the most Common CSC Marker CD133

The quantitative RT-PCR assay revealed that ALDH1A1 mRNA was expressed at detectable levels in seven out of nine SCLC cell lines (77.8%), three of which expressed it at unequivocally high levels (33.3%), while it was expressed in four of the 18 NSCLC cell lines, two of which expressed it at high levels (11.1%) (Figure 2). On the other hand, ALDH2 was expressed in eight of the nine SCLC cell lines and 17 of the 18 NSCLC cell lines. The levels were lower on the whole than those of ALDH1A1 and did not remarkably differ among the cell lines. mRNA of CD133, most commonly used CSC marker, was expressed only in SCLC cell lines (66.7%, six out of nine cell lines), and its level in SCLC cell lines tended to be associated with the level of ALDH1A1, but not ALDH2. The findings suggested ALDH1A1 to have an important significance in the maintenance of stemness in lung cancer cells, and might account for the highly malignant activity of SCLCs.

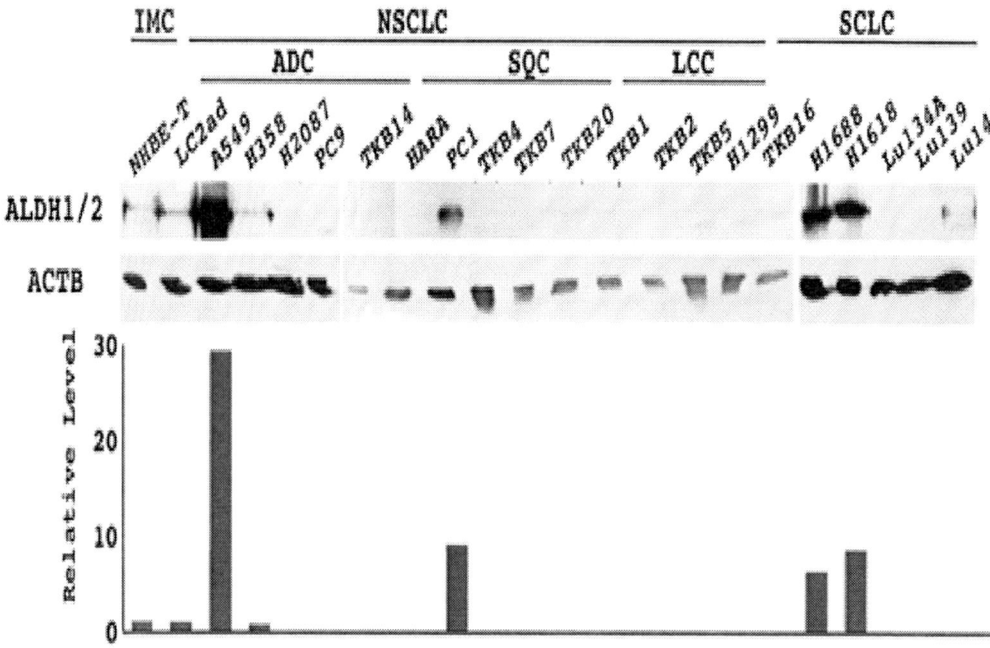

Figure 3. Expression of ALDH1A1/ALDH2 (ALDH1/2) protein in lung cancer cell lines. ALDH1/2 (top panel) and β-actin (ACTB) (second panel) protein expressions were analyzed by Western blotting. Levels of ALDH1/2 and ACTB protein were semi-quantified with a densitometer (NIH Image; National Institute of Mental Health at Bethesda, MD). The level of ALDH1/2 normalized to that of ACTB is presented in a graph (third panel). IMC, immortalized human airway epithelial cell lines; ADC, adenocarcinoma cell lines; SQC, squamous cell carcinoma cell lines; LCC, large cell carcinoma cell lines; NSCLC, non-small cell lung carcinoma cell lines; SCLC, small cell lung carcinoma cell lines. The experimental materials and methods are as follows. The cell lines (the details of the experimental materials are described in the legend for Figure 2) grown to sub-confluence were solved with extraction buffer, as described elsewhere [104]. After centrifugation, supernatants were recovered as protein extracts. The extracts were mixed with equal volumes of 2×sample buffer [104], and then boiled. The samples were subjected to sodium dodecyl sulfate-polyacrylamide gel electrophoresis, and transferred onto PVDF membranes (Amersham, Arlington Heights, IL). The membranes were incubated with nonfat dry milk in 0.01 M Tris-buffered saline containing 0.1% Tween-20 (TBS-T) to block non-immunospecific protein binding, and then with 0.1 μg/ml of a primary antibody which non-selectively binds to both ALDH1A1 and ALDH2 (clone 44, BD Transduction, San Jones, CA) or a primary antibody against ACTB (Sigma). After washing with TBS-T, the membranes were incubated with animal-matched horseradish peroxidase-conjugated secondary antibodies (Amersham). Immunoreactivity was visualized with the enhanced chemiluminescence system (ECL, Amersham).

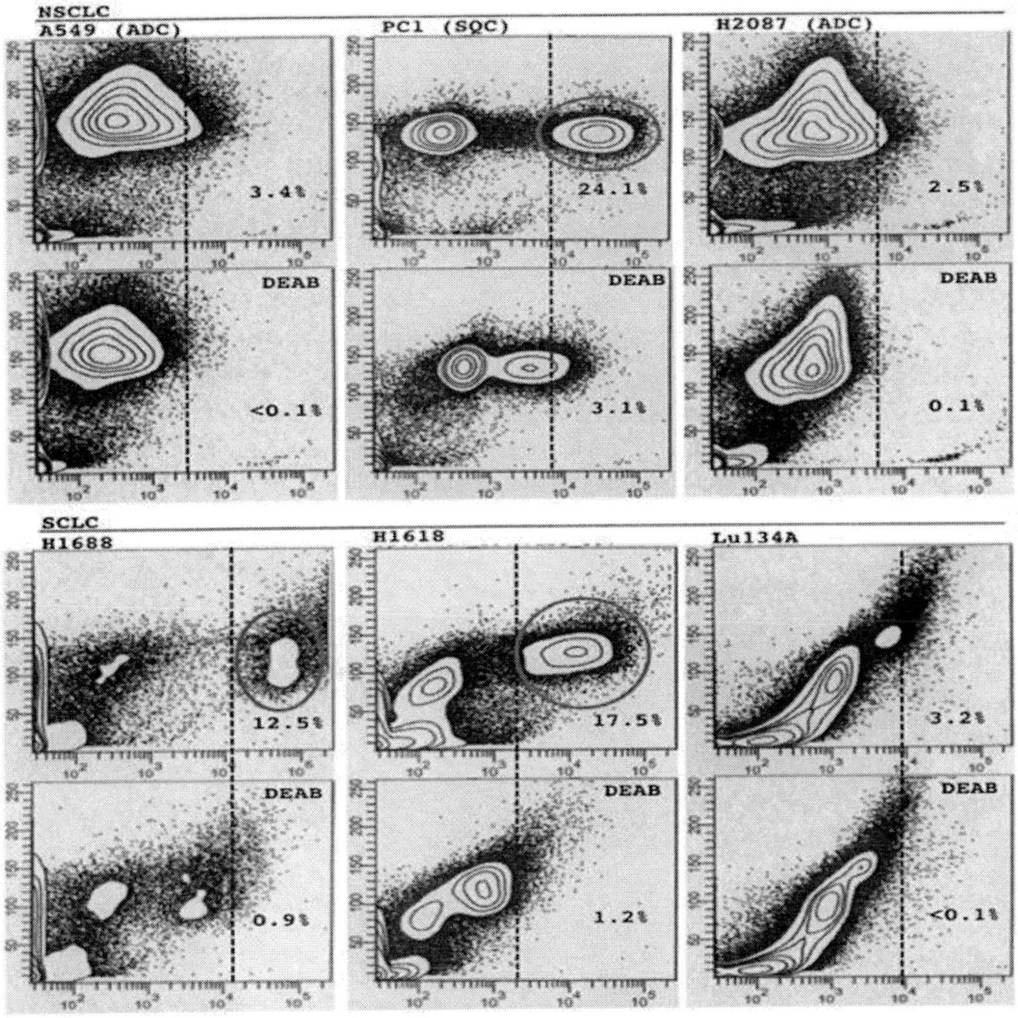

Figure 4. Measurement of fraction of cells with ALDH activity (Aldefluor assay) in lung cancer cell lines. Cells were labeled with Aldefluor (BODIPY-aminoacetaldehyde [BAAA]) (Stem cell technology Inc., Vancouver, Canada) with or without the ALDH inhibitor diethylaminobenzaldehyde (DEAB) (Stem cell technology). The proportion of fraction of cells with ALDH activity was measured by flow cytometer. The X-axis is fluorescence intensity (log scale), and the Y-axis is forward scatter level (linear scale). The fraction of cells with strong ALDH activity is shown (red circle). NSCLC, non-small cell lung carcinoma cell lines; ADC, adenocarcinoma cell lines; SQC, squamous cell carcinoma cell lines; SCLC, small cell lung carcinoma cell lines. The experimental materials and methods are as follows. The details of the cell lines examined are described in the legend for Figure 1. Cells with ALDH activity was labeled using Aldefluor assay kit (Stem cell technology) according to the manufacturer's instructions. Briefly, 1.0×10^6 cells in 1 ml of Aldefluor assay buffer with BAAA at a concentration of 1.5 mM were incubated for 45 min at 37C. In each experiment, a sample of cells was treated under identical conditions with 50 mM of a specific ALDH inhibitor (DEAB) to serve as a negative control. The fraction of cells with ALDH activity labeled by Aldefluor was measured with a flow cytometer (BD Science, San Jose, CA) (excitation wave length 488 nm and emission wave length 525 nm (green fluorescence)). Data for 1.0×10^5 cells were collected.

ALDH Protein Expression in Lung Cancer Cell Lines

ALDH protein was detected by Western blotting using a non-selective antibody, which binds both ALDH1A1 and ALDH2 proteins (clone 44, BD transduction, Palo Alto, CA). The protein was expressed at high levels in two of the nine SCLC cell lines (22.2%), and two of the 18 NSCLC cell lines (11.1%) (Figure 3). The level of protein paralleled well the level of ALDH1A1 mRNA, but not ALDH2 mRNA, in NSCLC cell lines, suggesting that the protein detected by the Western blot analysis was ALDH1A1 rather than ALDH2 (Figure 2 and Figure 3). Thus, we describe the protein detected here by the Western blot analysis as ALDH1A1. Interestingly, one SCLC cell line (Lu134) with a high level of ALDH1A1 mRNA did not express ALDH1A1 (either ALDH1A1 or ALDH2) (Figure 2). This result is similar to a previous observation that a SCLC cell line, SW210.5, expressed ALDH1 mRNA, but only a very small amount of protein [93]. These findings suggest a potential post-translational mechanism to be involved in ALDH1A1 protein expression in some SCLC cells.

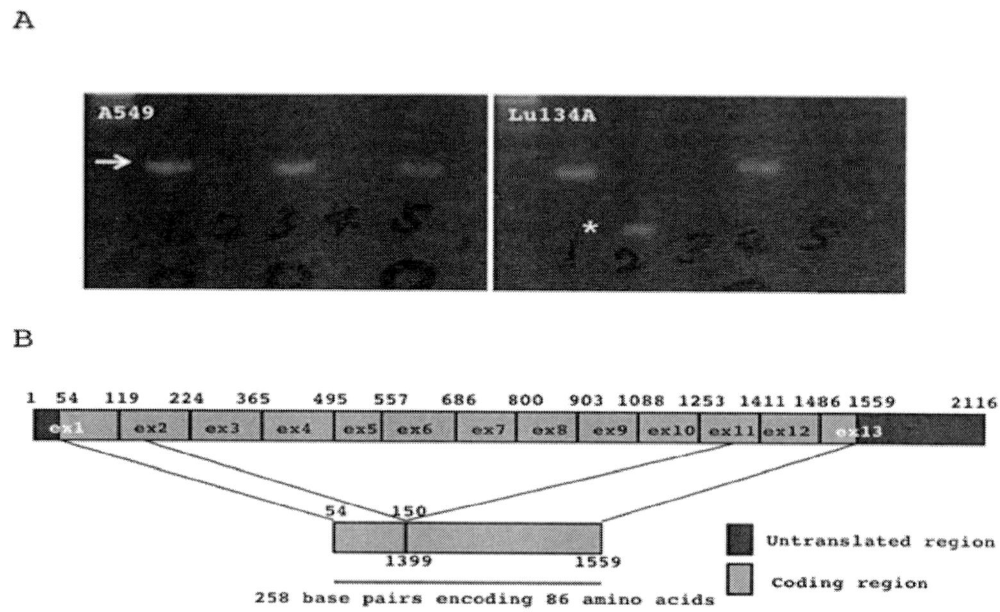

Figure 5. Analysis of primary structure of mRNA of ALDH1A1. The protein-coding sequence in ALDH1A1 mRNA was amplified by RT-PCR using primers, forward, 5'-aggagccgaatcagaaatgtc; reverse, 5'-aagagcttctctccactcttg, according to the method descried in the legend for Figure 2. The PCR product was sub-cloned into the plasmid vector pT7Blue (Novagen, Darmstadt, Germany), and then its size was checked by PCR using universal primers (T7 promoter primer and M13M4 primer (Novagen)). (A) A representative result from A549 (ADC) and Lu134A (SCLC) cells is shown. Shorter PCR products (faster migrating band (asterisk)) were found in some sub-clones from Lu134A. Bands of expected size with a full-length coding region of ALDH1A1 (NCBI accession # NM_000689) are indicated with an arrow. (B) Schema of the primary structure of the consensus mRNA and the shorter variant with their mRNA spliced sites in the *ALDH1A1* gene, is shown. The shorter novel variant consists of parts of exon 1, exon2, exon 11, exon 12, and exon 13. "ex" in figure means exon.

ALDH Activity in Lung Cancer Cell Lines

The fraction of cells with ALDH activity was measured with the Aldefluor assay. The two SCLC cell lines with high ALDH1A1 protein levels (H1688 and H1618) had fractions of cells with strong ALDH activity (Figure 4). All of the SCLC cell lines with very weak ALDH protein expression (the faint bands detected by Western blotting in these cell lines were presumably ALDH2, because these cell lines expressed only ALDH2, not ALDH1A1, mRNA) had only a small fraction (less than 10%) of cells with ALDH activityOn the other hand, among NSCLC cell lines examined (A549, PC1, H441, H2087 and H1299) (not all data shown), only one (PC1) had fraction of cells with strong ALDH activity (Figure 4). One cell line with high ALDH1A1 protein levels (A549) unexpectedly had only a very small fraction of cells with strong ALDH activity. Summarizing the findings, ALDH1A1 protein expression was closely associated with ALDH activity in SCLC cells, but not necessarily in NSCLC cells, suggesting the potential post-translational mechanism to be involved in activation of ALDH1A1 protein in NSCLCs.

Primary Structure of ALDH1A1 mRNA

To elucidate the possible involvement of a mutation (or polymorphism) or splicing disorder in the difference among the levels of mRNA, protein and activity, which was observed in Lu134 SCLC and A549 NSCLC cells, the nucleotide sequence of open reading frames of cDNA were analyzed.

No mutation (or polymorphism) causing an amino acid substitution was found in either cell line (data not shown). However, interestingly, short mRNA variant (258 base pairs in the open reading frame, encoding 86 amino acids: see Figure 5) was found in the Lu134A cell line. This variant was found in three of eight sub-clones (37.5%) in our sub-cloning experiment (part of the result is shown in Figure 5). The result suggested the possible involvement of such a variant in the post-transcriptional regulation of ALHD1A1 expression, and also implied a potential difference between SCLC and NSCLC, although further screening of a larger number of cell lines and primary lung cancers is required to test this idea.

Post-translational Modification of ALDH1A1 Protein

Since no mutation was found in the cell line with the lag between ALDH1/2 protein expression and ALDH activity (A549 cells), we next verified the possible involvement of a post-translational modification. To screen for such a modification, two-dimensional Western blot analysis was performed with A549 (NSCLC) and H1688 (SCLC) cells (Figure 6). While the results did not reveal unequivocal evidence of a modification, the ALDH1A1 protein migrated slightly faster in A549 cells (Figure 6). To elucidate the mechanism underlying the lag between ALDH1A1 protein expression and ALDH activity, further investigations of protein structure and modifications such as glycosylation, phosphorylation and acetylation status, are required.

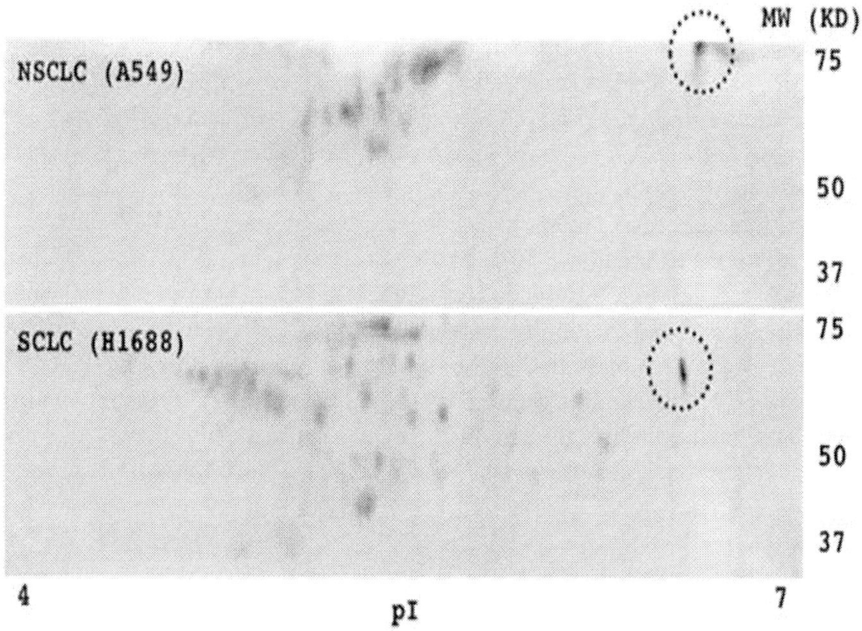

Figure 6. Two-dimensional Western blotting analysis of ALDH1A1/ALDH2 (ALDH1/2) protein in a NSCLC cell line (top panel; A549) and SCLC cell line (Bottom panel; H1688). Spots of ALDH1/2 protein were circulated with dashed lines. MW, molecular weight; KD, kilo-dalton; pI, isoelectric point plugin. The experimental materials and methods are as follows. Two-dimensional electrophoresis (2-DE) was carried out using a horizontal electrophoresis system (Maltiphor II; Amersham) according to the manufacture's instruction. Briefly, equal amount of protein sample was subjected to the first-dimensional isoelectric focusing, and followed by the second dimensional sodium dodecyl sulfate-polyacrylamide gel electrophoresis. The details of method are described elsewhere [105,106]. The separated proteins on the 2-DE gels were transferred onto a polyvinylidene difluoride membrane (FluoroTrans® PVDF Membrane, Nippon Genetics, Tokyo, Japan). The membranes were incubated with nonfat dry milk in 0.01 M Tris-buffered saline containing 0.1% Tween-20 (TBS-T) to block non-immunospecific protein binding, and then with 0.1 μg/ml of a primary antibody, which non-selectively binds to both ALDH1A1 and ALDH2 (clone 44, BD Transduction). After washing with TBS-T, the membranes were incubated with animal-matched horseradish peroxidase-conjugated secondary antibodies (Amersham). Immunoreactivity was visualized with the enhanced chemiluminescence system (ECL, Amersham).

ALDH Protein Expression in Primary Lung Cancers

ALDH protein expression in primary lung tumors was examined by immunohistochemistry using a non-selective antibody (clone 44, BD transduction, Palo Alto, CA), which binds both ALDH1A1 and ALHD2 proteins (ALDH1/2). The protein expression was detected in three of nine SCLCs (33.3%) and in 41 of 70 NSCLCs (58.6%) (Table 2). The levels tended to be higher in NSCLC, especially SQC, than in SCLC (Figure 5). The results were similar to those reported by Patel, *et al.* [96], who found in their immunohistochemical analysis that the ALDH isozymes 1A1 and 1A3 were expressed at significantly higher levels in NSCLC than in SCLC [96]. However, we have found that there is a discrepancy between the results of Western blotting for cancer cell lines and immunohistochemistry for primary lung cancers. The frequency of ALDH1/2 protein expression was considerably higher in primary cancers than in cell lines among NSCLCs, whereas it was similar between the two among SCLCs (Figure 3 and Table 2). Moreover, non-cancerous airway cells *in vivo*, i.e., both the bronchial, bronchiole and alveolar epithelial cells, exhibited high levels of immunohistochemical expression of ALHD1/2 protein compared to cancer cells in all cases examined (Figure 7 and Table 2).

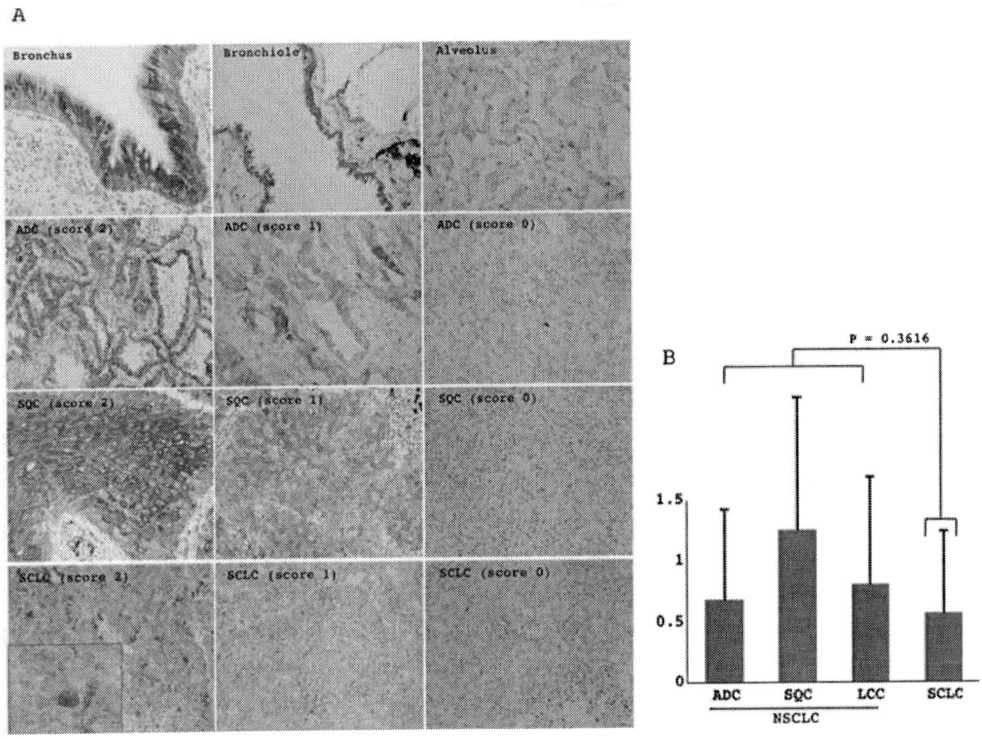

Figure 7. Expression of ALDH1A1/ALDH2 (ALDH1/2) protein in non-cancerous airway epithelia and primary lung cancers. (A) Representative photographs of immunohistochemistry of surgical specimens of non-cancerous airway epithelia (top panels) and lung cancers (the other panels) are shown. Magnifications are ×200 in, non-cancerous airway epithelia (bronchus, bronchiole and alveolus), adenocarcinoma (ADC), squamous cell carcinoma (SQC) and small cell lung carcinoma (SCLC), and ×400 in the inset of SCLC. Levels of ALDH1/2 expression were evaluated according to a scoring system; negative (score 0), unequivocally strong (score 2), and positive but weaker than a score of 2 (score 1). (B) Seventy-nine tumors (49 ADCs, 16 SQCs, 5 large cell carcinomas, and 9 SCLCs) were examined. The mean and standard deviation (error bar) among each histological type are shown in graph. Differences were analyzed with Student's t-test, and P value is indicated. The experimental materials and methods are as follows. All cases examined were of lung cancer patients who underwent surgical resection at the Kanagawa Prefectural Cardiovascular and Respiratory Disease Center Hospital (Yokohama, Japan) between 2001 and 2008. Informed consent for research use was obtained from all the subjects providing materials. Tissue sections (4 μm thick), cut from the formalin-fixed and paraffin-embedded tissue block with largest tumor dimension, were deparaffinized and rehydrated, and incubated with 3% hydrogen peroxide to block endogenous peroxidase activities. The sections were incubated with 5% goat serum to block non-immunospecific protein binding. After antigen retrieval treatment, boiling in citrated buffer (0.01 M, pH6.0) to restore the masked epitope, the sections were incubated with a primary antibody, which non-selectively binds to both ALDH1A1 and ALDH2 (clone 44, BD Transduction). Immunoreactivity was visualized with an Envision detection system (DAKOcytomation, Carpinteria, CA), and the nuclei were counterstained with hematoxylin.

Table 2. Positive rate of immunohistochemical ALDH1/2 expression among NSCLC and SCLC

		NSCLC		SCLC
No. of cases analyzed	ADC [49]	SQC [16]	LCC [5]	[9]
Positive rate % [No.]	51.0% [25]	87.5% [14]	40.0% [2]	33.3% [3]

NSCLC, non-small cell lung carcinoma; SCLC, small cell lung carcinoma; ADC, adenocarcinoma. SQC, squamous cell carcinoma; LCC, large cell carcinoma.

Chi-square test (among all, $P = 0.0254$; NSCLC versus SCLC, $P = 0.154$).

Immunohistochemical analysis was performed in formalin-fixed tumor sections using a primary antibody against ALDH (BD transduction, Palo Alto, CA).

Immunoreactivity was visualized with an Envision detection system (DAKO).

If 5% or more of neoplastic cells in a tumor showed immunohistochemical expression of ALDH, it was judged as positive.

Interestingly, the two non-cancerous immortalized airway epithelial cell lines (NHBE-T and HPL1D) showed very weak expression of ALDH1/2 protein *in vitro*. The ALDH family is expressed in response to toxic stress [99-101]. The marked expression of ALDH1/2 protein in non-cancerous airway epithelial cells *in vivo* is supposed to be induced by external stimuli such as dust, cigarette smoke and so on. In NSCLCs, ALDH1/2 protein tended to be expressed more strongly among *in situ* parts than invasive parts (data not shown), in support of our supposition. Furthermore ALDH1/2 protein expression tended to decrease in parallel with the dedifferentiation process, as a large proportion of poorly differentiated NSCLCs expressed the protein only faintly (data not shown). In well-differentiated and *in situ* NSCLCs, ALDH1/2 expression may still be regulated by the physiological system (it may be lost during progression process to develop poorly differentiated ones). Although further investigation is required to elucidate the mechanism and significance of such a downregulation of ALDH1/2 protein expression in primary lung cancers, the results obtained here imply that ALDH1/2 protein plays diverse roles in different situations is not a universal stem cell marker. The mechanism to induce ALDH1/2 protein expression and its significance are likely to differ among the non-cancerous airway epithelia, NSCLCs and SCLCs.

CONCLUSION

As is widely accepted, among lung cancers, SCLC and NSCLC are distinctly different in terms of biological behavior and pathogenesis. We have hypothesized that the CSCs of these two major subtypes of lung cancer possess different biological properties and that the abundance of CSCs population differs between the two. We have here focused upon ALDH to confirm such a potential difference.

The proportion of cells with strong ALDH activity tended to be associated with the CD133 mRNA level especially in SCLC cell lines (Figure 2). Recently, Jiang, *et al.* [52] demonstrated, in SCLC cell lines, that the ALDH1A1^{high}-CD133^{high}-ASCL1^{high} subpopulation exhibits the features of CSCs and that ASCL1 directly regulates ALDH1A1 and CD133 both *in vitro* and *in vivo*. Previous observations [60] are consistent with our results and also support the hypothesis that the size of the CSC fraction (population) could be one causes of highly malignant activity of SCLC. Importantly, however, not all SCLCs among cell lines and primary tumors were found to have either protein expression or a fraction of cells with high ALDH activity (Figure 4, Figure 7 and Table 2). We thus speculate that the ALDH activity is only one of the factors determining the stemness of CSCs in SCLCs. Alternatively, ALDH1A1 protein expression or ALDH activity is just part of the machinery to maintain stemness and might have significance only in some fractions of SCLCs. On the other hand, Ucar, *et al.* [95] proposed ALDH activity to be a CSC marker in a NSCLC cell line (NIH-H522 LCC cell line). Moreover, Jiang, *et al.* [49] reported that, in NSCLCs, cancer cells with strong ALDH1A1 activity, which were isolated using the Aldefluor assay followed by fluorescence-activated cell sorting, showed CSC features and CD133 expression. They proposed that ALDH1A1 is a lung cancer stem cell-associated marker, being a potential prognostic factor and therapeutic target for the treatment of patients with lung cancer. In our experiments, one NSCLC cell line (PC1 [SQC]) had a high ALDH1A1 protein level and a large fraction of cells with strong ALDH activity (Figure 3 and Figure 5), but did not express CD133 mRNA. Taken together, it is supposed that there is considerable heterogeneity in the mechanism maintaining the stemness of CSCs of SCLCs and NSCLCs.

Aside from the maintenance of stemness, another interesting finding of our experiments was that the level of ALDH1A1 mRNA did not always parallel the level of protein in SCLC cell lines, whereas, in NSCLC cell lines (Figure 3 and Figure 4), the level of protein was not always consistent with that of activity. Furthermore, the *in vivo* findings revealed that either non-cancerous airway epithelia or low-grade neoplasms such as well-differentiated or *in situ* NSCLCs showed stronger immunohistochemical expression of ALDH1A1 (possibly ALDH2 too) protein than less-differentiated cancer cells.

From the current findings, the mechanism and pathway which regulate the expression of ALDH1A1 mRNA and its protein as well as its enzymatic activity, and its role vary in different situations and among non-cancerous airway cells, NSCLCs and SCLCs, as well as among individual tumors. We speculate that ALDH1A1, its expression and/or activity, is only one of the factors determining the stemness in lung cancers.

In conclusion, the CSCs in SCLC and NSCLC differ distinctly from each other in terms not only of their abundance (suggested by CD133 mRNA levels) but also of the regulatory mechanism of ALDH1A1 expression and its activity, as well as its role in the maintenance/ activation of stemness. The investigation of the mechanism of ALDH activation and its role in the maintenance of the stemness not only of CSCs but also of normal stem cells would provide a novel paradigm for stem cell biology and the development of a molecular targeting therapy for lung cancer.

ACKNOWLEDGMENTS

This work was supported by the Japanese Ministry of Education, Culture, Sports, and Science (Tokyo Japan), Smoking Research Foundation (Tokyo, Japan), and by a grant from Yokohama Medical Facility (Yokohama, Japan). We especially thank Hideaki Mitsui (Department of Pathology, Yokohama City University Graduate School of Medicine, Yokohama, Japan), Shigeko Iwanade (Division of Pathology, Kanagawa Prefectural

Cardiovascular and Respiratory Center Hospital, Yokohama, Japan), and Tetsukan Woo (Department of General Thoracic Surgery, Kanagawa Prefectural Cardiovascular and Respiratory Center Hospital, Yokohama, Japan) for assistance.

REFERENCES

[1] Parkin, M., Tyczynski, JE., Boffetta, P., Samet, J., Shields, P., Caporaso, N. Lung cancer epidemiology and etiology. In: Travis, W.D., Brambilla, E., Muller-Hermelink, H.K., Harris, C.C. (eds). *Tumours of the lung. Tumours of the lung, pleura, thymus and heart. World Health Organization Classification of Tumours. Pathology & Genetics.* Lyon, IARC Press 2004; 12-15.

[2] Travis, W.D., Brambilla, E., Muller-Hermelink, H.K., Harris, C.C. (eds). IARC Press: Lyon, 2004; 9-124. Working group that convened for an editorial and consensus conference in Lyon, France, March 12-16, 2003. Tumours of the Lung. In: *World Health Organization Classification of Tumours. Pathology and Genetics of Tumours of the Lung, Pleura, Thymus and Heart.*

[3] Otto, W.R. (2002) Lung epithelial stem cells. *J Pathol, 197*, 527-535.

[4] Giangreco, A., Groot, K.R., Janes, S.M. (2007) Lung cancer and lung stem cells: strange bedfellows? *Am J Respir Crit Care Med, 175*, 547-553.

[5] Giangreco, A., Arwert, E.N., Rosewell, I.R., Snyder, J., Watt, F.M., Stripp, B.R. (2009) Stem cells are dispensable for lung homeostasis but restore airways after injury. *Proc Natl Acad Sci USA, 106,* 9286-9291.

[6] Blanpain, C., Horsley, V., Fuchs, E. Epithelial stem cells: turning over new leaves. (2007) *Cell, 128*, 445-458.

[7] Kitamura, H., Yazawa, T., Shimoyamada, H., Okudela, K., Sato, H. (2008) Molecular and genetic pathogenesis of lung cancer: differences between small-cell and non-small-cell carcinomas. *Open Pathol J, 2,* 106-114. Doi:10.2174/1874375700802010106

[8] Kitamura, H., Yazawa, T., Sato, H., Okudela, K., Shimoyamada, H. (2009) Small cell lung cancer: significance of RB alterations and TTF-1 expression in its carcinogenesis, phenotype, and biology. *Endcr Pathol, 20,* 101-107.

[9] Nuciforo, P., Fraggetta, F. (2004) Cancer stem cell theory: pathologists' considerations and ruminations about wasting time and wrong evaluations. *J Clin Patho1, 7,* 782-783.

[10] Clarke, M.F., Dick, J.E., Dirks, P.B., Eaves, C.J., Jamieson, C.H., Jones, D.L. (2006) Cancer stem cells--perspectives on current status and future directions: AACR Workshop on cancer stem cells. *Cancer Res, 66,* 9339-9344.

[11] Lobo, N.A., Shimono, Y., Qian, D., Clarke, M.F. (2007) The biology of cancer stem cells. *Annu Rev Cell Dev Biol, 23,* 675-699.

[12] Rapp, U.R., Ceteci, F., Schreck, R. (2008) Oncogene-induced plasticity and cancer stem cells. *Cell Cycle, 7,* 45-51.

[13] Kim, C.F., Dirks, P.B. (2008) Cancer and stem cell biology: how tightly intertwined? *Cell Stem Cell, 3,* 147-150.

[14] Yang, Y.M., Chang, J.W. (2008) Current status and issues in cancer stem cell study. *Cancer Invest, 26,* 741-755.

[15] Li, X., Lewis, M.T., Huang, J., Gutierrez, C., Osborne, C.K., Wu, M.F. (2008) Intrinsic resistance of tumorigenic breast cancer cells to chemotherapy. *J Natl Cancer Inst, 100,* 672-679.

[16] Li, L., Borodyansky, L., Yang, Y. (2009) Genomic instability en route to and from cancer stem cells. *Cell Cycle, 8,* 1000-1002.

[17] Hill, R.P. (2006) Identifying cancer stem cells in solid tumors: case not proven. *Cancer Res, 66,* 1883-1890.

[18] Kelly, P.N., Dakic, A., Adams, J.M., Nutt, S.L., Strasser, A. (2007) Tumor growth need not be driven by rare cancer stem cells. *Science, 317,* 337.

[19] Lewis, M.T. (2008) Faith, heresy and the cancer stem cell hypothesis. *Future Oncol, 4,* 585-589.

[20] Yoo, M.H., Hatfield, D.L. (2008) The cancer stem cell theory: is it correct? *Mol Cells, 26,* 514-516.

[21] Vezzoni, L., Parmiani, G. (2008) Limitations of the cancer stem cell theory. *Cytotechnology, 58,* 3-9.

[22] Rowan, K. (2009) Are cancer stem cells real? After four decades, debate still simmers. *J Natl Cancer Inst, 101,* 546-547.

[23] Sneddon, J.B., Werb, Z. (2007) Location, location, location: the cancer stem cell niche. *Cell Stem Cell, 1,* 607-611.

[24] Kitamura, H., Okudela, K., Yazawa, T., Sato, H., Shimoyamada, H. (2009) Cancer stem cell: implications in cancer biology and therapy with special reference to lung cancer. *Lung Cancer, 66,* 275-281.

[25] Sung, J.M., Cho, H.J., Yi, H., Lee, C.H., Kim, H.S., Kim, D.K. (2008) Characterization of a stem cell population in lung cancer A549 cells. *Biochem Biophys Res Commun, 371,* 163-167.

[26] Feldmann, G., Dhara, S., Fendrich, V., Bedja, D., Beaty, R., Mullendore, M., Karikari, C., Alvarez, H., Iacobuzio-Donahue, C., Jimeno, A., Gabrielson, K.L., Matsui, W., Maitra, A. (2007) Blockade of hedgehog signaling pancreatic cancer invasion and metastases: a new paradigm for combination therapy in solid cancers. *Cancer Res, 67,* 2187-96.

[27] Besson, A., Hwang, H.C., Cicero, S., Donovan, S.L., Gurian-West, M., Johnson, D. (2007) Discovery of an oncogenic activity in p27Kip1 that causes stem cell expansion and a multiple tumor phenotype. *Genes Dev, 21,* 1731-1746.

[28] Yin, A.H., Miraglia, S., Zanjani, E.D., Almeida-Porada, G., Ogawa, M., Leary, A.G., et *al.* (1997) AC133, a novel marker for human hematopoietic stem and progenitor cells. *Blood, 90,* 5002-5012.

[29] Wuchter, C., Ratei, R., Spahn, G., Schoch, C., Harbott, J., Schnittger, S., *et al.* (2001) Impact of CD133 (AC133) and CD90 expression analysis for acute leukemia immunophenotyping. *Haematologica, 86,* 154-161.

[30] Shmelkov, S.V., St. Clair, R., Lyden, D., Rafii, S. (2005) AC133/CD133/Prominin-1. *Int J Biochem Cell Biol, 37,* 715-719.

[31] Uchida, N., Buck, D.W., He, D., Reitsma, M.J., Masek, M., Phan, T.V., *et al.* (2000) Direct isolation of human central nervous system stem cells. *Proc Natl Acad Sci USA, 97,* 14720-14725.

[32] Pötgens, A.J., Bolte, M., Huppertz, B., Kaufmann, P., Frank, H.G. (2001) Human trophoblast contains an intracellular protein reactive with an antibody against CD133--a novel marker for trophoblast. *Placenta, 22,* 39-645.

[33] Salven, P., Mustjoki, S., Alitalo, R., Alitalo, K., Rafii, S. (2003) VEGFR-3 and CD133 identify a population of CD34+ lymphatic/vascular endothelial precursor cells. *Blood, 101,* 168-172.

[34] Richardson, G.D., Robson, C.N., Lang, S.H., Neal, D.E., Maitland, N.J., Collins, A.T. (2004) CD133, a novel marker for human prostatic epithelial stem cells. *Cell Science, 117 pt16,* 3539-3545.

[35] Piechaczek, C. (2001) CD133. *J Biol Regul Homeost Agents, 15,* 101-102.

[36] Yu, Y., Flint, A., Dvorin, E.L., Bischoff, J. (2002) AC133-2, a novel isoform of human AC133 stem cell antigen. *J Biol Chem, 277,* 20711-20716.

[37] Marzesco, A.M., Janich, P., Wilsch-Bräuninger, M., Dubreuil, V., Langenfeld, K., Corbeil, D., *et al.* Release of extracellular membrane particles carrying the stem cell marker prominin-1 (CD133) from neural progenitors and other epithelial cells *J Cell Science, 118 pt13,* 2849-2858.

[38] Taïeb, N., Maresca, M., Guo, X.J., Garmy, N., Fantini, J., Yahi, N. (2009) The first extracellular domain of the tumour stem cell marker CD133 contains an antigenic ganglioside-binding motif. *Cancer Lett, 278,* 164-173.

[39] Choi, D., Lee, H.W., Hur, K.Y., Kim, J.J., Park, G.S., Jang, S.H., et al. Cancer stem cell markers CD133 and CD24 correlate with invasiveness and differentiation in colorectal adenocarcinoma. *World J Gastroenterol, 15,* 2258-2264.

[40] Ahn, S.M., Goode, R.J., Simpson, R.J. (2008) Stem cell markers: insights from membrane proteomics? *Proteomics, 8,* 4946-4957.

[41] Klonisch, T., Wiechec, E., Hombach-Klonisch, S., Ande, S.R., Wesselborg, S., Schulze-Osthoff, K., *et al.* Cancer stem cell markers in common cancers - therapeutic implications. *Trends Mol Med, 14,* 450-460.

[42] Eramo, A., Lotti, F., Sette, G., Pilozzi, E., Biffoni, M., Di Virgilio. A., *et al.* (2008), Identification and expansion of the tumorigenic lung cancer stem cell population. *Cell Death Differ, 15,* 504-514.

[43] Wang, J., Sakariassen, P.Ø., Tsinkalovsky, O., Immervoll, H., Bøe, S.O., Svendsen, A., *et al.* (2008) CD133 negative glioma cells form tumors in nude rats and give rise to CD133 positive cells. *Int J Cancer, 122,* 761-768.

[44] Ogden, A.T., Waziri, A.E., Lochhead, R.A., Fusco, D., Lopez, K., Ellis, J.A., *et al.* (2008) Identification of A2B5+CD133- tumor-initiating cells in adult human gliomas. *Neurosurgery, 60,* 505-514.

[45] Shmelkov, S.V., Butler, J.M., Hooper, A.T., Hormigo, A., Kushner, J., Milde, T., *et al.* (2008) CD133 expression is not restricted to stem cells, and both CD133+ and CD133- metastatic colon cancer cells initiate tumors. *J Clin Invest, 188,* 2111-2120.

[46] Mizrak, D., Brittan, M., Alison, M.R. CD133: molecule of the moment. *J Pathol, 214,* 3-9.

[47] Bidlingmaier, S., Zhu, X., Liu, B. (2008) The utility and limitations of glycosylated human CD133 epitopes in defining cancer stem cells. *J Mol Med, 86,* 1025-1032.

[48] Meng, X., Wang, X., Wang, Y. (2009) More than 45% of A549 and H446 cells are cancer initiating cells: evidence from cloning and tumorigenic analyses. *Oncol Rep, 12,* 995-1000.

[49] Jiang, F., Qiu, Q., Khanna, A., Todd, N.W., Deepak, J., Xing, L, *et al.* (2009) Aldehyde dehydrogenase 1 is a tumor stem cell-associated marker in lung cancer. *Mol Cancer Res, 7,* 330-338

[50] Levina, V., Marrangoni, A.M., DeMarco, R., Gorelik, E., Lokshin, A.E. (2008) Drug-selected human lung cancer stem cells: cytokine network, tumorigenic and metastatic properties. *PLoS ONE, 2,* e3077.

[51] Chen, Y.C., Hsu, H.S., Chen, Y.W., Tsai, T.H., How, C.K., Wang, C.Y., *et al.* (2008) Oct-4 expression maintained cancer stem-like properties in lung cancer-derived CD133-positive cells. *PLoS ONE, 3,* e2637.

[52] Jiang, T., Collins, B.J., Jin, N., Watkins, D.N., Brock, M.V., Matsui, W., *et al.* (2009) Achaete-scute complex homologue 1 regulates tumor-initiating capacity in human small cell lung cancer. *Cancer Res, 69,* 845-854.

[53] Ito, T., Udaka, N., Okudela, K., Yazawa, T., Kitamura, H. (2003) Mechanisms of neuroendocrine differentiation in pulmonary neuroendocrine cells and small cell carcinoma. *Endocr Pathol, 14,* 133-139.

[54] Goodell, M.A., Brose, K., Paradis, G., Conner, A.S., Mulligan, R.C. (1996) Isolation and functional properties of murine hematopoietic stem cells that are replicating in vivo. *J Exp Med, 183,* 1797-1806.

[55] Wu, C., Alman, B.A. Side population cells in human cancers. *Cancer Lett, 268,* 1-9.

[56] Hirschmann-Jax, C., Foster, A.E., Wulf, G.G., Nuchtern, J.G., Jax, T.W., Gobel, U., *et al.* (2004) A distinct "side population" of cells with high drug efflux capacity in human tumor cells. *Proc Natl Acad Sci USA, 101,* 14228-14233.

[57] Hirschmann-Jax, C., Foster, A.E., Wulf, G.G., Goodell, M.A., Brenner, M.K. (2005) A distinct "side population" of cells in human tumor cells: implications for tumor biology and therapy. *Cell Cycl*e, 4, 203-205

[58] Zhou, S., Schuetz, J.D., Bunting, K.D., Colapietro, A.M., Sampath, J., Morris, J.J., *et al.* (2001) The ATP binding cassette transporter Bcrp1/ABCG2 is expressed in a wide variety of stem cells and is a molecular determinant of the side-population phenotype. *Nat Med, 7,* 1028-1034.

[59] Telford, W.G., Bradford, J., Godfrey, W., Robey, R.W., Bates, S.E. (2007) Side population analysis using a violet-excited cell-permeable DNA dye. *Stem Cells, 25,* 1029-1036.

[60] Ho MM, Ng AV, Lam S, Hung JY. Side population in human lung cancer cell lines and tumors is enriched with stem-like cancer cells. *Cancer Res* 2007; 67:4827-4833.

[61] Sophos, N.A., Vasiliou, V. (2003) Aldehyde dehydrogenase gene superfamily: the 2009 update. *Chem Biol Interact, 143-144, 5-22.*

[62] Huang, E.H., Hynes, M.J., Zhang, T., Ginestier, C., Dontu, G., Appelman, H., *et al.* (2009) Aldehyde dehydrogenase 1 is a marker for normal and malignant human colonic stem cells (SC) and tracks SC overpopulation during colon tumorigenesis. *Cancer Res, 69,* 3382-3389.

[63] Jones, R.J., Barber, J.P., Vala, M.S., Collector, M.I., Kaufmann, S.H., Ludeman, S.M., *et al.* (1995) Assessment of aldehyde dehydrogenase in viable cells. *Blood, 85,* 2742-2746.

[64] Armstrong, L., Stojkovic, M., Dimmick, I., Ahmad, S., Stojkovic, P., Hole, N., *et al.* (2004) Phenotypic characterization of murine primitive hematopoietic progenitor cells isolated on basis of aldehyde dehydroganse activity. *Stem Cells, 22,* 1142-1151.

[65] Corti, S., Locatelli, F., Papadimitriou, D., Donadoni, C., Salani, S., Del Bo, R., *et al.* (2006) Identification of a primitive brain-derived neural stem cell population based on aldehyde dehydrogenase activity. *Stem Cells, 24,* 975-985.

[66] Ginestier, C., Hur, M.H., Charafe-Jauffret, E., Monville, F., Dutcher, J., Brown, M., et *al.* (2007) ALDH1 is a marker of normal and malignant human mammary stem cells and a predictor of poor clinical outcome. *Cell Stem Cell, 1,* 555-567.

[67] Dylla, S.J., Beviglia, L., Park, I.K., Chartier, C., Raval, J., Ngan, L., *et al.* (2008) Colorectal cancer stem cells are enriched in xenogeneic tumors following chemotherapy. *PLoS ONE, 3,* e2428.

[68] Storms, R.W., Trujillo, A.P., Springer, J.B., Shah, L., Colvin, O.M., Ludeman, S.M., *et al.* (1999) Isolation of primitive human hematopoietic progenitors on the basis of aldehyde dehydrogenase activity. *Proc Natl Acad Sci USA, 96,* 9118-9123.

[69] Koch, L.K., Zhou, H., Ellinger, J., Biermann, K., Höller, T., von Rücker, A., *et al.* (2008) Stem cell marker expression in small cell lung carcinoma and developing lung tissue. *Hum Pathol, 39,* 1597-1605.

[70] Lanza, F., Healy, L., Sutherland, D.R. Structural and functional features of the CD34 antigen: an update. *J Biol Regul Homeost Agents, 15,* 1-13.

[71] Nielsen, J.S., McNagny, K.M. (2008) Novel functions of the CD34 family. *J Cell Sci, 121pt22,* 3683-92.

[72] Doyonnas, R., Nielsen, J.S., Chelliah, S., Drew, E., Hara, T., Miyajima, A., McNagny, K.M. (2005) *Blood, 105,* 4170-4178.

[73] Gutova, M., Najbauer, J., Gevorgyan, A., Metz, M.Z., Weng, Y., Shih, C.C., *et al.* (2007) Identification of uPAR-positive chemoresistant cells in small cell lung cancer. *PLoS ONE, 2,* e243.

[74] Alfano, D., Franco, P., Vocca, I., Gambi, N., Pisa, V., Mancini, A., Caputi, M., Carriero, M.V., Iaccarino, I., Stoppelli, M.P. (2009) The urokinase plasminogen activator and its receptor: role in cell growth and apoptosis. *Thromb Haemost, 93,* 205-211.

[75] Van der Flier, L.G., Clevers, H. (2009) Stem cells, self-renewal, and differentiation in the intestinal epithelium. *Annu Rev Physiol, 71,* 5.1-5.20.

[76] Liao, X., Siu, M.K., Au, C.W., Chan, Q.K., Chan, H.Y., Wong, E.S., et al. (2009) Aberrant activation of hedgehog signaling pathway contributes to endometrial carcinogenesis through β-catenin. *Mod Pathol, 22,* 839-847.

[77] Watkins, D.N., Berman, D.M., Burkholder, S.G., Wang, B., Beachy, P.A., Baylin, S.B. (2003) Hedgehog signalling within airway epithelial progenitors and in small-cell lung cancer. *Nature, 422,* 313-317.

[78] Yagui-Beltrán, A., He, B., Jablons, D.M. (2008) The role of cancer stem cells in neoplasia of the lung: past, present and future. *Clin Transl Oncol, 10,* 719-725.

[79] Peacock, C.D., Watkins, D.N. (2008) Cancer stem cells and the ontogeny of lung cancer. *J Clin Oncol, 26,* 2883-2889.

[80] Lemjabbar-Alaoui, H., Dasari, V., Sidhu, S.S., Mengistab, A., Finkbeiner, W., Gallup, M., *et al.* (2006) Wnt and Hedgehog are critical mediators of cigarette smoke-induced lung cancer. *PLoS ONE, 1,* e93.

[81] Alison, M.R., Islam, S. (2009) Attributes of adult stem cells. *J Pathol, 217,* 144-160.

[82] Polakis, P. (2000) Wnt signaling and cancer. *Genes Dev, 14,* 1837-1851.

[83] Reya, T., Clevers, H. (2005) Wnt signalling in stem cells and cancer. *Nature, 434,* 843-850.

[84] Valk-Lingbeek, M.E., Bruggenman, S.W.M., van Lohuizen, M. (2004) Stem cell and cancer: poly-comb connection. *Cell, 118,* 409-418.

[85] Dovey, J.S., Zacharek, S.J., Kim, C.F., Lees, J.A. (2008) Bmi1 is critical for lung tumorigenesis and bronchioalveolar stem cell expansion. *Proc Natl Acad Sci USA. 105,* 11857-11862.

[86] Ovitt, C.E., Schöler, H.R. (1998) The molecular biology of Oct-4 in the early mouse embryo. *Mol Hum Reprod, 4,* 1021-1031.

[87] Basak, S.K., Veena, M.S., Oh, S., Huang, G., Srivatsan, E., Huang, M., Sharma, S., Batra, R.K. (2009) The malignant pleural effusion as a model to investigate intratumoral heterogeneity in lung cancer. *PLoS One, 4,* e5884.

[88] Collins, A.T., Berry, P.A., Hyde, C., Stower, M.J., Maitland, N.J. (2005) Prospective identification of tumorigenic prostate cancer stem cells. *Cancer Res, 65,* 10946-10951.

[89] Annabi, B., Lachambre, M.P., Plouffe, K., Sartelet, H., Béliveau, R. (2009) Modulation of invasive properties of CD133(+) glioblastoma stem cells: a role for MT1-MMP in bioactive lysophospholipid signaling. *Mol Carcinog, 48,* 910-919.

[90] Li, L., Neaves, W.B. (2006) Normal stem cells and cancer stem cells: the niche matters. *Cancer Res, 66,* 4553-4557.

[91] Hilbe, W., Dirnhofer, S., Oberwasserlechner, F., Schmid, T., Gunsilius, E., Hilbe, G., *et al.* (2004) CD133 positive endothelial progenitor cells contribute to the tumour vasculature in non-small cell lung cancer. *J Clin Pathol, 57,* 965-969.

[92] Moreb, J.S., Baker, H.V., Chang, L.J., Amaya, M., Lopez, M.C., Ostmark, B., Chou, W. (2008) ALDH isozymes downregulation affects cell growth, cell motility and gene expression in lung cancer cells. *Mol Cancer, 7*, 87.

[93] Moreb, J.S., Zucali, J.R., Ostmark, B., Benson, N.A. (2007) Heterogeneity of aldehyde dehydrogenase expression in lung cancer cell lines is revealed by Aldefluor flow cytometry-based assay. *Cytometry B Clin Cytom, 72,* 281-9.

[94] Moreb, J.S. (2008) Aldehyde dehydrogenase as a marker for stem cells. *Curr Stem Cell Res Ther, 3,* 237-46.

[95] Ucar, D., Cogle, C.R., Zucali, J.R., Ostmark, B., Scott, E.W., Zori, R., *et al.* (2009) Aldehyde dehydrogenase activity as a functional marker for lung cancer. *Chem Biol Interact, 178,* 48-55.

[96] Patel, M., Lu, L., Zander, D.S., Sreerama, L., Coco, D., Moreb, J.S. (2008) ALDH1A1 and ALDH3A1 expression in lung cancers: correlation with histologic type and potential precursors. *Lung Cancer, 59,* 340-349.

[97] Carpentino, J.E., Hynes, M.J., Appelman, H.D., Zheng, T., Steindler, D.A., Scott, E.W., Huang, E.H. (2008) Aldehyde dehydrogenase-expressing colon stem cells contribute to tumorigenesis in the transition from colitis to cancer. *Cancer Res, 69,* 8208-8215.

[98] Christ, O., Lucke, K., Imren, S., Leung, K., Hamilton, M., Eaves, A., Smith, C., Eaves, C. (2007) Improved purification of hematopoietic stem cells based on their elevated aldehyde dehydrogenase activity. *Haematologica, 92,* 1165-1172.

[99] Sisson, J.H. (2007) Alcohol and airways function in health and disease. *Alcohol, 41,* 293-307.

[100] Moriwaki, Y., Yamamoto, T., Higashino, K. (1997) Distribution and pathophysiologic role of molybdenum-containing enzymes. *Histol Histopathol, 12,* 513-524.

[101] Yin SJ. Alcohol dehydrogenase: enzymology and metabolism. Alcohol Alcohol Suppl. 1994;2:113-9.

[102] Cozens, A.L., Yezzi, M.J., Kunzelmann, K., Ohrui, T., Chin, L., Eng, K., Finkbeiner, W.E., Widdicombe, J.H., Gruenert, D.C. CFTR expression and chloride secretion in polarized immortal human bronchial epithelial cells. *Am J Respir Cell Mol Biol, 10,* 38-47.

[103] Masuda, A., Kondo, M., Saito, T., Yatabe, Y., Kobayashi, T., Okamoto, M., Suyama, M., Takahashi, T., Takahashi, T. (1997) Establishment of human peripheral lung epithelial cell lines (HPL1) retaining differentiated characteristics and responsiveness to epidermal growth factor, hepatocyte growth factor, and transforming growth factor β1. *Cancer Res, 57,* 4898-4904.

[104] Okudela, K., Hayashi, H., Ito, T., Yazawa, T., Suzuki, T., Nakane, Y., Sato, H., Ishi, H., KeQin, X., Masuda, A., Takahashi, T., Kitamura, H. (2004) K-ras gene mutation enhances motility of immortalized airway cells and lung adenocarcinoma cells via Akt activation: possible contribution to non-invasive expansion of lung adenocarcinoma. *Am J Pathol, 164,* 91-100.

[105] Deshusses JM, Burgess JA, Scherl A, Wenger Y, Walter N, Converset V, Paesano S, Corthals GL, Hochstrasser DF, Sanchez JC. (2003) Exploitation of specific properties of trifluoroethanol for extraction and separation of membrane proteins. *Proteomics, 3,* 1418-1424.

[106] Zhan X, Desiderio DM. (2003) Spot volume vs. amount of protein loaded onto a gel: a detailed, statistical comparison of two gel electrophoresis systems. *Electrophoresis, 24,* 1818-1833.

In: Stem Cell Research: New Developments
Editors: Hiroshi Tanaka and Michael C. F. Chang
ISBN: 978-1-61942-081-6

Chapter 9

STEM CELLS IN HEAD AND NECK CANCER: A KEY TO THE FUTURE?

Chiara Bianchini[1], Andrea Ciorba[1], Roberta Piva[2], Stefano Pelucchi[1] and Antonio Pastore[1]
[1]ENT Department, University Hospital of Ferrara, Italy
[2]Department of Biochemistry and Molecular Biology, University of Ferrara, Italy

ABSTRACT

The biology of stem cells and their properties have already been recognized as integral to tumour pathogenesis in several types of cancer. A role for stem cells has been demonstrated, so far, for the hematopoietic system diseases, as well as for several solid tumours such as breast, brain and lung cancer. There is a rising interest in the field of oncology in order to understand if cancer stem cells can play a key role also in the pathogenesis of head and neck tumours. It is likely that cancer stem cells are a minor population of tumour cells that possess the stem cell property of self-renewal. The evidence that the development of a tumour comes from a small number of cells with stem-like characteristic, could bring to the identification of therapies against these cellular targets, fundamental for maintenance and progression of the lesion. This new model for cancer will have significant implications for the way we will study and treat tumours.

Head and neck cancer is still the sixth most common cancer type worldwide. Disappointingly, despite significant advances in surgical and other treatments that enhance quality of life, survival rates have only moderately improved during the last 20 years.

Aim of this chapter is to discuss among this new model of cancerogenesis.

INTRODUCTION

Understanding the biological mechanisms of cancer development and spreading, represents a primary purpose in order to eradicate the disease. In the last years, the existence as well as the pathological meaning of cancer stem cells has been matter of discussion and a large number of articles have been published about the role that these cells play in the development and maintenance of the tumours. Cancer stem cells are neoplastic cells which have stem features such as self-renewal, high migration capacity, drug resistance, high proliferation abilities.

The existence of cancer stem cells has been supported by numerous researches. In specific tumor models such as acute myeloid leukemia, it has been demonstrated that definite cellular subsets express antigenic markers similar to hematopoietic stem cells, showing clonogenic activity (Lapidot et al. T, 1994; Bonnet D et al, 1997; Graziano A et al 2008). Nonetheless, it has been reported that cells with staminal properties (such as high proliferation rate, ability of expansion and growth in tissue environments different from the original one) could reside also in solid tumours built by heterogeneous cellular populations (Reya et al., 2001; Graziano A et al 2008).

Particularly, it seems to be evidence of stem-like cells within solid tumors of brain, lung, breast, ovarian, prostate, colon cancer and also larynx (Dontu G et al., 2005; Graziano A et al 2008; Ferrandina G et al 2009; Li CY et al, 2009; McDonald SA, et al 2009; Tirino V, et al 2009; Ailles L et al 2009; Wei XD et al 2009). Therefore, the development of a tumour seems related to the growth and to the spreading of a small cluster of cells with stem-like characteristic. In the future, only the comprehension of the biology of these cell types could provide specific therapeutic targets, in order to hamper cancer progression.

Head and neck cancer is still the sixth most common cancer type worldwide. Disappointingly, despite significant advances in surgical and other treatments that enhance quality of life, survival rates have only moderately improved during the last 20 years (Braakhuis BJ et al 2005; Forastiere A et al 2001). Moreover, head and neck cancer has a severe impact on patients' quality of life and the significant morbidity subsequent to treatment often require long term multidisciplinary care (Bianchini C et al 2008).

Concerning Stem Cells and Cancer Cells

One key feature of cancer cells is their unlimited cell division capacity, reminiscent of the self-renewing proliferation of stem cells. However, there are differences that set cancer cells apart from stem cells. Firstly, the self-renewing mechanism in stem cells responds to a feedback system that senses the number of mature cells and regulates the rate of division, whereas in cancer cells this feedback mechanism is disrupted. Secondly, high-grade tumour cells lack the ability to properly differentiate into mature cells, suggesting aberrant differentiation programs. Thus, only understanding the molecular differences between stem cells and cancer cells may help provide us with new insights into the mechanism of tumorogenesis (Bianchini C et al 2008; Cabanillas R et al 2009; Graziano A et al 2008; Zhou ZT et al 2008).

At the molecular level, some recent studies have evidenced that maintenance of stem cells and tumour cells may involve some common pathways (Pardal R et al 2005). One example is the polycomb gene bmi-1. In mice, this gene was recently shown to be essential for maintaining both the hematopoietic stem cell state as well as the leukemic activity (Lessard J, et al 2003). Also Wnt signaling cascade as well as sonic hedgehog (Shh) have been reported to be involved in both neoplastic tissue/cell maintenance and tumorigenesis (Polakis P 2000; Reya T el al 2003; Watkins DN et al 2003).

Isolation of Cancer Stem Cells to Study the Biology of the Tumour

So far, rare subpopulations of cancer stem cells have been identified for leukemia and other solid tumours (Lapidot et al. T, 1994; Bonnet D et al, 1997). Within these tumours, these rare fractions of cancer stem cells are in large part responsible for maintaining the tumour mass, as they have the capacity to self-renew and to generate a high number of progeny via differentiation program.

Recent studies of cell lines derived from oral squamous cell carcinoma indicate the presence of subpopulations of cells with phenotypic and behavioral characteristics corresponding to both normal epithelial stem cells and to cells capable of initiating tumours in vivo (Costea et al., 2006; Chiou SH et al 2008).

Recently, also in human laryngeal tumours, chinese investigators have characterized a cluster of CD 133+ stem cells of the Hep-2 cell line, suggesting that this subset population could own a strong selected tumorigenic ability (Wei XD et al 2009). A population of highly malignant cells in a head and neck squamous cell carcinoma cell line has also been established from primary head and neck tumours using sequential rounds of xenotransplantation. These cells named SASVO3, possess enhanced tumorigenic ability both in vitro and in vivo; it has been reported that SASVO3 cells exhibits properties of cancer stem cells, including increased abilities of sphere-forming, potential of transplanted tumor growth and elevated expression of stem cell markers such as Bmi1 (Chen CY et al 2009).

Cancer Progression: A "Staminal" Point of View

For cancer development it has been proposed that, a stem cell acquires one (or more) genetic alterations, and forms an area in the mucosal epithelium with genetically altered daughter cells. As cancer stem cells escape the normal control mechanisms and gain growth advantage, the patch starts to expand developing a malignant clone (Bianchini C et al 2008).

Hirata offered a specific point of view concerning this topic. In his papers he supports the idea that carcinoma progression originates in the "hetero-duplication mitosis" that divides non-maturable stem cells into two different types of daughter cells: maturable and non-maturable cancerous stem cells. The divided nonmaturable daughter stem cell, repeats the original mitosis while reproducing the above two types of daughter stem cells, thus continuing hetero-duplication mitotic progression of the cancer. The maturable daughter cells become terminally mature cancer cells (Hirata Y 1999).

The application of these stem cell concepts could explain many important neoplastic features including the clonal origin and heterogeneity of tumours, the occasional formation of tumours from the transit amplifying cells or progenitor cells, the formation of precancerous ''patches'' as well as the concept of "field cancerization". Slaughter firstly proposed this term in order to describe a situation in which: (1) oral cancer develops in multifocal areas of precancerous change; (2) histologically abnormal tissue surrounds the tumour; (3) oral cancer often consists of multiple independent lesions that sometimes coalesce; and (4) the persistence of abnormal tissue after surgery may explain second primary tumours and local recurrences (Slaughter DP et al 1953). Since the Slaughter proposal, within head and neck cancers, many investigators have found cancer cells associated to genetic alterations in tumour adjacent macroscopically normal tissue and surgical margins (Braakhuis BJ et al 2005). Analyses of loss of heterozygosity, microsatellite instability, chromosomal instability and mutations in the p53 gene have been used to detect these alterations and to identify a "field at risk" (Bianchini C et al 2008; Braakhuis BJ et al 2005; Hittelman WN, 2001; Cheng ZG, 2009).

These observations may lead to consider that also head and neck tumours should originate from aberrant stem cells, and that carcinogenesis should be considered as a multistep process, in which an accumulation of genetic and epigenetic alterations forms the basis for the progression from a normal cell to a cancer one.

Gene Expression and Markers of Head and Neck Cancer Stem Cells

Understanding the molecular biology of cancer stem cells would help not only in identifying the mechanism of tumorogenesis, but could also offer the possibility to detect cellular indicators of malignant conversion and progression, thus helping in early identification of cancer stem cells in a specific tissue. This could represent a powerful tool for early diagnosis of particular interest for clinical practice.

So far, only very few "staminal markers" have been identified in head and neck tumours (see also Table 1). Particularly in head and neck squamous cell carcinomas, cells expressing specific antigens, such as the surface CD 44+, as well as high levels of nuclear BMI1, have been reported to be capable of initiating tumor growth and to be involved in the spreading (Ailles L et al 2009). Also Aldehyde dehydrogenase 1 (ALDH1) has been considered as a marker for cancer stem cells. Even if the role of ALDH1 in head and neck squamous cell carcinoma has yet to be determined, it has been reported that ALDH1+ cells displayed radioresistance and represented a reservoir for tumor growth (Chen YC et al 2009; Clay MR et al 2010). In the same way, also in nasopharingeal cell lines at least two genes, gp96 and GDF15, have been described to be involved in radioresistance as it has been reported that knockdown of these genes enhances radiosensitivity (Chang JT et al 2007).

Sterz CM et al, using immunohistochemical analysis, found antigens CD44 and MMP-9 to co-localize tumour cells at the invasive front within head and neck squamous cell carcinomas; particularly at the western blot analysis they pointed to a role of a MMP-9 positive basal-cell-like cell layer in the process of HNSCC invasiveness (Sterz CM et al, 2009).

Table 1. Putative markers in Head and Neck Cancers

Markers	Tumour Type	References
CD 133+	Squamous Cell Carcinoma	Wei XD et al 2009
CD 44+	Squamous Cell Carcinoma	Ailles L et al 2009
ALDH1	Squamous Cell Carcinoma	Chen YC et al 2009; Clay MR et al 2010
MPP-9	Squamous Cell Carcinoma	Sterz CM et al, 2009
GDF 15	Nasopharyngeal Carcinoma	Chang JT et al 2007

Conclusion

It is likely that stem cell biology already had an impact in the cancer research field since it seems increasingly evident that cancer can be considered a stem-cell disorder. The stem-cell model for cancer probably could have an impact also on the identification of future therapeutic targets.

Particularly, in a near future, among head and neck tumours will be necessary to (1) further elucidate the critical molecular events involved in head and neck carcinogenesis, and (2) identify possible cellular/molecular markers or cellular site of intervention.

Acknowledgments

The oncological project of the ENT Clinic and of the Molecular Biology Section at the University of Ferrara is also supported by a grant for scientific research from the CARIFE Foundation and by a grant for scientific research from the University of Ferrara and the Emilia Romagna Region.

References

Ailles L, Prince M. Cancer stem cells in head and neck squamous cell carcinoma. *Methods Mol Biol.* 2009;568:175-93.

Bianchini C, Ciorba A, Pelucchi S, Piva R, Pastore A. Head and neck cancer: the possible role of stem cells. *Eur Arch Otorhinolaryngol.* 2008 Jan;265(1):17-20.

Bonnet D, Dick JE. 1997. Human acute myeloid leukemia is organized as a hierarchy that originates from a primitive hematopoietic cell. *Nat Med 3*:730–737.

Braakhuis BJ, Leemans CR, BrakenhoV RH (2005) Expanding fields of genetically altered cells in head and neck squamous carcinogenesis. *Semin Cancer Biol 15*:113–120

Cabanillas R, Llorente JL. The Stem Cell Network model: clinical implications in cancer. *Eur Arch Otorhinolaryngol.* 2009 Feb;266(2):161-70.

Chang JT, Chan SH, Lin CY, Lin TY, Wang HM, Liao CT, Wang TH, Lee LY, Cheng AJ. Differentially expressed genes in radioresistant nasopharyngeal cancer cells: gp96 and GDF15. *Mol Cancer Ther.* 2007 Aug;6(8):2271-9.

Chen CY, Chiou SH, Huang CY, Jan CI, Lin SC, Tsai ML, Lo JF. Distinct population of highly malignant cells in a head and neck squamous cell carcinoma cell line established by xenograft model. *J Biomed Sci*. 2009 Nov 16;16:100.

Chen YC, Chen YW, Hsu HS, Tseng LM, Huang PI, Lu KH, Chen DT, Tai LK, Yung MC, Chang SC, Ku HH, Chiou SH, Lo WL. Aldehyde dehydrogenase 1 is a putative marker for cancer stem cells in head and neck squamous cancer. *Biochem Biophys Res Commun*. 2009 Jul 31;385(3):307-13.

Chen ZG. The cancer stem cell concept in progression of head and neck cancer. *J Oncol*. 2009;2009:894064. Epub 2009 Dec 3.

Chiou SH, Yu CC, Huang CY, Lin SC, Liu CJ, Tsai TH, Chou SH, Chien CS, Ku HH, Lo JF. Positive correlations of Oct-4 and Nanog in oral cancer stem-like cells and high-grade oral squamous cell carcinoma. *Clin Cancer Res*. 2008 Jul 1;14(13):4085-95.

Clay MR, Tabor M, Owen JH, Carey TE, Bradford CR, Wolf GT, Wicha MS, Prince ME. Single-marker identification of head and neck squamous cell carcinoma cancer stem cells with aldehyde dehydrogenase. *Head Neck*. 2010 Jan 13.

Costea DE, Tsinkalovsky O, Vintermyr OK, Johannessen AC, Mackenzie IC. 2006. Cancer stem cells—new and potentially important targets for the therapy of oral squamous cell carcinoma. *Oral Dis 12*:443–454.

Dontu G, Liu S, Wicha MS. 2005. Stem cells in mammary development and carcinogenesis: Implications for prevention and treatment. *Stem Cell Rev 1*:207–213.

Ferrandina G, Martinelli E, Petrillo M, Prisco MG, Zannoni G, Sioletic S, Scambia G. CD133 antigen expression in ovarian cancer. *BMC Cancer*. 2009 Jul 7;9(1):221.

Forastiere A, Koch W, Trotti A, Sidransky D (2001) Medical progress–head and neck cancer. *N Engl J Med 345*:1890–1900

Graziano A, d'Aquino R, Tirino V, Desiderio V, Rossi A, Pirozzi G. The stem cell hypothesis in head and neck cancer. *J Cell Biochem*. 2008 Feb 1;103(2):408-12.

Hirata Y (1999) Progression of cancer. Med Hypotheses 52(6):51–13

Hittelman WN (2001) Genetic instability in epithelial tissues at risk for cancer. *Ann N Y Acad Sci 952*:1–12

Lapidot T, Sirard C, Vormoor J, Murdoch B, Hoang T, Caceres-Cortes J, Minden M, Paterson B, Caligiuri MA, Dick JE. 1994. A cell initiating human acute myeloid leukaemia after transplantation into SCIDmice. *Nature 367*:645–648.

Lessard J, Sauvageau G (2003) Bmi-1 determines the proliferative capacity of normal and leukaemic stem cells. *Nature 423*(6937):255–260

Li CY, Li BX, Liang Y, Peng RQ, Ding Y, Xu DZ, Zhang X, Pan ZZ, Wan DS, Zeng YX, Zhu XF, Zhang XS. Higher percentage of CD133+ cells is associated with poor prognosis in colon carcinoma patients with stage IIIB. *J Transl Med*. 2009 Jul 7;7(1):56.

McDonald SA, Graham TA, Schier S, Wright NA, Alison MR. Stem cells and solid cancers. *Virchows Arch*. 2009 Jul;455(1):1-13. Epub 2009 Jun 5.

Pardal R, Molofsky AV, He S, Morrison SJ (2005) Stem cell selfrenewal and cancer stem cells proliferation are regulated by common networks that balance the activation of proto-oncogenes and tumor suppressors. *Cold Spring Harb Symp Quant Biol 70*:177–185.

Polakis P (2000) Wnt signaling and cancer. *Genes Dev 14*(15):1837–1851

Reya T, Morrison SJ, Clarke MF, Weissman IL. 2001. Stem cells, cancer, and cancer stem cells. *Nature 414*:105–111.

Reya T, Duncan AW, Ailles L, Domen J, Scherer DC, Willert K, Hintz L, Nusse R, Weissman IL (2003) A role for wnt signalling in self-renewal of haematopoietic stem cells. *Nature 423*(6938):409–414

Slaughter DP, Southwick HW, Smejkal W (1953) "Field cancerization" in oral stratified squamous epithelium. *Cancer 6*:963–968

Sterz CM, Kulle C, Dakic B, Makarova G, Böttcher MC, Bette M, Werner JA, Mandic R. A basal-cell-like compartment in head and neck squamous cell carcinomas represents the invasive front of the tumor and is expressing MMP-9. *Oral Oncol.* 2010 Feb;46(2):116-22.

Tirino V, Camerlingo R, Franco R, Malanga D, La Rocca A, Viglietto G, Rocco G, Pirozzi G. The role of CD133 in the identification and characterisation of tumour-initiating cells in non-small-cell lung cancer. *Eur J Cardiothorac Surg.* 2009 May 21.

Watkins DN, Berman DM, Burkholder SG, Wang B, Beachy PA, Baylin SB (2003) Hedgehog signalling within airway epithelial progenitors and in small-cell lung cancer. *Nature 422*(6929):313– 317

Wei XD, Zhou L, Cheng L, Tian J, Jiang JJ, Maccallum J. In vivo investigation of CD133 as a putative marker of cancer stem cells in Hep-2 cell line. *Head Neck.* 2009 Jan;31(1):94-101.

Zhou ZT, Jiang WW. Cancer stem cell model in oral squamous cell carcinoma. *Curr Stem Cell Res Ther.* 2008 Jan;3(1):17-20.

In: Stem Cell Research: New Developments
Editors: Hiroshi Tanaka and Michael C. F. Chang
ISBN: 978-1-61942-081-6

Chapter 10

GENETIC AND EPIGENETIC ALTERATIONS THAT DRIVE LEUKEMIC STEM CELL SELF-RENEWAL

***Vincent van den Boom*[*]*, Sarah J. Horton*[*]**
***and Jan Jacob Schuringa*[†]**
University of Groningen, University Medical Center Groningen, Groningen, The Netherlands

ABSTRACT

Acute myeloid leukemia has emerged as a paradigm for the concept of the cancer stem cell. This hypothesis presumes that the disease is maintained by a rare population of leukemia-initiating stem cells which have acquired genetic or epigenetic changes. It is most likely that a single (epi)genetic event will not be sufficient to cause leukemia, but that a number of sequential events are required. Similar to normal hematopoietic stem cells, both intrinsic as well as extrinsic factors that arise from the bone marrow niche, provide essential cues that regulate cell fate decisions such as leukemic stem cell self-renewal and differentiation. In this chapter, we will review the genetic and epigenetic abnormalities that underlie the process of leukemic transformation, and will discuss which events potentially co-operate to induce leukemia.

INTRODUCTION

Acute myeloid leukemia (AML) arises from genetic defects in the hematopoietic stem cell (HSC). HSCs can undergo self-renewal divisions to ensure maintenance of the stem cell pool as well as generate large numbers of mature functional blood cells via migration, differentiation, proliferation and (anti-) apoptotic events. Complex processes such as self-renewal and differentiation must be tightly controlled as a shift in the balance towards self-

---

* These authors contributed equally.

† Correspondence concerning this article should be addressed to: Jan Jacob Schuringa, Tel: +31 50 3619391; Fax: +31 50 3614862; Email: j.schuringa@int.umcg.nl.

renewal severely impairs the hematopoietic process and might ultimately lead to the development of AML [1]. Thus a thorough understanding of the mechanisms involved in the regulation of self-renewal divisions of normal and leukemic stem cells are pivotal in tackling the highly malignant disorder of AML.

AML is in most cases a stem cell disease [2-4]. The malignant clone is hierarchically organized – strikingly similar to the normal hematopoietic system [5]- and consists of rare leukemic stem cells (LSC) that have the exclusive capacity to transfer disease into irradiated recipients. The more committed blast population within the leukemic clone lacks these properties. The most convincing evidence comes from transplantation studies in which the SCID leukemia-initiating cells (SL-IC) of all subtypes of AML, regardless of the heterogeneity in maturation characteristics of the leukemic blasts, resided exclusively in the immature $CD34^{+}/CD38^{-}$ compartment [2,4]. However, this finding was challenged recently by a study which demonstrated that most SL-ICs were present in the $CD34^{+}/CD38^{+}$ fraction of AML samples when the immune mediated clearance of anti-CD38 coated cells was prevented [6]. Thus a multipotent progenitor (MPP) rather than an HSC may serve as the cell of origin in some AMLs and this will be discussed in more detail in part I.

Leukemic transformation is regarded as a multistep process in which a number of sequential events ultimately induce the full spectrum of leukemia [7,8]. These transformation steps include chromosomal translocations such as t(8;21), inv(16) and t(15;17), as well as mutations in tyrosine kinase receptors (FLT3, C-KIT) or signal transduction molecules such as RAS, JAK2 and NPM1 (reviewed in [8,9]). Multiple events ultimately lead to enhanced self-renewal and differentiation defects of the LSC. A number of studies have indeed elegantly shown that oncogenes such as AML1-ETO and FLT3-ITDs do not result in leukemic transformation individually, but act synergistically when expressed within the same stem cell [7]. Furthermore, the fact that the incidence of AML increases with age (approximately half of AML patients are more than 65 years of age) further strengthens the notion that an accumulation of genetic and/or epigenetic alterations makes the stem cell compartment more prone to the development of AML. In this chapter we will review the current understanding of how genetic and epigenetic events might affect stem cell self-renewal properties and how these hits might collaborate in the process of leukemic transformation.

I. Genetic Alterations in LSCs that Affect Self-renewal and/or Differentiation

Translocations

CBF Fusion Genes

The genes encoding the heterodimeric transcription factor complex AML1/CBFβ are among the most frequently mutated in human acute leukemia. CBFβ enhances the DNA binding capacity of AML1, whose target genes play critical roles in hematopoiesis. Conditional gene targeting studies in mice have demonstrated that while both subunits are essential for fetal HSC development, CBFβ but not AML1 is essential for the maintenance of adult HSCs [10]. The most common chromosomal rearrangements involving the *AML1/CBFβ* genes are the t(8;21)(q22;q22) translocation which generates the *AML1-ETO* fusion gene and inv(16)(p13q22) which generates the *CBFβ-MYH11* fusion gene. Various mouse models have been generated in an attempt to model disease induced by these fusion proteins. A myeloproliferative disorder resulted when AML1-ETO expression was targeted to the HSC compartment using the *SCA1* promoter (Table 1, [11]). However, other AML1-ETO models did not result in the development of AML unless the animals were treated with mutagenic agents [12].

Although AML1-ETO conditional knock-in mice did not develop AML, myeloid progenitors isolated from these mice displayed enhanced re-plating potential *in vitro* [13]. Furthermore, elevated numbers of HSCs and abnormal myeloid cells were observed in the bone marrow of mice transplanted with AML1-ETO retrovirally transduced murine HSCs [14]. Retroviral delivery of AML1-ETO to human $CD34^+$ cord blood cells resulted in HSC expansion in stromal co-culture assays and enhanced proliferation in cytokine driven liquid cultures. However, transplantation of these cultured cells into NOD/SCID mice did not result in leukemia [15-17]. Taken together these studies suggest that AML1-ETO expression promotes the self-renewal of HSCs but requires co-operating mutations to induce overt leukemia.

The mechanisms by which AML1-ETO promotes the self-renewal of HSCs remain unclear although up-regulation of survivin expression may be a contributing factor [18]. The finding that the *AML1-ETO* translocation can be detected in neonatal Guthrie card spots suggests that the translocation occurs *in utero* as the initiating event and results in the generation of a pre-leukemic clone. Secondary genetic or epigenetic events are then required for the development of clinically overt leukemia [19]. A recent report found that AML1-ETO expressing cells displayed an enhanced mutation rate *in vivo* and suggested that AML1-ETO may directly facilitate the acquisition of secondary events by suppressing endogenous DNA repair pathways [20].

In contrast to AML1-ETO, CBFβ-MYH11 conditional knock-in mice spontaneously developed AML in the absence of mutagen treatment [21]. Interestingly the genes *Plag1* or *Plag2*, which were previously shown to co-operate with CBFβ-MYH11 in AML development [22], were over-expressed in many of the AML samples in this conditional model. Retroviral over-expression of CBFβ-MYH11 increased the proliferative capacity of human $CD34^+$ CB cells but did not result in leukemia upon transplantation into NOD/SCID mice [23]. These studies suggest that like AML1-ETO, expression of CBFβ-MYH11 confers a pre-leukemic status to the cells by enhancing their self-renewal. Subsequent alterations which will be discussed later on are required for the transition to overt leukemia.

Table 1. Summary of the models for the most common genetic events in myeloid leukemia

Translocations			
Gene	**Model**	**Phenotype**	**Ref.**
AML1-ETO	**Mouse** Transgenic-*Sca1*	Myeloproliferative disorder.	[11]
	Mouse Knock-in	Embryonic lethal. Abnormal myeloid cells in fetal liver with increased self-renewal potential.	[194]
	Mouse Conditional knock-in	Enhanced re-plating *in vitro*. AML upon ENU treatment.	[13]

Table 1. (Continued)

Translocations			
Gene	**Model**	**Phenotype**	**Ref.**
	Mouse Retroviral transduction	Increased numbers of abnormal cells in the BM. No AML.	[14]
	Human (CD34$^+$ CB) Retroviral transduction	Long-term proliferation *in vitro*. No AML.	[15,17]
CBFβ-SMMHC	**Mouse** Knock-in	Embryonic lethal. Lack of definitive hematopoiesis.	[195]
	Mouse Knock-in chimera	Block in myeloid and lymphoid differentiation. AML after ENU treatment.	[196]
	Mouse Conditional knock-in	AML with median latency of 5 months.	[21]
	Human (CD34+ CB) Retroviral transduction	Increased proliferation *in vitro*. No leukemia.	[23]
PML-RARα	**Mouse** Transgenic- *hCathepsin G*	Myeloproliferative disorder, low frequency of APL with long latency.	[26,27]
	Mouse Transgenic- *hMRP8*	Low frequency of APL with long latency.	[25]
	Mouse Transgenic – *hCD11b*	Slight impairment in hematopoiesis. No leukemia.	[28]
	Mouse (lin$^-$ BM) Retroviral transduction	Short latency, high penetrance APL. Impaired neutrophil differentiation.	[30]
	Human (lin$^-$ PB) Retroviral transduction	Enhanced promyelocytic differentiation but subsequent block in vitro.	[29]
NUP98-Hoxa9	**Mouse** Transgenic - *hCathepsin G*	Myeloproliferative disorder, eventual progression to AML.	[197]
	Mouse (whole BM) Retroviral transduction	Myeloproliferative disorder, eventual progression to AML.	[35]
	Human (CD34$^+$ CB) Retroviral transduction	Increased proliferation and HSC self-renewal *in vitro* and *in vivo*.	[36]
MLL-AF9	**Mouse** Knock-in	AML within 6-9 months preceded by myeloproliferation. Small number of ALL cases.	[198,199]
	Mouse (cKit$^+$ BM) Retroviral transduction	Myeloid immortalisation *in vitro*, AML *in vivo*.	[42]
	Human (Lin$^-$ CB) Retroviral transduction	Enhanced proliferation *in vitro*. ALL upon transplantation into NOD/SCID mice.	[43]
	Human (CD34$^+$ CB) Retroviral transduction	Immortalisation *in vitro*. AML or ALL *in vivo*.	[44]
MLL-ENL	**Mouse** Translocator	Rapid AML within 4 months.	[48]
	Mouse (Lin$^-$ BM) Retroviral transduction	Myeloid immortalisation *in vitro*, AML *in vivo*.	[41]
BCR-ABL (p210)	**Human** (Lin$^-$ CB) Retroviral transduction	Enhanced proliferation in vitro. ALL in NOD/SCID mice.	[43]
	Mouse Transgenic - *metallothionein*	T, B or myeloid acute leukemia	[200,201]
	Mouse Transgenic - *Tec*	ALL in founder mice. CML in transgenic progeny.	[202]
	Mouse Transgenic inducible (Tet-Off system)	Acute pre-B cell leukemia reversible upon tetracycline treatment.	[203]
	Mouse Transgenic-*Sca1*	CML with longer latency (4-18 months). Progression to either myeloid or lymphoid blast crisis.	[59]
	Mouse (whole BM) Retroviral transduction	CML with short latency and high penetrance. T lymphoid lymphoma or CML in secondarys.	[56,57]
	Human (Lin$^-$ CB) Retroviral transduction	Enhanced erythroid differentiation *in vitro*, myeloproliferative disease *in vivo*.	[58,204]

Translocations			
Gene	**Model**	**Phenotype**	**Ref.**
CEBPα	**Mouse** N-terminal knock-in mutant (p42 deficient)	AML with complete penetrance. Latency 6 months – 1 year.	[74]
	Mouse Knock-in mutant chimeras	C-terminal mutant: Immature erythroid leukemia. N-terminal mutant: AML with shorter latency than C-terminal. Combined mutants: AML with shorter latency than either mutant alone.	[75]
	Mouse (Lin- BM) Retroviral transduction N-terminal mutant	Altered kinetics but no differentiation block *in vitro*.	[205]
	Human (CD34+ CB) Retroviral transduction N-terminal mutant	Block in differentiation at abnormal promyelocytic stage *in vitro*.	[205]
FLT3-ITD	**Mouse** Knock-in	Fatal myeloproliferative disorder. Median latency 10 months.	[82]
	Mouse (BM) Retroviral transduction	Lethal myeloproliferative disorder. Latency 40 – 60 days.	[81]
	Human ($CD34^+$ CB) Retroviral transduction	Enhanced proliferation and self-renewal *in vitro*.	[83]
Flt3-TKD	**Mouse** (BM) Retroviral transduction	Lymphoid disease with long latency. T cell lymphoma or B-ALL.	[88]
$cKit^{V814}$	**Mouse** Transgenic – $H\text{-}2L^d$	ALL or lymphoma in 4/15 mice.	[89]
	Mouse (BM) Retroviral transduction.	Factor-independent growth *in vitro*. Lymphoid leukemia *in vivo*. Latency 6-19 weeks.	[89]
$NPMc^+$	**Mouse** Transgenic – *hMRP8*	Non-fatal myeloproliferative disease from 6 months of age.	[93]
$KRas^{G12D}$	**Mouse** Conditional Knock-in	Fatal myeloproliferative disorder with complete penetrance.	[99]
	Mouse – Conditional knock-in. BM chimeras.	T cell malignancies and JMML depending on cell dosage used.	[103]
$KRas^{G12D}$	**Mouse** (BM) Retroviral transduction	CMML. Median latency 64 days.	[97]
$NRas^{G12D}$	**Mouse** (BM) Retroviral transduction	AML (latency 49.5 days) or CMML (latency 62.5 days).	[97]
$NRAS^{G13C}$	**Human** ($CD34^+$ CB) Retroviral transduction	Enhanced myeloid proliferation and monocytic differentiation *in vitro* and *in vivo*.	[98]

RARα Fusion Genes

The promyelocytic leukemia – retinoic acid receptor alpha (PML-RARα) fusion protein, which is expressed as a result of the t(15;17)(q22;q21) translocation, is found in > 95% of cases of acute promyelocytic leukemia (APL). Unlike other types of AML in which disease is thought to originate from an HSC, numerous studies suggest that APL arises from a committed progenitor. This theory is supported by the lack of PML-RARα expression in the HSC ($CD34^+CD38^-$) compartment isolated from APL patients [24] and the inability of these cells to transplant leukemia into NOD/SCID mice [2].

Transgenic mice in which PML-RARα expression was driven from promoters expressed during the myeloid- promyelocytic stages of differentiation (*Cathepsin G* and *MRP8*), developed APL after long latency and low penetrance [25-27]. In contrast, mice in which PML-RARα expression was directed from a promoter expressed at a later stage of myeloid differentiation (*CD11b*), did not develop leukemia [28]. These studies highlight the importance of proper targeting of PML-RARα expression. The hMRP8-PML-RARα transgenic mice displayed a pre-leukemic phase which was associated with impaired neutrophil differentiation [25]. Impaired differentiation was also observed upon retroviral delivery of PML-RARα expression to both murine and human hematopoietic stem and progenitor cells (HSPCs) [29,30]. In contrast to the transgenic mice, the murine transduction/ transplantation model gave rise to short latency APL with high penetrance. It is possible that retroviral insertional mutagenesis rapidly met the requirement for co-operating mutations in this model. Alternatively, the targeting of PML-RARα expression to more primitive hematopoietic progenitor cells rather than committed myeloid cells may explain the difference in penetrance and latencies.

The mechanism underlying the differentiation block induced by PML-RARα has been the subject of intense investigations. Both wild-type retinoic acid receptor (RARα) and PML-RARα mediate the transcriptional repression of retinoic acid (RA) target genes by binding the nuclear co-repressors NCOR and SMRT which recruit histone deacetylases (HDACs) – these are described in more detail in part II. During normal myeloid differentiation, physiological concentrations of retinoic acid (RA) induce the dissociation of the co-repressors and associated HDACs from RARα allowing the recruitment of transcriptional activators and normal myeloid differentiation. However, physiological concentrations of RA do not permit the dissociation of co-repressors and HDACs from the PML-RARα complex thus resulting in a block in differentiation [31]. This block is alleviated by higher concentrations of RA which is used in the clinic in combination with chemotherapy to achieve remission in the majority of patients.

Many AML cells exhibit enhanced survival upon genotoxic stress yet do not carry mutations of the *p53* tumour suppressor gene. In many cases the leukemic cells have acquired more subtle ways to inhibit p53 function. For example, the PML-RARα fusion protein retains the ability to interact with the product of the remaining wild-type *PML* allele which normally associates with p53. Recruitment of p53 to the PML-RARα/HDAC complex results in the inhibition of p53 acetylation and subsequent inactivation [32]. An alternative mechanism is proposed for AMLs with the t(8;21) translocation in which AML1-ETO has been shown to directly repress transcription of the p53 checkpoint mediator *p14ARF* [33].

NUP98 Fusion Genes

The *NUP98* gene undergoes reciprocal chromosomal translocations with many other partner genes and is hence one of the most promiscuous fusion partner genes in leukemia. *NUP98*-fusion genes are found in patients with AML, myelodysplastic syndrome, or blast crisis CML [34]. The *NUP98* nucleoporin gene encodes an important component of the nuclear pore complex. To date 21 fusion partners of NUP98 have been described of which the most common and extensively studied is NUP98-Hoxa9. Retroviral transduction of murine HSPCs with NUP98-HOXA9 enhanced the proliferation of myeloid progenitors *in vitro* and induced a myeloproliferative disorder *in vivo* which eventually progressed to AML. The latency of AML progression was markedly decreased upon co-expression of MEIS1 which also co-operates with wild-type HOXA9 to induce AML [35]. Retroviral transduction of human $CD34^+$ cells with NUP98-HOXA9 enhanced HSC proliferation and expansion *in vitro* and *in vivo*. Impaired neutrophil differentiation in response to G-CSF was also observed [36]. Gene expression profiling revealed that the Hox genes *Hoxa7*, *Hoxa9* and their co-factor *Meis1*, well recognized for their ability to induce AML in animal models [37], were upregulated upon NUP98-HOXA9 expression in both murine and human models [36,38]. Several genes including *CEBPα* were also down-regulated upon NUP98-HOXA9 expression in human CD34^{+} cells. Interestingly, restoration of *CEBPα* expression impaired the proliferation of NUP98-HOXA9 transduced cells suggesting that down-modulation of *CEBPα* expression by this fusion protein contributes to enhanced HSC proliferation and impaired differentiation [36]. A recent study using a transgenic Notch reporter mouse very elegantly demonstrated that NUP98-HOXA9 enhanced HSC self-renewal by increasing the number of HSCs undergoing symmetrical cell divisions. In contrast, the *BCR-ABL* fusion gene promoted proliferation but did not alter the ratio of symmetric versus asymmetric cell division [39].

MLL Fusion Genes

Like many of the genes involved in chromosomal translocations in acute leukemia, MLL plays an important role in normal hematopoietic development and is essential for definitive hematopoiesis [40]. Over 50 fusion partner genes of *MLL* have been identified so far of which the most common are *AF9*, *ENL* and *AF4*. Immortalized myeloid cell lines were efficiently generated following retroviral transduction of murine HSPCs with either MLL-ENL or MLL-AF9. Retrovirally transduced cells were able to induce AML with short latency and high penetrance upon transfer into mice [41,42]. Both fusion proteins were also able to enhance the proliferation of human cord blood cells and induce ALL upon transplantation into NOD/SCID mice [43]. However, the skew towards ALL in this model did not faithfully recapitulate the disease in humans. In patients the *MLL-ENL* fusion gene is found in both acute myeloid and lymphoid leukemia, while *MLL-AF9* is primarily associated with myeloid leukemia. Another study using human cord blood cells demonstrated that MLL-AF9 was able to give rise to either AML or ALL and this depended on the recipient strain of mice. AML was observed if the cells were transplanted into NOD/SCID-SGM3 (which are engineered to produce human SCF, GM-SCF and IL3) and ALL was observed if the mice were transplanted into NOD/SCID/β2m$^{-/-}$ mice [44]. These results suggest that the microenvironment plays an important role in the lineage of the leukemia.

Retroviral delivery of MLL-ENL to purified populations of murine HSCs, committed myeloid progenitors (CMPs) or granulocyte-macrophage progenitors (GMPs) followed by transplantation into recipient mice resulted in AML from all three populations [45]. This study demonstrated that MLL-fusions are able to impose self-renewal activity on committed progenitors which normally lack this ability. Using an MLL-AF9 retroviral transduction/ transplantation model LSCs were identified which shared the same phenotype as the GMP from which they arose and expressed a self-renewal signature normally only observed in HSCs [46]. However, a recent study using MLL-AF9 'knock-in' mice in which MLL-AF9 expression was directed from the endogenous *MLL* promoter revealed that physiological levels of MLL-AF9 expression were not sufficient to transform GMPs [47].

The inter-chromosomal recombination model is perhaps the most elegant model to study the role of chromosomal translocations in leukemia. Gene targeting in mice was used to engineer *loxP* sites into the murine *MLL* and *ENL* loci. When these mice were crossed with *Lmo2-Cre* mice, the *de novo* translocation of *MLL* and *ENL* loci occurred specifically in hematopoietic cells and resulted in the generation of both reciprocal translocation products. The resultant MLL-ENL translocator mice developed AML rapidly within 4 months of birth suggesting that secondary alterations are not required in this model [48].

The models described above indicate that MLL-fusions promote the proliferation and self-renewal of hematopoietic progenitor cells. The mechanisms by which MLL-fusion proteins transform cells remain elusive although *HOX* genes and their associated co-factors play an important role. Multiple *HOXA* genes, the HOX co-factors *MEIS1* and *PBX3* and *FLT3* are up-regulated in patients with MLL translocations [49]. Several studies have shown that both wild-type MLL and MLL-fusion proteins directly regulate the expression of a subset of 5'*HoxA* genes [50-52]. Recent studies have shown that both HOXA9 and MEIS1 are required for the maintenance of immortalisation by MLL-fusion proteins and loss of expression of either gene induces growth arrest, apoptosis or differentiation of leukemic or immortalised cells [53-55].

BCR-ABL

The p210 BCR-ABL fusion protein is expressed as a result of the t(9;22)(q34;q11) chromosomal translocation. This translocation is found in the vast majority of CML patients and results in the generation of a constitutively active tyrosine kinase. Many murine retroviral transduction/

transplantation models have been described which model the human disease with variable efficiency. Most of the studies demonstrated that BCR-ABL expression was sufficient to induce CML with a very short latency in recipient mice [56,57]. However, these studies were not very efficient at modeling the progression to myeloid blast crisis, which is eventually observed in CML patients if left untreated. Retroviral transduction of human Lin^- cord blood cells with BCR-ABL resulted in enhanced erythroid differentiation *in vitro* and a low incidence of myeloproliferative disease upon transplantation into NOD/SCID/$\beta 2m^{-/-}$ mice [58]. Targeting of BCR-ABL expression to the HSC compartment using the Sca1 promoter resulted in the most faithful model of CML so far although in this model BCR-ABL expression was limited to HSCs and was not expressed in more mature cells [59]. These mice developed CML with relatively long latency which progressed to either myeloid or lymphoid blast crisis. The CML cells from these mice displayed genomic instability as previously reported in CML patient samples [60]. Interestingly, the CML was reversible upon elimination of LSCs thus providing proof that elimination of LSCs is of therapeutic benefit [59].

It is assumed that transition to blast crisis is associated with the acquisition of secondary events. In support of this, activation of the Wnt signaling pathway through increased nuclear localization of β-catenin was observed in patients with accelerated phase and blast crisis CML. Furthermore, activation of the Wnt pathway endowed granulocyte-macrophage progenitors (GMPs) isolated from CML patients with self-renewal activity [61]. Although there are multiple lines of evidence to suggest that CML arises as a result of BCR-ABL expression in an HSC [62,63], this data suggests that during disease progression to blast crisis the LSC may evolve from an HSC to a GMP as a result of secondary genetic or epigenetic events. The study outlined previously by Wu et al showed that BCR-ABL acts to enhance proliferation rather than self-renewal of HSCs. Several studies showed that the Stat5 transcription factor is an important mediator of this effect [64-67]. In addition to STAT5, BCR-ABL is known to regulate several other signaling networks including RAS, ERK and CRKL [68]. In addition, RAC and Hedgehog signaling play an important part in leukemogenesis mediated by BCR-ABL. BCR-ABL hyper-activates RAC1 and RAC2 and both genes are required for BCR-ABL induced CML in mouse models [69]. Loss of

Smoothened, an important component of the Hedgehog pathway also impairs CML induction by BCR-ABL [70].

Point Mutations/Insertions

CEBPα

AML patients without detectable chromosomal aberrations often harbor point mutations or insertions/deletions involving *CEBPα*, *FLT3*, *cKIT* or *NPM*. CEBPα is a transcription factor required for the CMP-GMP transition in normal hematopoiesis [71]. It is translated into two major polypeptides of 42 kDa (p42) and 30 kDa (p30) due to alternative translation initiation. Two major groups of *CEBPα* mutations are observed in AML; N-terminal and C-terminal mutations. Leukemic cells often possess mutations in both alleles of *CEBPα*; 1 allele harbors an N-terminal mutation and the other a C-terminal mutation [72]. Homozygous N- or C- terminal mutations are almost never observed in AML suggesting that there is selection for both types of mutation during leukemic progression. N-terminal mutations cause a frame shift leading to loss of the p42 isoform whereas C-terminal mutations involve insertions/deletions within the DNA binding domain of CEBPα [73]. The N-terminal mutation was very elegantly modeled by engineering the mouse *Cebp* locus to only express the p30 isoform. These mice uniformly developed AML within 1 year of birth. Interestingly, committed myeloid cells were capable of transferring disease to secondary recipients in this model implying that the CEBPα mutant confers self-renewal to this population [74]. The *Cebp* locus was also modified such that only the C-terminal CEBPα mutation was expressed. Since *CEBPα* mutations often result in embryonic lethality the combined effects of both N- and C-terminal mutations were studied in chimeric mice. Mice engrafted with fetal liver cells expressing only the C-terminal CEBPα mutation displayed an expansion of pre-malignant HSCs and developed leukemia which had an immature erythroid phenotype and a longer latency than chimeric mice expressing only the N-terminal mutation. Chimeric mice engrafted with cells expressing both N- and C-terminal mutations developed AML more rapidly than mice expressing either mutation alone suggesting that these mutations co-operate in AML progression [75]. Other mutations also result in the de-regulation of CEBPα function. The NUP98-HOXA9 and AML1-ETO fusion proteins down-regulate its expression [36,76]. Also PML-RARα can bind to CEBPα and prevent it from binding to its target gene promoters [77]. Therefore, alterations in CEBPα function may be a very common event in leukemogenesis and are thought to contribute to the differentiation block observed in AML.

FLT3 and cKIT

Mutations resulting in constitutive activation of receptor tyrosine kinases are frequently observed in AML. The FLT3 and cKIT receptors are normally activated by the ligands FLT3L and SCF respectively and are required for the survival, proliferation and normal differentiation of HSPCs [78,79]. *FLT3*-internal tandem duplications (ITDs) are frequently found in AML patients and are associated with a particularly poor prognosis. Point mutations in the tyrosine kinase domain (TKD) of *FLT3* are less common in AML. They are often observed in pediatric ALL patients with *MLL*-rearrangements and T-ALL [80]. Several models have provided insight into the role of these activated kinases in leukemia. Overexpression of FLT3-ITD in murine HSPCs resulted in a lethal myeloproliferative disorder when transplanted into mice [81]. The same outcome was observed when FLT3-ITD expression was directed from the endogenous *Flt3* promoter using a knock-in approach [82]. Retroviral delivery of FLT3-ITD to human $CD34^+$ cord blood cells resulted in enhanced progenitor self-renewal, proliferation and erythroid differentiation [83]. These effects were not observed upon over-expression of wild-type FLT3 in these models. This may be because FLT3-ITD, but not wild-type FLT3, is able to activate STAT5 [84] and several studies have demonstrated that this transcription factor is a critical mediator of FLT3-ITD activity. Co-expression of a dominant-negative STAT5 mutant in human cord blood cells abrogated FLT3-ITD-induced progenitor proliferation [83]. Furthermore, mice which expressed a mutated FLT3-ITD incapable of activating Stat5 failed to develop myeloproliferative disease (MPD) [85]. FLT3-ITD not only enhances proliferation but also survival of leukemic cells by up-regulating the expression of MCL1 and SURVIVIN [86,87].

Interestingly, FLT3-TKD mutants are much less effective at activating STAT5 and also display a distinct biology to FLT3-ITD mutants. Whereas mice expressing FLT3-ITD developed MPD, mice expressing FLT3-TKD developed lymphoid disorders (T cell lymphoma or B-ALL) instead [88]. A similar phenotype was observed upon over-expression of the $cKIT^{V814}$ mutant in murine HSPCs. This mutant conferred growth factor independence to these cells and induced lymphoid leukemia with incomplete penetrance when transplanted into mice [89]. The lack of AML in these models suggests that by themselves these mutations are not sufficient to transform the myeloid lineage and require co-operating mutations to do so. This is consistent with the finding that *cKIT* mutations are frequently observed in AML patients expressing the *AML1-ETO* or *CBFβ-MYH11* fusion genes [90].

NPM

Mutations of the *Nucleophosmin1* gene (*NPM1*) occur in approximately 60% of AML cases with normal karyotype. NPM normally shuttles between the nucleus and the cytoplasm to fulfill its role in centrosome duplication and ribosome biogenesis. All NPM1 mutations lead to common alterations of the C-terminus, which result in exclusive cytoplasmic localization of the mutant ($NPMc^+$) protein [91]. Transformation assays have demonstrated that $NPMc^+$ behaves as an oncogene and antagonizes the tumor suppressor function of ARF [92]. Recently a transgenic mouse model was reported in which expression of $NPMc^+$ was directed from the human *MRP8* promoter. Although these mice developed a myeloproliferative disorder, they did not progress to AML [93].

RAS

Oncogenic *NRAS* and *KRAS* point mutations have been identified in myeloid and T cell disorders. Aberrant RAS signaling is particularly prevalent in juvenile myelomonocytic leukemia (JMML) [94]. RAS proteins are small GTPases which normally cycle between an active GTP-bound state and an inactive GDP-bound state. Activating *RAS* mutations prevent the hydrolysis of RAS-GTP and result in constitutive activation of the protein [95]. RAS proteins play a role in regulating multiple processes including proliferation, differentiation and survival [96]. Various models have successfully recapitulated the disorders associated with these mutations in humans. Murine HSPCs over-expressing $KRAS^{G12D}$ or $NRAS^{G12D}$ gave rise to CMML or AML upon transplantation into mice [97]. $NRAS^{G12D}$ over-expression in human $CD34^+$ cord blood cells enhanced proliferation and monocytic differentiation but did not induce disease in NOD/SCID mice [98]. Conditional expression of the $KRAS^{G12D}$ mutant from the endogenous *Ras* promoter resulted in a lethal myeloproliferative disease with complete penetrance [99,100]. The disease was found to originate from the HSC compartment in which elevated levels of pSTAT5, pERK and pS6 were induced by $KRAS^{G12D}$ [101]. Due to possible non cell-autonomous effects in this model, bone marrow cells conditionally expressing $KRAS^{G12D}$ from the endogenous promoter were used in competitive transplantation assays. Recipient mice developed T-cell leukemia, T cell lymphoma or a disease resembling JMML. Limiting dilution experiments revealed that the *Kras* mutation was insufficient for frank malignancy and co-operating events were acquired during the course of the experiment [102,103]. In addition to direct mutation of the *RAS* genes, the RAS signaling pathway is activated by a variety of other mechanisms including mutation of the *NF1* or *PTPN11* genes which regulate RAS-GTP levels but also by the BCR-ABL fusion protein [104] and mutant FLT3 [105].

II. Epigenetic Alterations in LSCs that Affect Self-renewal and/or Differentiation

Apart from genetic alterations acting as one of the steps in development of leukemia, epigenetic events have gained much interest for their role in leukemogenesis. The term epigenetics was coined by Sir Conrad Hall Waddington in 1942 but its definition in biology has been revisited and was recently described as: "an epigenetic trait is a stably heritable phenotype resulting from changes in a chromosome without alteration in the DNA sequence" [106,107]. This means that the phenotypical outcome of a genotype is not static, but can be modified by epigenetic processes. Epigenetic regulation of gene expression is regulated at the chromatin level. Microscopically, in interphase cell nuclei two types of chromatin can be observed: condensed chromatin (heterochromatin) and open chromatin (euchromatin). Heterochromatin is associated with silent genes whereas euchromatin contains mainly actively transcribed genes. The regulation of the chromatin structure is orchestrated at the level of the nucleosome, the structural unit of chromatin. A nucleosome is comprised of 146 bp DNA wrapped around a histone octamer, containing four different histones (H2A, H2B, H3 and H4) all present in duplicate. The amino-termini of the histones are unstructured and protrude from the nucleosomal core structure. These can be chemically altered by specific histone-modifying enzymes at various residues in several ways (acetylation, methylation, phosphorylation, ubiquitination etc.) [108]. Different modifications are involved in inducing either open or condensed chromatin. For example, acetylated histones are found in active chromatin and acetyl groups can be added to histones by histone acetyl transferases (HATs) and removed by histone deacetylases (HDACs). Histone methylation is present in both active and repressed chromatin, depending on the residue that is modified in the histone tail. DNA methylation is another well-known epigenetic modification which directly targets the genomic DNA. In mammals, cytosine residues in the context of CpG dinucleotides can be methylated by DNA methyltransferases (DNMTs). Methylation of CpG-dense regions (CpG islands, CGIs) in the promoters of genes causes repression of the transcriptional activity. Mechanistically, DNA methylation can act in two different ways. First, CpG methylation can interfere with the binding of activating transcription factors to CpG-containing sequences.

Secondly, methylated CpGs can be targeted by methyl-CpG-binding proteins (i.e. MBDs), which can recruit HDACs resulting in deacetylation of genes that are targeted by DNA methylases [109,110]. In normal cells only a small fraction of the CGIs are methylated and the majority (~85%) are hypomethylated. In contrast, outside promoter regions and CGIs the genomic DNA is globally hypermethylated [111,112]. Data from multiple model organisms suggest a role for intra- and intergenic DNA methylation in maintenance of genome integrity, silencing of transposons and inhibition of cryptic transcription initiation.

Aberrant Epigenetic Regulation in AML

Given the fact that epigenetic regulation can induce a stable heritable gene expression profile in cells, a role for epigenetic events in generation and clonal expansion of cancer cells is very likely. Increasing knowledge about aberrant epigenetic activation of oncogenes and/or silencing of tumor suppressor genes underlines the importance of epigenetic events in tumor formation. Here we will discuss the role of abnormal epigenetic regulation in the process of leukemogenesis and more specifically in acute myeloid leukemia (AML). We will discuss important epigenetic pathways affected in AML and how this might contribute to development and progression of the disease.

DNA Methylation

DNA methylation was the first epigenetic modification found to be dramatically changed in cancer cells. Despite a reduction in global methylation levels in cancer cells, promoter-specific hypermethylation is observed. Together, this leads to unwanted transcription of repeats, activation of genes and abnormal silencing of tumor suppressor genes [113]. Inactivation of tumor suppressors is known to provide a major contribution to cancerous growth of cells and is suggested to take place in the initial steps of cancer development [114]. These tumor-suppressor genes are referred to as "epigenetic gatekeepers" and a classical example, which is commonly hypermethylated in various types of solid tumors, is the *p16INK4A* gene. Down-regulation of the p16INK4A transcript is known to result in increased self-renewal of stem cells and progenitors allowing more time for cells to develop secondary genetic abnormalities like mutations or translocations. In AML, *p16INK4A* hypermethylation is observed less frequently. In contrast, AML and myelodysplastic syndrome (MDS) patients often display hypermethylation of *p15INK4B*, a gene located directly upstream of *p16INK4A* in the genome [115-118]. p15INK4B is highly homologous to p16INK4A and most likely plays an important role in hematopoietic cell lineages. AML patients in clinical remission with a methylated *p15INK4B* show an increased risk of relapse and a significant reduction in survival [119]. Although *p15Ink4B*$^{-/-}$ mouse models do not spontaneously develop myeloid leukemias, they do display extramedullary hematopoiesis and lymphoid hyperplasia in the spleen and reactive lymph nodes [120]. Furthermore, heterozygous deletion of *p15Ink4B* increases the frequency of retrovirus-induced myeloid leukemia in mice [121]. Apart from *p15INK4B* other frequently hypermethylated genes in AML include, among others, *CALCITONIN*, *E-CADHERIN*, *ER* and *MDR1*. Genome-wide analyses of DNA hypermethylation in AML patients at diagnosis and relapse showed an increase in DNA methylation at relapse, indicating that in myeloid malignancies DNA hypermethylation is not only involved in the initiation of disease but also during disease progression [122]. Very recently, genome-wide DNA methylation profiles of 344 AML patients were generated [123]. Clustering analysis identified 16 groups with distinct methylation profiles. Some of these groups correlated with known mutations (*CEBPα*) or translocations (*e.g. AML-ETO* and *PML-RARα*). Interestingly, 5 groups did not correlate with a specific genetic abnormality but did predict clinical outcome, underlining the biological and clinical relevance of these DNA methylation profiles in AML. Clinical intervention in aberrant DNA hypermethylation became possible with the approval of 5-azacytidine and 5-aza-2'-deoxycytidine (decitabine), which induce global hypomethylation. Decatibine treatment of MDS patients induces re-expression of the p15INK4B transcript and critically improved the survival of MDS patients [124,125].

Histone Acetylation

Histone acetylation is a chromatin mark associated with actively transcribed genes. Several lysine residues on the tails of histone H3 and H4 can be acetylated by histone acetyl transferases (HATs). The identified HATs can be categorized in three different families: GCN5/PCAF, MYST and p300/CBP. Within the MYST family, two members have been reported to be translocated in AML: MOZ (MYST3) and MORF (MYST4). Many different translocations producing *MOZ* fusions have been identified, including t(8;16)(p11;p13) [126] resulting in *MOZ-CBP* and t(8;22)(p11;q13) [127,128], inv(8)(p11;q13) [129,130] and t(8; 20)(p11;q13) [131] generating *MOZ-p300, MOZ-TIF2* and *MOZ-NcoA3* respectively. For the *MORF* gene only the t(10;16)(q22;p13) translocation has been identified which generates a *MORF-p300* fusion [132,133]. It is proposed that expression of these fusions leads to aberrant histone acetylation, thereby inducing leukemogenesis. Interestingly, HAT activity was dispensable for leukemic transformation by MOZ-TIF2 in mouse bone marrow transplants [134]. However, it was shown that MOZ-TIF2 expression leads to aberrant recruitment of CBP and p300 to target genes of nuclear receptors and p53 [135,136]. Gene targeting studies in mice revealed that MOZ is very important for maintenance of the HSC pool during early hematopoiesis and important for proper reconstitution of recipient mice in transplantation experiments [128,137]. Mice carrying a single point mutation in the HAT catalytic domain also display reduced numbers of HSCs and progenitors underlining the importance of HAT activity in normal hematopoiesis [138]. Gene expression analysis of AML patients with the *MOZ-CBP* t(8;16)(p11;p13) translocation showed increased expression of *HOXA9*, *HOXA10* and *MEIS1* [139]. Over-expression of these genes has been associated with leukemogenesis [37]. Up-regulation of *HOX* genes by MOZ-CBP does not reflect aberrant targeting of the fusion product since the wild-type MOZ protein is known to regulate *HOX* gene expression during development, but rather is a result of deregulation of HAT activity of the fusion protein [140-142].

Histone Methylation

Histone methylation is a chromatin modification that is found on both active and silent genes. Depending on the specific residue being methylated the mark poises activation or repression of a gene. A large group of highly conserved methyltransferases has been identified that target lysine or arginine residues on amino-termini of histone H3 and H4 [108]. The specificity of methyltransferases is much higher than that of histone acetyl transferases and in general they are specific for a single residue. In addition, residues can be either mono-, di- or tri-methylated, which cause different outcomes in terms of gene regulatory activity. In this chapter we will focus on two specific types of histone methylation, which are both involved in tumor formation and progression, despite their opposing activities in modulating gene activity.

H3K4 Methylation

A classical histone methyltransferase gene affected in leukemia is *Mixed Lineage Leukemia* (*MLL*). A number of translocations generating *MLL* fusions have been introduced in this chapter already. The *MLL* gene was initially identified as a member of the Trithorax family of transcriptional activators in *Drosophila* [143]. The Su(var)3-9, Enhancer-of-zeste, Trithorax (SET) domain at the C-terminus of MLL possesses methyltransferase activity specific for lysine 4 on histone H3 (H3K4), a modification associated with transcriptional activation. Wild-type MLL resides in a multi-protein complex which regulates the maintenance, but not the initiation of *HOX* gene expression during early development [51,144]. Since *Mll* knockout mice are embryonic lethal, much attention has been directed to the role of *Mll* in fetal hematopoiesis. *Mll*$^{-/-}$ mice display defects in HSC maintenance and progenitor differentiation, which is at least in part dependent on correct expression of *Hox* genes, since re-expression of some *HOX* genes (*HOXA9*, *HOXA10* and *HOXB4*) can revert the progenitor phenotype [40,145,146]. Conditional *Mll*-null models revealed that MLL plays an important role in adult hematopoiesis since it is required to maintain the quiescence of the HSC pool [147,148].

Interestingly, MLL fusion proteins all lack a functional SET domain, since the part of the *MLL* gene encoding the SET domain is lost in the fusion gene [149]. However, they are still targeted to genes regulated by wild-type MLL and induce their aberrant activation. [50-52]. This activation is likely due to the fact that at least a set of MLL fusion proteins (*i.e.* MLL-ENL, MLL-AF4 and MLL-AF10) are capable of recruiting the non-SET domain containing histone methyltranferase DOT1L, which can methylate histone H3 at lysine 79 (H3K79), a modification associated with active transcription [150,151]. In addition, genome-wide analysis of MLL-AF4 induced histone modification patterns in a cell line model showed a dramatically changed chromatin interaction profile at target genes compared to wild-type MLL, which also likely contributes to aberrant gene expression [152]. The interaction between MLL fusions and DOT1L takes place via the ENL, AF4 or AF10 moiety of the fusion. This may imply that H3K79 methylation renders MLL target genes active (*e.g. HOX* genes), even in the absence of a functional MLL SET domain, thereby compensating for the loss of MLL H3K4 methyltransferase activity.

Although for a long time histone methylation was thought of as a stable epigenetic mark, the identification of a large family of histone demethylases showed that regulation of histone methylation is much more dynamic [153]. Recently, a translocation, t(11;21;12) (p15;p13;p13), was identified in AML patients generating a NUP98-JARID1A fusion, the latter being a H3K4 demethylase [154]. The fusion encodes the C-terminus of JARID1A, which contains a plant homeodomain (PHD) motif, which is known to 'read' the histone code and can bind di- and tri-methylated H3K4. Mice transplanted with retrovirally transduced lineage-negative bone marrow cells over-expressing the fusion protein quickly developed leukemia, which was dependent on the functionality of the PHD motif [155]. The authors show that NUP98-JARID1A prevents demethylation of H3K4 thereby interfering with down-regulation of transcription factors during lineage-commitment, including the *Hox* genes, *Meis1* and *Pbx1*. Taken together these data underline the importance of correct regulation of H3K4 methylation in prevention of leukemogenesis.

H3K27 Methylation

H3K4 methylation-dependent activation of transcription by the Trithorax family of transcriptional activators (including MLL) is counteracted by the Polycomb group family of transcriptional repressors, which were first identified in *Drosophila*, and are responsible for silencing the expression of many developmental genes [143,156]. The Polycomb group proteins are found in different multi-protein complexes, which together operate in initiating and maintaining silencing of their target genes. The complex believed to initiate Polycomb-mediated repression is the Polycomb repressive complex 2 (PRC2), consisting of the core components EZH2, EED, SUZ12 and RbAp46/48. EZH2 was found to be a SET-domain containing histone methyltransferase specific for lysine 27 on histone H3 (H3K27) [157]. Methylation of H3K27 is thought to be the initiating event in Polycomb silencing. PRC1, another Polycomb repressive complex consisting of RING1A/B, HPC, HPH, BMI1 and SCMH can recognize trimethylated H3K27 though the HPC protein [158]. PRC1 recruitment to promoters was shown to block chromatin remodeling and prevent initiation, but not binding, of RNA polymerase II [159,160]. The RING1 subunit of the PRC1 is capable of ubiquitinating lysine 119 at histone H2A (H2AK119) [161,162]. To what extent ubiquitination of H2AK119 is a key process in Polycomb-mediated silencing is not completely resolved. *Bmi1*$^{-/-}$ mice display loss of H2A ubiquitination at almost 700 gene promoters and leads to their increased expression (*i.e. Hox* genes), suggesting that H2A ubiquitination is important for Polycomb silencing [163,164]. Genome-wide localization analysis of PRC components have shown that not all Polycomb target genes are bound by both PRC1 and PRC2 complexes, indicating the existence of multiple modes of Polycomb-mediated repression [165-167].

Both the PRC1 and PRC2 complexes have been linked to tumor formation. A role for *EZH2* in cancer was suggested from work on both prostate and breast tumors showing over-expression of EZH2 correlates with a poor prognosis [168-170]. AML cell survival was shown to be significantly impaired when cells were treated with an EZH2 inhibitor, indicating that also in AML cells EZH2 plays an important role in disease progression. In addition, EZH2 over-expression prevents HSC exhaustion in a murine transplantation models, indicating that the protein is involved in dealing with replicative stress in HSPCs [171]. In the specific case of *PML-RARα* translocations, it was shown that EZH2 can be recruited by the fusion protein and represses its target genes, thereby contributing to the leukemogenic phenotype [172]

Another Polycomb group protein whose high expression correlates with poor prognosis in AML and other hematological diseases is BMI1 [173-175]. BMI1 was initially observed to be oncogenic in a retroviral integration site screen where it was identified as a collaborating hit in MMLV-induced B-cell lymphomas in E*μ-myc* transgenic mice [176,177]. Knocking out the *Bmi1* gene results in reduced numbers of hematopoietic progenitors and more differentiated cells, eventually leading to hematopoietic failure [178]. More detailed analysis showed that BMI1 has a central regulatory role in self-renewal of HSCs by inducing symmetrical cell division both in mouse and human model systems [179-182]. Accordingly, *Bmi1*$^{-/-}$ mice display dramatically reduced HSC frequencies. BMI1 is also required for self-renewal of LSCs [181]. Over-expression of HOXA9 and MEIS1 in *Bmi1*$^{-/-}$ fetal liver cells and subsequent transplantation to irradiated recipients led to the development of AML. However, the leukemic cells could not repopulate secondary recipients suggesting that in the absence of Bmi1 the LSCs became exhausted. RNAi-mediated knockdown of BMI1 in both human cord blood and primary AML cells resulted in decreased self-renewal and led to induction of apoptosis [183]. Mechanistically, the role of BMI1 in regulating HSC self-renewal is partially explained by its ability to repress the *INK4A/ARF* locus [179,184]. Expression of p16INK4A and p19ARF in HSCs induces cell cycle arrest and p53-mediated cell death. Loss of BMI1 expression most likely results in a decreased H2AK119 ubiquitinating activity of the PRC1 complex at the *INK4A/ARF* locus, inducing expression of p16INK4A and p19ARF expression. Importantly, the hematopoietic phenotype of *Bmi1*$^{-/-}$ mice is not only dependent on the induction of *INK4A/ARF*. *Bmi1*$^{-/-}$ *Ink4A/Arf*$^{-/-}$ double knockout mice showed a partial recovery of hematopoietic cell counts but did not show a complete reversal of the Bmi1 null phenotype, suggesting that other pathways are also involved [185]. A candidate *INK4A/ARF*-independent pathway for BMI1 in controlling HSC and LSC self-renewal is regulation of reactive oxygen species (ROS) in the cell. Recently, it was shown that *Bmi1*$^{-/-}$ mice display impaired mitochondrial function due to increased expression of Polycomb target genes involved in ROS metabolism [186]. Long-term HSCs from *Bmi1*$^{-/-}$ mice showed increased levels of ROS and treatment of mice with the antioxidant N-acetylcysteine (NAC) resulted in a rescue of thymocyte cell numbers compared to non-treated *Bmi1*$^{-/-}$ mice. Furthermore, de-regulated ROS metabolism induced activation of the DNA damage response pathway. Knockout of *Chk2*, a component of the DNA damage response pathway, in a *Bmi*$^{-/-}$ background resulted in partial reversal of the thymocyte phenotype observed in *Bmi1*$^{-/-}$ mice. In addition, knockdown of BMI1 in human cord blood also induces increased ROS levels and apoptosis [183]. These data clearly show that apart from the well known role of BMI1 in regulating cell cycle and senescence through the *INK4A/ARF* locus, BMI1 is also implicated in other pathways regulating oxygen metabolism. It is clear that up-regulation of BMI1 in leukemic cells undoubtedly will give an advantage for these cells to cope with high oxygen levels. This is certainly advantageous for LSCs which are most likely not located in the oxygen-poor HSC niche and suffer from increased oxygen stress compared to normal HSCs.

III. Multiple (Epi) Genetic Defects are Required for Leukemic Transformation

It is clear from the models summarized in part I that many if not all of the genetic events described are not sufficient to induce AML by themselves but require co-operating events to do so. The original two-step model of leukemogenesis was first proposed by Dash and Gilliland who postulated that two types of mutations (class I and class II) are required for the development of AML. Class I mutations are thought to confer a proliferative or survival advantage to the cell and class II mutations impair differentiation and enhance self-renewal. It has been generally considered that *FLT3*, *cKIT*, and *N-RAS* mutations are class I mutations and balanced translocations including *AML1/ETO*, *CBFB/MYH11*, *PML/RARA*, and *MLL* abnormalities are class II mutations [187]. This hypothesis has gained support from the findings that co-expression of various class I and class II mutations do indeed co-operate to induce leukemia in animal models. For example, the incidence of mice developing APL upon expression of PML-RARα was dramatically increased and the latency shortened following co-expression of FLT3-ITD or KRAS [188,189]. Furthermore, co-expression of FLT3-ITD and AML1-ETO, which individually are insufficient to cause disease, resulted in fatal acute leukemia [190]. These models are clinically relevant since the FLT3-ITD mutation is frequently found in patients harboring the t(8;21) or t(15;17) translocations. Activating cKIT mutations are frequently observed in patients with the t(8;21) or inv(16) translocations [90]. Consistent with this activated c-KIT co-operates with AML1-ETO to induce leukemia in a murine transduction/transplantation model [191]. The frequent co-existence of NPM1 and FLT3-ITD mutations in AML patients [192] suggests (according to the classical two-hit model) that NPM1 mutations block differentiation or enhance self-renewal.

However, as yet there is no evidence to support the idea that genetic mutations exclusively affect either the proliferation/survival (class I) or differentiation (class II). In fact, various genetic mutations often affect both of these pathways. Furthermore, many other cell biological properties of leukemic cells are frequently altered, including interactions with the bone marrow microenvironment, regulation of oxidative stress and DNA repair, and the process of self-renewal whereby the symmetry of stem cell divisions might be affected. Also, we hypothesize that leukemogenesis does not necessarily result as a consequence of two or more genetic events but may be mediated by a combination of genetic and epigenetic events.

Clearly, in some instances epigenetic changes can occur as a consequence of genetic abnormalities. Some epigenetic modifiers are directly targeted by a translocation (e.g. *MLL*, *MOZ*, *JARID1A*), which leads to aberrant epigenetic signaling. This could be due to either mis-targeting of a functional epigenetic modifier (including an active catalytic domain) or correct targeting of an inactive form which blocks other chromatin modifying enzymes or sequesters other epigenetic modifiers. A classical example of the latter situation is the *MLL-AF9* translocation which leads to deregulated *HOX* gene expression due to aberrant targeting of DOT1L to its target genes [150,151]. Another example of translocations affecting the epigenetic state of genes are the PML-RARα and PLZF-RARα fusions, which are capable of recruiting the PRC2 and PRC1 complex respectively, leading to Polycomb-mediated silencing of their target genes [172,193].

On the other hand, epigenetic changes might be viewed as autonomous processes independent of genetic instability. Aging has dominant affects on the epigenetic landscape of hematopoietic stem cells, and myeloid leukemias arise particularly in elderly patients. Thus, it seems plausible that changes in epigenetic landscapes, for instance associated with aging, might contribute to the leukemic transformation process as well. The possibility to perform genome-wide analyses of epigenetic landscapes has set the stage for in depth analysis of epigenetic profiles in AML patients with known translocations or normal karyotypes. The recent publication by Figuero and colleagues is an example of how genome-wide analysis of DNA methylation levels in AML patients provides valuable information on the relation between DNA methylation and AML disease progression and how methylation profiles correlate with genetic hits [123]. Genome-wide DNA methylation analysis of 344 patients showed the existence of 16 distinct methylation profiles. A number of these profiles correlated with the presence of known translocations like *CBFB-MYH11*, *AML1-ETO*, *PML-RARα* or mutations in *NPM1* or *CEPBα*. Surprisingly, 5 clusters were identified in a group of

AMLs that did not share a common translocation or mutation. Most likely, AMLs clustered within these groups share unidentified mutations or deregulated expression of wild type epigenetic modifiers causing deregulated cell cycle control or a block in differentiation. A striking difference in clinical outcome was observed between these different groups, underlining the role of epigenetic regulation in disease progression and the importance of epigenetic analysis as a prognostic tool. The role of epigenetic analysis in survival prediction in AML was emphasized with the identification of a 15 gene methylation classifier which was predictive for clinical outcome in an independent patient cohort.

Most likely, in the near future more genome-wide epigenetic profiling studies on AML samples will be performed, leading to a better understanding of the contributing role of epigenetic hits in AML. As an example, genome-wide occupation analysis of over-expressed epigenetic modifiers like EZH2 and BMI1 and their associated epigenetic modification will be highly informative in elucidating the molecular mechanisms underlying the poor prognosis upon their over-expression. Identification of AML-specific target genes compared to normal hematopoietic cells will inevitably increase our knowledge of the role of epigenetic hits in the process of leukemogenesis, at what stage during disease progression they act and how they collaborate with genetic hits.

Conclusion

The generation of various genetic models using mouse or human cells has helped tremendously in gaining further insight into the process of leukemic transformation. From these models we have learned how genetic mutations might contribute to the development of hematological malignancies, but also that a single genetic alteration is most often not sufficient to induce overt leukemia. Besides genetic changes, epigenetic alterations, for instance as the consequence of aging, are likely to contribute as well. The challenge in the near future lies in establishing models in which these multiple hits are integrated in order to faithfully recapitulate leukemic development. These models will then provide excellent platforms to study molecular mechanisms involved in leukemic transformation and in which new drug entities can be tested.

References

[1] Passegue E, Jamieson CH, Ailles LE, Weissman IL. Normal and leukemic hematopoiesis: are leukemias a stem cell disorder or a reacquisition of stem cell characteristics? *Proc Natl Acad Sci USA*. 2003;100 Suppl 111842-11849.

[2] Bonnet D and Dick JE. Human acute myeloid leukemia is organized as a hierarchy that originates from a primitive hematopoietic cell. *Nat Med*. 1997;3(7):730-737.

[3] Hope KJ, Jin L, Dick JE. Acute myeloid leukemia originates from a hierarchy of leukemic stem cell classes that differ in self-renewal capacity. *Nat Immunol*. 2004;5(7):738-743.

[4] Lapidot T, Sirard C, Vormoor J, et al. A cell initiating human acute myeloid leukaemia after transplantation into SCID mice. *Nature*. 1994;367(6464):645-648.

[5] Bhatia M, Wang JC, Kapp U, Bonnet D, Dick JE. Purification of primitive human hematopoietic cells capable of repopulating immune-deficient mice. *Proc Natl Acad Sci USA*. 1997;94(10):5320-5325.

[6] Taussig DC, Miraki-Moud F, Anjos-Afonso F, et al. Anti-CD38 antibody-mediated clearance of human repopulating cells masks the heterogeneity of leukemia-initiating cells. *Blood*. 2008;112(3):568-575.

[7] Kelly LM and Gilliland DG. Genetics of myeloid leukemias. *Annu Rev Genomics Hum Genet*. 2002;3179-198.

[8] Warner JK, Wang JC, Hope KJ, Jin L, Dick JE. Concepts of human leukemic development. *Oncogene*. 2004;23(43):7164-7177.

[9] Jordan CT and Guzman ML. Mechanisms controlling pathogenesis and survival of leukemic stem cells. *Oncogene*. 2004;23(43):7178-7187.

[10] Link KA, Chou FS, Mulloy JC. Core binding factor at the crossroads: determining the fate of the HSC. *J Cell Physiol*. 2010;222(1):50-56.

[11] Fenske TS, Pengue G, Mathews V, et al. Stem cell expression of the AML1/ETO fusion protein induces a myeloproliferative disorder in mice. *Proc Natl Acad Sci USA*. 2004;101(42):15184-15189.

[12] Downing JR, Higuchi M, Lenny N, Yeoh AE. Alterations of the AML1 transcription factor in human leukemia. *Semin Cell Dev Biol*. 2000;11(5):347-360.

[13] Higuchi M, O'Brien D, Kumaravelu P, Lenny N, Yeoh EJ, Downing JR. Expression of a conditional AML1-ETO oncogene bypasses embryonic lethality and establishes a murine model of human t(8;21) acute myeloid leukemia. *Cancer Cell*. 2002;1(1):63-74.

[14] de Guzman CG, Warren AJ, Zhang Z, et al. Hematopoietic stem cell expansion and distinct myeloid developmental abnormalities in a murine model of the AML1-ETO translocation. *Mol Cell Biol*. 2002;22(15):5506-5517.

[15] Basecke J, Schwieger M, Griesinger F, et al. AML1/ETO promotes the maintenance of early hematopoietic progenitors in NOD/SCID mice but does not abrogate their lineage specific differentiation. *Leuk Lymphoma*. 2005;46(2):265-272.

[16] Mulloy JC, Cammenga J, MacKenzie KL, Berguido FJ, Moore MA, Nimer SD. The AML1-ETO fusion protein promotes the expansion of human hematopoietic stem cells. *Blood*. 2002;99(1):15-23.

[17] Mulloy JC, Cammenga J, Berguido FJ, et al. Maintaining the self-renewal and differentiation potential of human CD34+ hematopoietic cells using a single genetic element. *Blood*. 2003;102(13):4369-4376.

[18] Balkhi MY, Christopeit M, Chen Y, Geletu M, Behre G. AML1/ETO-induced survivin expression inhibits transcriptional regulation of myeloid differentiation. *Exp Hematol*. 2008;36(11):1449-1460.

[19] Mori H, Colman SM, Xiao Z, et al. Chromosome translocations and covert leukemic clones are generated during normal fetal development. *Proc Natl Acad Sci USA*. 2002;99(12):8242-8247.

[20] Krejci O, Wunderlich M, Geiger H, et al. p53 signaling in response to increased DNA damage sensitizes AML1-ETO cells to stress-induced death. *Blood*. 2008;111(4):2190-2199.

[21] Kuo YH, Landrette SF, Heilman SA, et al. Cbf beta-SMMHC induces distinct abnormal myeloid progenitors able to develop acute myeloid leukemia. *Cancer Cell*. 2006;9(1):57-68.

[22] Landrette SF, Kuo YH, Hensen K, et al. Plagl and Plagl2 are oncogenes that induce acute myeloid leukemia in cooperation with Cbfb-MYH11. *Blood.* 2005;105(7):2900-2907.

[23] Wunderlich M, Krejci O, Wei J, Mulloy JC. Human CD34+ cells expressing the inv(16) fusion protein exhibit a myelomonocytic phenotype with greatly enhanced proliferative ability. *Blood.* 2006;108(5):1690-1697.

[24] Turhan AG, Lemoine FM, Debert C, et al. Highly purified primitive hematopoietic stem cells are PML-RARA negative and generate nonclonal progenitors in acute promyelocytic leukemia. *Blood.* 1995;85(8):2154-2161.

[25] Brown D, Kogan S, Lagasse E, et al. A PMLRARalpha transgene initiates murine acute promyelocytic leukemia. *Proc Natl Acad Sci USA.* 1997;94(6):2551-2556.

[26] Grisolano JL, Wesselschmidt RL, Pelicci PG, Ley TJ. Altered myeloid development and acute leukemia in transgenic mice expressing PML-RAR alpha under control of cathepsin G regulatory sequences. *Blood.* 1997;89(2):376-387.

[27] He LZ, Tribioli C, Rivi R, et al. Acute leukemia with promyelocytic features in PML/RARalpha transgenic mice. *Proc Natl Acad Sci USA.* 1997;94(10):5302-5307.

[28] Early E, Moore MA, Kakizuka A, et al. Transgenic expression of PML/RARalpha impairs myelopoiesis. *Proc Natl Acad Sci USA.* 1996;93(15):7900-7904.

[29] Grignani F, Valtieri M, Gabbianelli M, et al. PML/RAR alpha fusion protein expression in normal human hematopoietic progenitors dictates myeloid commitment and the promyelocytic phenotype. *Blood.* 2000;96(4):1531-1537.

[30] Minucci S, Monestiroli S, Giavara S, et al. PML-RAR induces promyelocytic leukemias with high efficiency following retroviral gene transfer into purified murine hematopoietic progenitors. *Blood.* 2002;100(8):2989-2995.

[31] Minucci S, Nervi C, Lo Coco F, Pelicci PG. Histone deacetylases: a common molecular target for differentiation treatment of acute myeloid leukemias? *Oncogene.* 2001;20(24):3110-3115.

[32] Insinga A, Monestiroli S, Ronzoni S, et al. Impairment of p53 acetylation, stability and function by an oncogenic transcription factor. *EMBO J.* 2004;23(5):1144-1154.

[33] Linggi B, Muller-Tidow C, van de Locht L, et al. The t(8;21) fusion protein, AML1 ETO, specifically represses the transcription of the p14(ARF) tumor suppressor in acute myeloid leukemia. *Nat Med.* 2002;8(7):743-750.

[34] Moore MA, Chung KY, Plasilova M, et al. NUP98 dysregulation in myeloid leukemogenesis. *Ann N Y Acad Sci.* 2007;1106114-142.

[35] Kroon E, Thorsteinsdottir U, Mayotte N, Nakamura T, Sauvageau G. NUP98-HOXA9 expression in hemopoietic stem cells induces chronic and acute myeloid leukemias in mice. *EMBO J.* 2001;20(3):350-361.

[36] Chung KY, Morrone G, Schuringa JJ, et al. Enforced expression of NUP98-HOXA9 in human CD34(+) cells enhances stem cell proliferation. *Cancer Res.* 2006; 66(24):11781-11791.

[37] Argiropoulos B and Humphries RK. Hox genes in hematopoiesis and leukemogenesis. *Oncogene.* 2007;26(47):6766-6776.

[38] Calvo KR, Sykes DB, Pasillas MP, Kamps MP. Nup98-HoxA9 immortalizes myeloid progenitors, enforces expression of Hoxa9, Hoxa7 and Meis1, and alters cytokine-specific responses in a manner similar to that induced by retroviral co-expression of Hoxa9 and Meis1. *Oncogene.* 2002;21(27):4247-4256.

[39] Wu M, Kwon HY, Rattis F, et al. Imaging hematopoietic precursor division in real time. *Cell Stem Cell*. 2007;1(5):541-554.

[40] Ernst P, Mabon M, Davidson AJ, Zon LI, Korsmeyer SJ. An Mll-dependent Hox program drives hematopoietic progenitor expansion. *Curr Biol*. 2004;14(22):2063-2069.

[41] Lavau C, Szilvassy SJ, Slany R, Cleary ML. Immortalization and leukemic transformation of a myelomonocytic precursor by retrovirally transduced HRX-ENL. *EMBO J*. 1997;16(14):4226-4237.

[42] Somervaille TC and Cleary ML. Identification and characterization of leukemia stem cells in murine MLL-AF9 acute myeloid leukemia. *Cancer Cell*. 2006;10(4):257-268.

[43] Barabe F, Kennedy JA, Hope KJ, Dick JE. Modeling the initiation and progression of human acute leukemia in mice. *Science*. 2007;316(5824):600-604.

[44] Wei J, Wunderlich M, Fox C, et al. Microenvironment determines lineage fate in a human model of MLL-AF9 leukemia. *Cancer Cell*. 2008;13(6):483-495.

[45] Cozzio A, Passegue E, Ayton PM, Karsunky H, Cleary ML, Weissman IL. Similar MLL-associated leukemias arising from self-renewing stem cells and short-lived myeloid progenitors. *Genes Dev*. 2003;17(24):3029-3035.

[46] Krivtsov AV, Twomey D, Feng Z, et al. Transformation from committed progenitor to leukaemia stem cell initiated by MLL-AF9. *Nature*. 2006;442(7104):818-822.

[47] Chen W, Kumar AR, Hudson WA, et al. Malignant transformation initiated by Mll-AF9: gene dosage and critical target cells. *Cancer Cell*. 2008;13(5):432-440.

[48] Forster A, Pannell R, Drynan LF, et al. Engineering de novo reciprocal chromosomal translocations associated with Mll to replicate primary events of human cancer. *Cancer Cell*. 2003;3(5):449-458.

[49] Kohlmann A, Schoch C, Dugas M, et al. New insights into MLL gene rearranged acute leukemias using gene expression profiling: shared pathways, lineage commitment, and partner genes. *Leukemia*. 2005;19(6):953-964.

[50] Horton SJ, Grier DG, McGonigle GJ, et al. Continuous MLL-ENL expression is necessary to establish a "Hox Code" and maintain immortalization of hematopoietic progenitor cells. *Cancer Res*. 2005;65(20):9245-9252.

[51] Milne TA, Briggs SD, Brock HW, et al. MLL targets SET domain methyltransferase activity to Hox gene promoters. *Mol Cell*. 2002;10(5):1107-1117.

[52] Milne TA, Martin ME, Brock HW, Slany RK, Hess JL. Leukemogenic MLL fusion proteins bind across a broad region of the Hox a9 locus, promoting transcription and multiple histone modifications. *Cancer Res*. 2005;65(24):11367-11374.

[53] Faber J, Krivtsov AV, Stubbs MC, et al. HOXA9 is required for survival in human MLL-rearranged acute leukemias. *Blood*. 2009;113(11):2375-2385.

[54] Kumar AR, Li Q, Hudson WA, et al. A role for MEIS1 in MLL-fusion gene leukemia. *Blood*. 2009;113(8):1756-1758.

[55] Wong P, Iwasaki M, Somervaille TC, So CW, Cleary ML. Meis1 is an essential and rate-limiting regulator of MLL leukemia stem cell potential. *Genes Dev*. 2007;21(21):2762-2774.

[56] Gishizky ML, Johnson-White J, Witte ON. Efficient transplantation of BCR-ABL-induced chronic myelogenous leukemia-like syndrome in mice. *Proc Natl Acad Sci USA*. 1993;90(8):3755-3759.

[57] Pear WS, Miller JP, Xu L, et al. Efficient and rapid induction of a chronic myelogenous leukemia-like myeloproliferative disease in mice receiving P210 bcr/abl-transduced bone marrow. *Blood.* 1998;92(10):3780-3792.
[58] Chalandon Y, Jiang X, Christ O, et al. BCR-ABL-transduced human cord blood cells produce abnormal populations in immunodeficient mice. *Leukemia.* 2005;19(3):442-448.
[59] Perez-Caro M, Cobaleda C, Gonzalez-Herrero I, et al. Cancer induction by restriction of oncogene expression to the stem cell compartment. *EMBO J.* 2009;28(1):8-20.
[60] Melo JV and Barnes DJ. Chronic myeloid leukaemia as a model of disease evolution in human cancer. *Nat Rev Cancer.* 2007;7(6):441-453.
[61] Jamieson CH, Ailles LE, Dylla SJ, et al. Granulocyte-macrophage progenitors as candidate leukemic stem cells in blast-crisis CML. *N Engl J Med.* 2004;351(7):657-667.
[62] Fialkow PJ, Singer JW, Raskind WH, et al. Clonal development, stem-cell differentiation, and clinical remissions in acute nonlymphocytic leukemia. *N Engl J Med.* 1987;317(8):468-473.
[63] Takahashi N, Miura I, Saitoh K, Miura AB. Lineage involvement of stem cells bearing the philadelphia chromosome in chronic myeloid leukemia in the chronic phase as shown by a combination of fluorescence-activated cell sorting and fluorescence in situ hybridization. *Blood.* 1998;92(12):4758-4763.
[64] de Groot RP, Raaijmakers JA, Lammers JW, Jove R, Koenderman L. STAT5 activation by BCR-Abl contributes to transformation of K562 leukemia cells. *Blood.* 1999;94(3):1108-1112.
[65] Scherr M, Chaturvedi A, Battmer K, et al. Enhanced sensitivity to inhibition of SHP2, STAT5, and Gab2 expression in chronic myeloid leukemia (CML). *Blood.* 2006;107(8):3279-3287.
[66] Sillaber C, Gesbert F, Frank DA, Sattler M, Griffin JD. STAT5 activation contributes to growth and viability in Bcr/Abl-transformed cells. *Blood.* 2000;95(6):2118-2125.
[67] Ye D, Wolff N, Li L, Zhang S, Ilaria RL, Jr. STAT5 signaling is required for the efficient induction and maintenance of CML in mice. *Blood.* 2006;107(12):4917-4925.
[68] Ren R. Mechanisms of BCR-ABL in the pathogenesis of chronic myelogenous leukaemia. *Nat Rev Cancer.* 2005;5(3):172-183.
[69] Thomas EK, Cancelas JA, Chae HD, et al. Rac guanosine triphosphatases represent integrating molecular therapeutic targets for BCR-ABL-induced myeloproliferative disease. *Cancer Cell.* 2007;12(5):467-478.
[70] Zhao C, Chen A, Jamieson CH, et al. Hedgehog signalling is essential for maintenance of cancer stem cells in myeloid leukaemia. *Nature.* 2009;458(7239):776-779.
[71] Zhang P, Iwasaki-Arai J, Iwasaki H, et al. Enhancement of hematopoietic stem cell repopulating capacity and self-renewal in the absence of the transcription factor C/EBP alpha. *Immunity.* 2004;21(6):853-863.
[72] Barjesteh van Waalwijk van Doorn-Khosrovani, Erpelinck C, Meijer J, et al. Biallelic mutations in the CEBPA gene and low CEBPA expression levels as prognostic markers in intermediate-risk AML. *Hematol J.* 2003;4(1):31-40.
[73] Leroy H, Roumier C, Huyghe P, Biggio V, Fenaux P, Preudhomme C. CEBPA point mutations in hematological malignancies. *Leukemia.* 2005;19(3):329-334.

[74] Kirstetter P, Schuster MB, Bereshchenko O, et al. Modeling of C/EBPalpha mutant acute myeloid leukemia reveals a common expression signature of committed myeloid leukemia-initiating cells. *Cancer Cell.* 2008;13(4):299-310.

[75] Bereshchenko O, Mancini E, Moore S, et al. Hematopoietic stem cell expansion precedes the generation of committed myeloid leukemia-initiating cells in C/EBPalpha mutant AML. *Cancer Cell.* 2009;16(5):390-400.

[76] Pabst T, Mueller BU, Harakawa N, et al. AML1-ETO downregulates the granulocytic differentiation factor C/EBPalpha in t(8;21) myeloid leukemia. *Nat Med.* 2001;7(4):444-451.

[77] Tenen DG. Abnormalities of the CEBP alpha transcription factor: a major target in acute myeloid leukemia. *Leukemia.* 2001;15(4):688-689.

[78] Lennartsson J, Jelacic T, Linnekin D, Shivakrupa R. Normal and oncogenic forms of the receptor tyrosine kinase kit. *Stem Cells.* 2005;23(1):16-43.

[79] Mackarehtschian K, Hardin JD, Moore KA, Boast S, Goff SP, Lemischka IR. Targeted disruption of the flk2/flt3 gene leads to deficiencies in primitive hematopoietic progenitors. *Immunity.* 1995;3(1):147-161.

[80] Stirewalt DL and Radich JP. The role of FLT3 in haematopoietic malignancies. *Nat Rev Cancer.* 2003;3(9):650-665.

[81] Kelly LM, Liu Q, Kutok JL, Williams IR, Boulton CL, Gilliland DG. FLT3 internal tandem duplication mutations associated with human acute myeloid leukemias induce myeloproliferative disease in a murine bone marrow transplant model. *Blood.* 2002;99(1):310-318.

[82] Li L, Piloto O, Nguyen HB, et al. Knock-in of an internal tandem duplication mutation into murine FLT3 confers myeloproliferative disease in a mouse model. *Blood.* 2008;111(7):3849-3858.

[83] Chung KY, Morrone G, Schuringa JJ, Wong B, Dorn DC, Moore MA. Enforced expression of an Flt3 internal tandem duplication in human CD34+ cells confers properties of self-renewal and enhanced erythropoiesis. *Blood.* 2005;105(1):77-84.

[84] Mizuki M, Fenski R, Halfter H, et al. Flt3 mutations from patients with acute myeloid leukemia induce transformation of 32D cells mediated by the Ras and STAT5 pathways. *Blood.* 2000;96(12):3907-3914.

[85] Rocnik JL, Okabe R, Yu JC, et al. Roles of tyrosine 589 and 591 in STAT5 activation and transformation mediated by FLT3-ITD. *Blood.* 2006;108(4):1339-1345.

[86] Fukuda S, Singh P, Moh A, et al. Survivin mediates aberrant hematopoietic progenitor cell proliferation and acute leukemia in mice induced by internal tandem duplication of Flt3. *Blood.* 2009;114(2):394-403.

[87] Yoshimoto G, Miyamoto T, Jabbarzadeh-Tabrizi S, et al. FLT3-ITD up-regulates MCL-1 to promote survival of stem cells in acute myeloid leukemia via FLT3-ITD-specific STAT5 activation. *Blood.* 2009;114(24):5034-5043.

[88] Grundler R, Miething C, Thiede C, Peschel C, Duyster J. FLT3-ITD and tyrosine kinase domain mutants induce 2 distinct phenotypes in a murine bone marrow transplantation model. *Blood.* 2005;105(12):4792-4799.

[89] Kitayama H, Tsujimura T, Matsumura I, et al. Neoplastic transformation of normal hematopoietic cells by constitutively activating mutations of c-kit receptor tyrosine kinase. *Blood.* 1996;88(3):995-1004.

[90] Frohling S, Scholl C, Gilliland DG, Levine RL. Genetics of myeloid malignancies: pathogenetic and clinical implications. *J Clin Oncol.* 2005;23(26):6285-6295.

[91] Falini B, Nicoletti I, Bolli N, et al. Translocations and mutations involving the nucleophosmin (NPM1) gene in lymphomas and leukemias. *Haematologica.* 2007;92(4):519-532.

[92] Cheng K, Grisendi S, Clohessy JG, et al. The leukemia-associated cytoplasmic nucleophosmin mutant is an oncogene with paradoxical functions: Arf inactivation and induction of cellular senescence. *Oncogene.* 2007;26(53):7391-7400.

[93] Cheng K, Sportoletti P, Ito K, et al. The cytoplasmic NPM mutant induces myeloproliferation in a transgenic mouse model. *Blood.* 2009.

[94] Tartaglia M, Niemeyer CM, Fragale A, et al. Somatic mutations in PTPN11 in juvenile myelomonocytic leukemia, myelodysplastic syndromes and acute myeloid leukemia. *Nat Genet.* 2003;34(2):148-150.

[95] Bos JL, Rehmann H, Wittinghofer A. GEFs and GAPs: critical elements in the control of small G proteins. *Cell.* 2007;129(5):865-877.

[96] Boguski MS and McCormick F. Proteins regulating Ras and its relatives. *Nature.* 1993;366(6456):643-654.

[97] Parikh C, Subrahmanyam R, Ren R. Oncogenic NRAS, KRAS, and HRAS exhibit different leukemogenic potentials in mice. *Cancer Res.* 2007;67(15):7139-7146.

[98] Shen SW, Dolnikov A, Passioura T, et al. Mutant N-ras preferentially drives human CD34+ hematopoietic progenitor cells into myeloid differentiation and proliferation both in vitro and in the NOD/SCID mouse. *Exp Hematol.* 2004;32(9):852-860.

[99] Braun BS, Tuveson DA, Kong N, et al. Somatic activation of oncogenic Kras in hematopoietic cells initiates a rapidly fatal myeloproliferative disorder. *Proc Natl Acad Sci USA.* 2004;101(2):597-602.

[100] Chan IT, Kutok JL, Williams IR, et al. Conditional expression of oncogenic K-ras from its endogenous promoter induces a myeloproliferative disease. *J Clin Invest.* 2004;113(4):528-538.

[101] Van Meter ME, Diaz-Flores E, Archard JA, et al. K-RasG12D expression induces hyperproliferation and aberrant signaling in primary hematopoietic stem/progenitor cells. *Blood.* 2007;109(9):3945-3952.

[102] Sabnis AJ, Cheung LS, Dail M, et al. Oncogenic Kras initiates leukemia in hematopoietic stem cells. *PLoS Biol.* 2009;7(3):e59.

[103] Zhang J, Wang J, Liu Y, et al. Oncogenic Kras-induced leukemogeneis: hematopoietic stem cells as the initial target and lineage-specific progenitors as the potential targets for final leukemic transformation. *Blood.* 2009;113(6):1304-1314.

[104] Alvarado Y and Giles FJ. Ras as a therapeutic target in hematologic malignancies. *Expert Opin Emerg Drugs.* 2007;12(2):271-284.

[105] Scholl C, Gilliland DG, Frohling S. Deregulation of signaling pathways in acute myeloid leukemia. *Semin Oncol.* 2008;35(4):336-345.

[106] Goldberg AD, Allis CD, Bernstein E. Epigenetics: a landscape takes shape. *Cell.* 2007;128(4):635-638.

[107] Berger SL, Kouzarides T, Shiekhattar R, Shilatifard A. An operational definition of epigenetics. *Genes Dev.* 2009;23(7):781-783.

[108] Kouzarides T. Chromatin modifications and their function. *Cell.* 2007;128(4):693-705.

[109] Bird A. DNA methylation patterns and epigenetic memory. *Genes Dev*. 2002;16(1):6-21.

[110] Jones PL, Veenstra GJ, Wade PA, et al. Methylated DNA and MeCP2 recruit histone deacetylase to repress transcription. *Nat Genet*. 1998;19(2):187-191.

[111] Suzuki MM and Bird A. DNA methylation landscapes: provocative insights from epigenomics. *Nat Rev Genet*. 2008;9(6):465-476.

[112] Weber M and Schubeler D. Genomic patterns of DNA methylation: targets and function of an epigenetic mark. *Curr Opin Cell Biol*. 2007;19(3):273-280.

[113] Ting AH, McGarvey KM, Baylin SB. The cancer epigenome--components and functional correlates. *Genes Dev*. 2006;20(23):3215-3231.

[114] Jones PA and Baylin SB. The epigenomics of cancer. *Cell*. 2007;128(4):683-692.

[115] Claus R and Lubbert M. Epigenetic targets in hematopoietic malignancies. *Oncogene*. 2003;22(42):6489-6496.

[116] Herman JG, Civin CI, Issa JP, Collector MI, Sharkis SJ, Baylin SB. Distinct patterns of inactivation of p15INK4B and p16INK4A characterize the major types of hematological malignancies. *Cancer Res*. 1997;57(5):837-841.

[117] Kim WY and Sharpless NE. The regulation of INK4/ARF in cancer and aging. *Cell*. 2006;127(2):265-275.

[118] Uchida T, Kinoshita T, Nagai H, et al. Hypermethylation of the p15INK4B gene in myelodysplastic syndromes. *Blood*. 1997;90(4):1403-1409.

[119] Agrawal S, Unterberg M, Koschmieder S, et al. DNA methylation of tumor suppressor genes in clinical remission predicts the relapse risk in acute myeloid leukemia. *Cancer Res*. 2007;67(3):1370-1377.

[120] Latres E, Malumbres M, Sotillo R, et al. Limited overlapping roles of P15(INK4b) and P18(INK4c) cell cycle inhibitors in proliferation and tumorigenesis. *EMBO J*. 2000; 19(13):3496-3506.

[121] Wolff L, Garin MT, Koller R, et al. Hypermethylation of the Ink4b locus in murine myeloid leukemia and increased susceptibility to leukemia in p15(Ink4b)-deficient mice. *Oncogene*. 2003;22(58):9265-9274.

[122] Kroeger H, Jelinek J, Estecio MR, et al. Aberrant CpG island methylation in acute myeloid leukemia is accentuated at relapse. *Blood*. 2008;112(4):1366-1373.

[123] Figueroa ME, Lugthart S, Li Y, et al. DNA Methylation Signatures Identify Biologically Distinct Subtypes in Acute Myeloid Leukemia. *Cancer Cell*. 2010.

[124] Daskalakis M, Nguyen TT, Nguyen C, et al. Demethylation of a hypermethylated P15/INK4B gene in patients with myelodysplastic syndrome by 5-Aza-2'-deoxycytidine (decitabine) treatment. *Blood*. 2002;100(8):2957-2964.

[125] Garcia-Manero G. Demethylating agents in myeloid malignancies. *Curr Opin Oncol*. 2008;20(6):705-710.

[126] Borrow J, Stanton VP, Jr., Andresen JM, et al. The translocation t(8;16)(p11;p13) of acute myeloid leukaemia fuses a putative acetyltransferase to the CREB-binding protein. *Nat Genet*. 1996;14(1):33-41.

[127] Chaffanet M, Gressin L, Preudhomme C, Soenen-Cornu V, Birnbaum D, Pebusque MJ. MOZ is fused to p300 in an acute monocytic leukemia with t(8;22). *Genes Chromosomes Cancer*. 2000;28(2):138-144.

[128] Kitabayashi I, Aikawa Y, Yokoyama A, et al. Fusion of MOZ and p300 histone acetyltransferases in acute monocytic leukemia with a t(8;22)(p11;q13) chromosome translocation. *Leukemia.* 2001;15(1):89-94.
[129] Carapeti M, Aguiar RC, Goldman JM, Cross NC. A novel fusion between MOZ and the nuclear receptor coactivator TIF2 in acute myeloid leukemia. *Blood.* 1998;91(9):3127-3133.
[130] Liang J, Prouty L, Williams BJ, Dayton MA, Blanchard KL. Acute mixed lineage leukemia with an inv(8)(p11q13) resulting in fusion of the genes for MOZ and TIF2. *Blood.* 1998;92(6):2118-2122.
[131] Esteyries S, Perot C, Adelaide J, et al. NCOA3, a new fusion partner for MOZ/MYST3 in M5 acute myeloid leukemia. *Leukemia.* 2008;22(3):663-665.
[132] Kojima K, Kaneda K, Yoshida C, et al. A novel fusion variant of the MORF and CBP genes detected in therapy-related myelodysplastic syndrome with t(10;16)(q22;p13). *Br J Haematol.* 2003;120(2):271-273.
[133] Panagopoulos I, Fioretos T, Isaksson M, et al. Fusion of the MORF and CBP genes in acute myeloid leukemia with the t(10;16)(q22;p13). *Hum Mol Genet.* 2001;10(4):395-404.
[134] Deguchi K, Ayton PM, Carapeti M, et al. MOZ-TIF2-induced acute myeloid leukemia requires the MOZ nucleosome binding motif and TIF2-mediated recruitment of CBP. *Cancer Cell.* 2003;3(3):259-271.
[135] Collins HM, Kindle KB, Matsuda S, et al. MOZ-TIF2 alters cofactor recruitment and histone modification at the RARbeta2 promoter: differential effects of MOZ fusion proteins on CBP- and MOZ-dependent activators. *J Biol Chem.* 2006;281(25):17124-17133.
[136] Kindle KB, Troke PJ, Collins HM, et al. MOZ-TIF2 inhibits transcription by nuclear receptors and p53 by impairment of CBP function. *Mol Cell Biol.* 2005;25(3):988-1002.
[137] Thomas T, Corcoran LM, Gugasyan R, et al. Monocytic leukemia zinc finger protein is essential for the development of long-term reconstituting hematopoietic stem cells. *Genes Dev.* 2006;20(9):1175-1186.
[138] Perez-Campo FM, Borrow J, Kouskoff V, Lacaud G. The histone acetyl transferase activity of monocytic leukemia zinc finger is critical for the proliferation of hematopoietic precursors. *Blood.* 2009;113(20):4866-4874.
[139] Camos M, Esteve J, Jares P, et al. Gene expression profiling of acute myeloid leukemia with translocation t(8;16)(p11;p13) and MYST3-CREBBP rearrangement reveals a distinctive signature with a specific pattern of HOX gene expression. *Cancer Res.* 2006;66(14):6947-6954.
[140] Crump JG, Swartz ME, Eberhart JK, Kimmel CB. Moz-dependent Hox expression controls segment-specific fate maps of skeletal precursors in the face. *Development.* 2006;133(14):2661-2669.
[141] Miller CT, Maves L, Kimmel CB. moz regulates Hox expression and pharyngeal segmental identity in zebrafish. *Development.* 2004;131(10):2443-2461.
[142] Voss AK, Collin C, Dixon MP, Thomas T. Moz and retinoic acid coordinately regulate H3K9 acetylation, Hox gene expression, and segment identity. *Dev Cell.* 2009;17(5):674-686.
[143] Schuettengruber B, Chourrout D, Vervoort M, Leblanc B, Cavalli G. Genome regulation by polycomb and trithorax proteins. *Cell.* 2007;128(4):735-745.

[144] Nakamura T, Mori T, Tada S, et al. ALL-1 is a histone methyltransferase that assembles a supercomplex of proteins involved in transcriptional regulation. *Mol Cell.* 2002;10(5):1119-1128.

[145] Hess JL, Yu BD, Li B, Hanson R, Korsmeyer SJ. Defects in yolk sac hematopoiesis in Mll-null embryos. *Blood.* 1997;90(5):1799-1806.

[146] Ernst P, Fisher JK, Avery W, Wade S, Foy D, Korsmeyer SJ. Definitive hematopoiesis requires the mixed-lineage leukemia gene. *Dev Cell.* 2004;6(3):437-443.

[147] Jude CD, Climer L, Xu D, Artinger E, Fisher JK, Ernst P. Unique and independent roles for MLL in adult hematopoietic stem cells and progenitors. *Cell Stem Cell.* 2007;1(3):324-337.

[148] McMahon KA, Hiew SY, Hadjur S, et al. Mll has a critical role in fetal and adult hematopoietic stem cell self-renewal. *Cell Stem Cell.* 2007;1(3):338-345.

[149] Krivtsov AV and Armstrong SA. MLL translocations, histone modifications and leukaemia stem-cell development. *Nat Rev Cancer.* 2007;7(11):823-833.

[150] Krivtsov AV, Feng Z, Lemieux ME, et al. H3K79 methylation profiles define murine and human MLL-AF4 leukemias. *Cancer Cell.* 2008;14(5):355-368.

[151] Okada Y, Feng Q, Lin Y, et al. hDOT1L links histone methylation to leukemogenesis. *Cell.* 2005;121(2):167-178.

[152] Guenther MG, Lawton LN, Rozovskaia T, et al. Aberrant chromatin at genes encoding stem cell regulators in human mixed-lineage leukemia. *Genes Dev.* 2008;22(24):3403-3408.

[153] Shi Y and Whetstine JR. Dynamic regulation of histone lysine methylation by demethylases. *Mol Cell.* 2007;25(1):1-14.

[154] van Zutven LJ, Onen E, Velthuizen SC, et al. Identification of NUP98 abnormalities in acute leukemia: JARID1A (12p13) as a new partner gene. *Genes Chromosomes Cancer.* 2006;45(5):437-446.

[155] Wang GG, Song J, Wang Z, et al. Haematopoietic malignancies caused by dysregulation of a chromatin-binding PHD finger. *Nature.* 2009;459(7248):847-851.

[156] Schwartz YB and Pirrotta V. Polycomb silencing mechanisms and the management of genomic programmes. *Nat Rev Genet.* 2007;8(1):9-22.

[157] Cao R, Wang L, Wang H, et al. Role of histone H3 lysine 27 methylation in Polycomb-group silencing. *Science.* 2002;298(5595):1039-1043.

[158] Cao R and Zhang Y. The functions of E(Z)/EZH2-mediated methylation of lysine 27 in histone H3. *Curr Opin Genet Dev.* 2004;14(2):155-164.

[159] Dellino GI, Schwartz YB, Farkas G, McCabe D, Elgin SC, Pirrotta V. Polycomb silencing blocks transcription initiation. *Mol Cell.* 2004;13(6):887-893.

[160] Shao Z, Raible F, Mollaaghababa R, et al. Stabilization of chromatin structure by PRC1, a Polycomb complex. *Cell.* 1999;98(1):37-46.

[161] Wang H, Wang L, Erdjument-Bromage H, et al. Role of histone H2A ubiquitination in Polycomb silencing. *Nature.* 2004;431(7010):873-878.

[162] de NM, Mermoud JE, Wakao R, et al. Polycomb group proteins Ring1A/B link ubiquitylation of histone H2A to heritable gene silencing and X inactivation. *Dev Cell.* 2004;7(5):663-676.

[163] Cao R, Tsukada Y, Zhang Y. Role of Bmi-1 and Ring1A in H2A ubiquitylation and Hox gene silencing. *Mol Cell.* 2005;20(6):845-854.

[164] Kallin EM, Cao R, Jothi R, et al. Genome-wide uH2A localization analysis highlights Bmi1-dependent deposition of the mark at repressed genes. *PLoS Genet.* 2009;5(6):e1000506.
[165] Boyer LA, Plath K, Zeitlinger J, et al. Polycomb complexes repress developmental regulators in murine embryonic stem cells. *Nature.* 2006;441(7091):349-353.
[166] Lee TI, Jenner RG, Boyer LA, et al. Control of developmental regulators by Polycomb in human embryonic stem cells. *Cell.* 2006;125(2):301-313.
[167] Bracken AP, Dietrich N, Pasini D, Hansen KH, Helin K. Genome-wide mapping of Polycomb target genes unravels their roles in cell fate transitions. *Genes Dev.* 2006;20(9):1123-1136.
[168] Varambally S, Dhanasekaran SM, Zhou M, et al. The polycomb group protein EZH2 is involved in progression of prostate cancer. *Nature.* 2002;419(6907):624-629.
[169] Kleer CG, Cao Q, Varambally S, et al. EZH2 is a marker of aggressive breast cancer and promotes neoplastic transformation of breast epithelial cells. *Proc Natl Acad Sci USA.* 2003;100(20):11606-11611.
[170] Bracken AP, Pasini D, Capra M, Prosperini E, Colli E, Helin K. EZH2 is downstream of the pRB-E2F pathway, essential for proliferation and amplified in cancer. *EMBO J.* 2003;22(20):5323-5335.
[171] Kamminga LM, Bystrykh LV, de BA, et al. The Polycomb group gene Ezh2 prevents hematopoietic stem cell exhaustion. *Blood.* 2006;107(5):2170-2179.
[172] Villa R, Pasini D, Gutierrez A, et al. Role of the polycomb repressive complex 2 in acute promyelocytic leukemia. *Cancer Cell.* 2007;11(6):513-525.
[173] Sawa M, Yamamoto K, Yokozawa T, et al. BMI-1 is highly expressed in M0-subtype acute myeloid leukemia. *Int J Hematol.* 2005;82(1):42-47.
[174] Bea S, Tort F, Pinyol M, et al. BMI-1 gene amplification and overexpression in hematological malignancies occur mainly in mantle cell lymphomas. *Cancer Res.* 2001;61(6):2409-2412.
[175] Chowdhury M, Mihara K, Yasunaga S, Ohtaki M, Takihara Y, Kimura A. Expression of Polycomb-group (PcG) protein BMI-1 predicts prognosis in patients with acute myeloid leukemia. *Leukemia.* 2007;21(5):1116-1122.
[176] Haupt Y, Alexander WS, Barri G, Klinken SP, Adams JM. Novel zinc finger gene implicated as myc collaborator by retrovirally accelerated lymphomagenesis in E mu-myc transgenic mice. *Cell.* 1991;65(5):753-763.
[177] van LM, Verbeek S, Scheijen B, Wientjens E, van der GH, Berns A. Identification of cooperating oncogenes in E mu-myc transgenic mice by provirus tagging. *Cell.* 1991;65(5):737-752.
[178] van der Lugt NM, Domen J, Linders K, et al. Posterior transformation, neurological abnormalities, and severe hematopoietic defects in mice with a targeted deletion of the bmi-1 proto-oncogene. *Genes Dev.* 1994;8(7):757-769.
[179] Park IK, Qian D, Kiel M, et al. Bmi-1 is required for maintenance of adult self-renewing haematopoietic stem cells. *Nature.* 2003;423(6937):302-305.
[180] Iwama A, Oguro H, Negishi M, et al. Enhanced self-renewal of hematopoietic stem cells mediated by the polycomb gene product Bmi-1. *Immunity.* 2004;21(6):843-851.
[181] Lessard J and Sauvageau G. Bmi-1 determines the proliferative capacity of normal and leukaemic stem cells. *Nature.* 2003;423(6937):255-260.

[182] Rizo A, Dontje B, Vellenga E, de HG, Schuringa JJ. Long-term maintenance of human hematopoietic stem/progenitor cells by expression of BMI1. *Blood.* 2008;111(5):2621-2630.

[183] Rizo A, Olthof S, Han L, Vellenga E, de HG, Schuringa JJ. Repression of BMI1 in normal and leukemic human CD34(+) cells impairs self-renewal and induces apoptosis. *Blood.* 2009;114(8):1498-1505.

[184] Jacobs JJ, Kieboom K, Marino S, DePinho RA, van LM. The oncogene and Polycomb-group gene bmi-1 regulates cell proliferation and senescence through the ink4a locus. *Nature.* 1999;397(6715):164-168.

[185] Bruggeman SW, Valk-Lingbeek ME, van der Stoop PP, et al. Ink4a and Arf differentially affect cell proliferation and neural stem cell self-renewal in Bmi1-deficient mice. *Genes Dev.* 2005;19(12):1438-1443.

[186] Liu J, Cao L, Chen J, et al. Bmi1 regulates mitochondrial function and the DNA damage response pathway. *Nature.* 2009;459(7245):387-392.

[187] Dash A and Gilliland DG. Molecular genetics of acute myeloid leukaemia. *Best Pract Res Clin Haematol.* 2001;14(1):49-64.

[188] Chan IT, Kutok JL, Williams IR, et al. Oncogenic K-ras cooperates with PML-RAR alpha to induce an acute promyelocytic leukemia-like disease. *Blood.* 2006; 108(5):1708-1715.

[189] Kelly LM, Kutok JL, Williams IR, et al. PML/RARalpha and FLT3-ITD induce an APL-like disease in a mouse model. *Proc Natl Acad Sci USA.* 2002;99(12):8283-8288.

[190] Schessl C, Rawat VP, Cusan M, et al. The AML1-ETO fusion gene and the FLT3 length mutation collaborate in inducing acute leukemia in mice. *J Clin Invest.* 2005;115(8):2159-2168.

[191] Zheng X, Oancea C, Henschler R, Ruthardt M. Cooperation between constitutively activated c-Kit signaling and leukemogenic transcription factors in the determination of the leukemic phenotype in murine hematopoietic stem cells. *Int J Oncol.* 2009; 34(6):1521-1531.

[192] Suzuki T, Kiyoi H, Ozeki K, et al. Clinical characteristics and prognostic implications of NPM1 mutations in acute myeloid leukemia. *Blood.* 2005;106(8):2854-2861.

[193] Boukarabila H, Saurin AJ, Batsche E, et al. The PRC1 Polycomb group complex interacts with PLZF/RARA to mediate leukemic transformation. *Genes Dev.* 2009;23(10):1195-1206.

[194] Yergeau DA, Hetherington CJ, Wang Q, et al. Embryonic lethality and impairment of haematopoiesis in mice heterozygous for an AML1-ETO fusion gene. *Nat Genet.* 1997;15(3):303-306.

[195] Castilla LH, Wijmenga C, Wang Q, et al. Failure of embryonic hematopoiesis and lethal hemorrhages in mouse embryos heterozygous for a knocked-in leukemia gene CBFB-MYH11. *Cell.* 1996;87(4):687-696.

[196] Castilla LH, Garrett L, Adya N, et al. The fusion gene Cbfb-MYH11 blocks myeloid differentiation and predisposes mice to acute myelomonocytic leukaemia. *Nat Genet.* 1999;23(2):144-146.

[197] Iwasaki M, Kuwata T, Yamazaki Y, et al. Identification of cooperative genes for NUP98-HOXA9 in myeloid leukemogenesis using a mouse model. *Blood.* 2005; 105(2):784-793.

[198] Corral J, Lavenir I, Impey H, et al. An Mll-AF9 fusion gene made by homologous recombination causes acute leukemia in chimeric mice: a method to create fusion oncogenes. *Cell.* 1996;85(6):853-861.

[199] Dobson CL, Warren AJ, Pannell R, et al. The mll-AF9 gene fusion in mice controls myeloproliferation and specifies acute myeloid leukaemogenesis. *EMBO J.* 1999;18(13):3564-3574.

[200] Honda H, Fujii T, Takatoku M, et al. Expression of p210bcr/abl by metallothionein promoter induced T-cell leukemia in transgenic mice. *Blood.* 1995;85(10):2853-2861.

[201] Voncken JW, Kaartinen V, Pattengale PK, Germeraad WT, Groffen J, Heisterkamp N. BCR/ABL P210 and P190 cause distinct leukemia in transgenic mice. *Blood.* 1995;86(12):4603-4611.

[202] Honda H, Oda H, Suzuki T, et al. Development of acute lymphoblastic leukemia and myeloproliferative disorder in transgenic mice expressing p210bcr/abl: a novel transgenic model for human Ph1-positive leukemias. *Blood.* 1998;91(6):2067-2075.

[203] Huettner CS, Zhang P, Van Etten RA, Tenen DG. Reversibility of acute B-cell leukaemia induced by BCR-ABL1. *Nat Genet.* 2000;24(1):57-60.

[204] Chalandon Y, Jiang X, Hazlewood G, et al. Modulation of p210(BCR-ABL) activity in transduced primary human hematopoietic cells controls lineage programming. *Blood.* 2002;99(9):3197-3204.

[205] Schwieger M, Lohler J, Fischer M, Herwig U, Tenen DG, Stocking C. A dominant-negative mutant of C/EBPalpha, associated with acute myeloid leukemias, inhibits differentiation of myeloid and erythroid progenitors of man but not mouse. *Blood.* 2004;103(7):2744-2752.

In: Stem Cell Research: New Developments
Editors: Hiroshi Tanaka and Michael C. F. Chang
ISBN: 978-1-61942-081-6

Chapter 11

MESENCHYMAL STEM CELLS AND THEIR ROLE IN TUMOR PROGRESSION

Jürgen Dittmer*
Clinic for Gynecology, University of Halle, Germany

ABSTRACT

Mesenchymal stem cells (MSCs) are adult stem cells that derive from the bone marrow. A major feature of these cells is their ability to differentiate into adipocytes, chondrocytes or osteocytes. They are also defined by the expression of certain markers, such as CD105, CD73 and CD90, and the lack of others (CD45, CD34, CD14, CD79a and HLA-DR). This expression profile makes them distinct from other bone-derived cells. Several functions have been attributed to MSCs. E.g., MSCs modulate immune responses by suppressing the activities of a number of immune cells. This function is thought to be important to prevent excessive inflammation in the wound healing process. MSCs are chemoattracted to wounds. Probably mistaking tumors for wounds, MSCs also enter solid tumors, where they modulate the activities of tumor cells by exposing them to a plethora of cyto- and chemokines. Recently, MSC-secreted CCL5 has been shown to trigger breast cancer cells to metastasize to lung. Moreover, MSCs are able to differentiate into carcinoma-associated fibroblasts (CAF) which are known to have tumor-promoting activity. This review will summarize the current knowledge on the functions of MSCs in tumor progression.

1. DEFINING MESENCHYMAL STEM CELLS

Mesenchymal stem cells (MSCs) or also called multipotent mesenchymal stromal cells were discovered by Alexander Friedenstein. Friedenstein found a population of bone marrow stromal cells that are distinct from haematopoietic progenitor cells in that they were able to form osseous tissues instead of giving rise to haematopoietic cells [1]. These osteogenic cells are clonogenic cells with fibroblast-like appearance. Owing to their capability of self-maintenance they were classified as stem cells [2,3]. These stem cells are able to differentiate to a number of mesenchymal cells, such as adipocytes, chondroblasts and osteoblasts [4]. MSCs are rare in the bone marrow (1 MSC per 34000 nucleated cells) [5] and are a heterogenous population of cells that show varying developmental potentials (reviewed in [6]). When maintained in vitro, they may quickly lose their potential to differentiate to chondrocytes and adipocytes. Up to now, there are no specific markers defined that allow to clearly identify a cell as an MSC. Instead, a list of minimal criteria has been proposed by the International Society for Cellular Therapy to be used to define an MSC [7]. These criteria include (i) adherence to plastic, (ii) capacity to differentiate to osteoblasts, adipocytes and chondroblasts and (iii) expression of the surface markers CD105 (endoglin), CD73 (ecto 5'-nucleotidase) and CD90 (Thy-1) and lack of the surface markers CD45 (pan-leukocyte marker), CD34 (marker for primitive haematopoietic progenitors and endothelial cells), CD14 and CD11 (markers for monocytes and macrophages), CD79α and CD19 (markers for B-cells) and HLA-DR (provided that MSCs are not stimulated by factors, such as IFN-γ). To isolate human (h)MSCs from bone marrow aspirates cells are grown in culture plastic ware to separate plastic adherent hMSCs from the other non-adherent bone marrow cells. For the verification of the hMSC characteristics, the plastic-adherent cells are tested for their ability to differentiate to osteoblasts, adipocytes and chondroblasts and examined for the expression or lack of expression of the above mentioned markers by FACS analysis [8]. In addition to bone marrow, a variety of other tissues, such as human adipose, can be used as a source for isolating hMSCs [9]. Interestingly, pericytes show characteristics of MSCs [10]. Pericytes isolated from skeletal muscles or non-muscle tissues have the potential to differentiate to osteobasts, adipocytes and chondroblasts and express typical MSC markers.

2. Immunomodulatory Effects of MSCs

There is growing evidence that MSCs modulate the activities of immune cells (reviewed in [11]). Immune cells of both types of immunity, innate and adaptive, are affected by MSCs (Table 1). Of the innate immunity, antigen-presenting dendritic cells (DCs), type I interferon-expression plasmacytoid dendritic cells (pDCs), anti-tumor acting natural killer (NK) cells and anti-bacterial acting neutrophils are targets of MSCs. Of the adaptive immunity, B-cells and different types of T-cells are susceptible to MSCs. Dendritic cells are important for antigen presentation. MSCs have been shown to block the maturation of monocytes to mature dendritic cells [12,13] suggesting that antigen presentation and, hence, immune responses are suppressed by MSCs. Also the expression levels of a number of cytokines in DCs are altered by MSCs [14]. Interestingly, while the secretion of the anti-inflammatory interleukin-10 is upregulated, the expression of the pro-inflammatory tumor necrosis factor is reduced [14,15] supporting the notion that MSCs have the potential to act immunosuppressive. MSCs' interference with the immune system is continued on the level of T-cells. First, as a consequence of MSCs negative effect of DC maturation the number of T-cells activated by

* Correspondence concerning this article should be addressed to: Jürgen Dittmer, Clinic for Gynecology, University of Halle, Ernst-Grube-Str. 40, 06120 Halle, Germany. Tel: +49-345-557-1338; Fax: +49-345-557-5261; e.mail: juergen.dittmer@medizin.uni-halle.de.

DC-dependent antigen presentation decline. Second, MSCs inhibit the proliferation of activated T-cells [16-19] by arresting them in the G1 phase [20]. The G1 arrest was accompanied by downregulation of cyclin D2 and upregulation of $p27^{kip1}$. In addition, in response to MSCs, a shift in the T-helper cell population from pro-inflammatory T_H1 to anti-inflammatory T_H2 cells and an expansion of suppressive regulatory $CD4^+$ T-cells are observed [14,51] which may reduce T-helper cell-dependent B-cell response and hence antibody production. This may further contribute to the immunosuppressive effect of MSCs. In respect to the immune response to tumor cells, it is striking that MSCs inhibit the activity of $CD8^+$ cytotoxic T-cells [22] as well as the proliferation of cytotoxic NK-cells [14,23,24]. Hence, MSCs attack anti-tumor effector cells of both the adaptive and innate immune system and may therefore reduce the ability of the immune system to recognize and eliminate tumor cells. It is interesting that MSCs can also be targeted NK cells as MSCs express low levels of MHC class I molecules [25]. In the presence of interferon γ which increases the expression level of the MHC class I molecules, MSCs are more protected against NK-mediating cytotoxicity [25]. The balance between MSCs and NK cells and hence the extent of the cytotoxic effect of NK cells on tumor cells may therefore be dependent upon the level of certain cytokines. The effect of MSCs on immune cells seems to be accomplished by direct cell-cell contact and by soluble factors that are secreted by MSCs. Among these MSC-released factors are prostaglandin E2, interleukin-6, indoleamine 2,3-dioxygenase (IDO) and sHLA-G5 [14,21,23,26]. The expression of CD90 seems to be important for the immunosuppressive activity of MSCs, as downregulation of CD90 resulted in loss of the inhibitory effect of MSCs on the proliferation of PHA-stimulated peripheral blood lymphocytes [27,28]. This was accompanied by reduced secretion of sHLA-G und interleukin-10.

3. MSCs and Injuries

Inflammation seems to attract MSCs [31]. MSCs have been suggested to "sense" injuries as they enter wounds to contribute to wound healing [32-37]. By using bioluminescent imaging, Kidd et al. showed that, when injected to injured mice, MSCs expressing the firefly luciferase were predominantly visible in wounds, whereas, in non-injured mice, MSCs were found in lungs, liver and spleen [38]. Facilitated wound healing by MSCs could be demonstrated, when the lungs of mice were injured by bleomycin. MSCs that colonized the injured lung differentiated to specific lung epithelium-like cell phenotypes and suppressed inflammation and collagen deposition [32,39]. Intravenously delivered MSCs into rats have been shown to ameliorate recovery from middle cerebral artery occlusion (MCAO)-evoked stroke [34,40]. This was accompanied by the presence of MSCs in the ischemic hemisphere. Differentiation of MSCs to cells expressing neuronal markers have also been observed [40]. The notion that MSCs are able to differentiate to neurons has been supported by experiments with MSCs derived from umbilical cord blood [41-43]. However, whether MSCs are in fact able to transdifferentiate into neurons is a matter of debate, since MSCs have been shown to spontaneously fuse with other cells [44,45]. MSCs have also been reported to enter lesions of chronic rejection in rats with cardiac grafts or to invade infarcted myocards where they differentiate to fibroblasts or even to cardiomyocytes [37,46,47]. In the presence of MSCs, rats showed better recovery from kidney damage (mesangiolysis) [48]. The regenerated glomeruli contained MSC-derived glomerular cells. Also, ischemically injured renal tubules in mice could be repaired by MSCs which differentiated to tubular epithelial cells [49,50]. In diabetic mice, intracardically infused or intravenously injected MSCs increased the number of pancreatic islets and insulin production [51,52]. Some of the pancreatic islets contained hMSC-derived insulin-producing cells.

Table 1. Effects of MSCs on immune cells

type of immunity	cell type	function	effects of MSCs	MSC-released factor(s) involved	references
innate	dendritic cells (DCs), plasmacytoid DCs (pDCs)	antigen-presenting, expression of type I interferon	impairment of antigen-presenting function, inhibition of tumor necrosis factor production, increased expression of anti-inflammatory cytokine IL-10	prostaglandin E2	[12-14]
innate	natural killer cells (NKs)	anti-viral and anti-tumor effector activities	inhibition of cytotoxic effects, anti-proliferative, inhibition of interferon γ production	prostaglandin E2	[14, 23, 24]
innate	neutrophils	defense against bacteria	inhibition of respiratory burst activity and apoptosis	interleukin-6	[26]
adaptive	T-cells	several effector functions	anti-proliferative, increased survival of quiescent cells, decreased interferon γ production, decreased cytotoxicity as mediated by cytotoxic T-cells (CTL)	prostaglandin E2 sHLA-GS indoleamine 2,3-dioxygenase (IDO)	[14, 16-22]
adaptive	B-cells	antibody productions	controversial, maybe anti-proliferative		[20, 29, 30]

The apparent plasticity of MSCs and their ability to predominantly colonizes wounds have fueled the hope that MSCs are ideal tools for tissue regeneration [31]. In particular, MSCs may be useful agents to treat neurological disorders and spinal cord injury [53] as well as the infarcted myocardium [35,54,55]. MSCs can potentially also be used as vehicles to administer drugs to sites of injuries. E.g., BDNF (brain-derived neurotrophic factor) expressing MSCs have been injected into rats to improve recovery from stroke [34]. Similarly, insulin-producing MSCs have been administered to mice to treat diabetes [56]. However, this enthusiasm has recently been dampened by the observation that hMSC frequently undergo sponteaneous malignant transformation *in vitro* [57]. The transformed hMSCs were shown to trigger the development of lung cancer in mice. In addition, hMSCs can be transformed into sarcoma cells [58-60]. Whether hMSCs injected in humans for therapeutic uses will also transform and induce cancer is not yet know.

4. MSCs and Cancer

MSCs are also attracted to tumors [38,61,62]. E.g., luciferase-loaden MSCs specifically accumulated in breast cancer xenografts in mice [38]. Tumors can be assumed to be wounds that never heal [63]. It is, therefore, thought that MSCs "mistake" tumors for normal wounds, probably as a result of similar inflammatory signals that are released by wounds and tumors [64]. A number of studies support this hypothesis. When prostate Capan-1 cancer cells were injected into SCID (severe combined immunodeficient) mice whose bone marrow was replaced by bone marrow from beta-galactosidase transgenic mice, X-gal positive cells were identified in the tumor [65]. The X-gal positive cells were mostly fibroblasts and to a lesser extent endothelial cells suggesting that X-gal positive MSCs entered the tumor and differentiated into various stromal cells. In a similar way, bone marrow of a GFP-positive mouse was transplanted into a GFP-negative mouse with pancreatic insulinoma. GFP-positive cells were found within the tumor [66]. Of the myofibroblasts in the tumor, 25% were GFP positive and, hence, derived from the donor bone marrow.

The ability to trace and invade tumors may make MSCs a good tool for delivering anti-tumor drugs to the tumors. A number of studies have been undertaken to analyze this interesting possibility. In these studies, MSCs loaded with chemokines, cytokines or oncolytic viruses were injected into tumor-bearing mice. In one study, MSCs was engineered to express the immunostimulatory chemokine CX3CL1. It was found that CX3CL1-expressing MSCs inhibited lung metastasis formation by B16.F10 murine melanoma and C26 murine colon carcinoma cells [62]. Likewise, the growth of malignant human A375SM melanoma cells in mice was decreased when mice were injected with hMSCs expressing interferon β [61]. Also, TRAIL (TNF-related apoptosis inducing ligand) expressing hMSCs inhibited growth of DLD-1 colorectal cancer cells and U87 glioma cells in mouse xenografts [67, 68]. Another study showed that interleukin-2 overexpressing rat MSCs home to tumors formed by 9L gliomas and reduce their growth [69]. Fritz et al. transfected murine MSCs with the uPA (urokinase plasminogen activator) inhibitor hATF, an amino-terminal fragment of uPA, and administered these cells to mice to successfully treat bone lesions as induced by metastatic prostate cancer cells [70]. Two groups used hMSCs as vehicles to specifically deliver the oncolytic Delta24-RGD or CRAd adenovirus to glioma xenografts formed by U87MG or U251-V121 glioma cells [71,72]. These adenovirus-infected hMSCs entered the tumors and induced tumor growth inhibition or even elimination. Another interesting approach is the use of MSCs for localized chemotherapy. hMSCs were forced to express cytosine deaminase (CD), a prodrug activating enzyme that converts 5-fluorocytosine (5-FC) into the commonly used drug 5-fluorouracil (5-FU), and injected into mice bearing gastric cancer xenografts [73]. When these mice were systemically treated with 5-FC, tumor volume significantly decreased compared to the control group which did not receive hMSCs. In contrast to CD-expressing hMSCs, control hMSCs had no effect on tumor growth suggesting that the hMSC-CD-dependent conversion of 5-FC to 5-FU was required for the tumor-inhibiting effect.

Even if not loaded with anti-tumor drugs, MSCs are capable of interfering with tumor progression, as they are able to directly interact with tumor cells and to expose tumor cells to the many chemokines and cytokines they secret. Among the factors that they secret are interleukins, such as IL-6 and IL-8, other cytokines, such as TGFβ (transforming growth factor β) 1 and 2 [74] and chemokines, such als CCL2, CCL5 and CXCL12 (SDF-1 = stromal cell derived factor 1). hMSC-derived CCL5 (Rantes) may play an important role in breast cancer metastasis. When hMSCs and MDA-MB-231 breast cancer cells were subcutaneously co-injected into mice, MSCs stimulated breast cancer cells to metastasize to lung, an effect that could be mimicked by CCL5 [75]. Knock-down of the CCL5 receptor CCR in MDA-MB-231 cells abrogated the response of these cells to hMSCs suggesting that the MDA-MB-

231/hMSC communication depended upon the interaction of CCL5 with CCR5. Effects of hMSCs on other types of breast cancer cells have also been reported. hMSCs have been found to promote the motility of MCF-7 cells [76], which, in contrast to the mesenchymal MDA-MB-231 cells, are epithelial-like breast cancer cells. As such they produce E-cadherin which causes these cells to form tight cell-cell contacts. Hence, the E-cadherin based cell-cell interaction needs to be interrupted to allow movement of MCF-7 cells. Consequently, E-cadherin expression in MCF-7 cells grown in conventional two-dimensional adherent cultures was found to be downregulated in the presence of MSCs [77,78]. In three-dimensional spheroid cultures, hMSCs caused the MCF-7 cell-cell contacts to be become less tight which was accompanied by E-cadherin shedding (removal of the extracellular E-cadherin domain) [76]. E-cadherin shedding in MCF-7 cells was demonstrated to be dependent on the metalloprotease ADAM10 (a disintegrin and metalloprotease 10). As inhibition of this enzyme by the specific inhibitor GI254023X blocked hMSC-induced motility of MCF-7 cells it is likely that hMSCs interfered with the activity of ADAM10 to increase the migratory activity of MCF-7. Unlike the effect of hMSCs on the metastasic activity of MDA-MB-231 cells, the hMSC effect on the migratory activity of MCF-7 cells could not be mimicked by CCL5 suggesting that hMSCs affect the behavior of mesenchymal and epithelial-like breast cancer cells by different factors. Besides migration, hMSCs have also been shown to increase breast cancer growth *in vivo* and *in vitro* [79, 80]. In SCID/beige mice, hMSCs allowed estrogen-receptor α (ERα)-expressing MCF-7 cells to grow independently of estrogen [79]. Interestingly, this was accompanied by an increased level of the progesterone receptor. These data may indicate that hMSCs play a role in the development of resistance towards anti-estrogens which are used to treat breast cancer patients with ERα-positive breast cancer. In three-dimensional *in vitro* cultures, hMSCs were found to promote the growth of MCF-7 cells and a number of other ERα-positive breast cancer cells (T47D, BT474 and ZR-75-1) [80]. It is noteworthy that the growth of the fast-growing MDA-MB-231 cells were not affected by hMSCs. Likewise, the effect of hMSCs on the migration of the fast-migrating MDA-MB-231 cells was much weaker than on slow-migrating MCF-7 cells [76]. It seems, therefore, that aggressive MDA-MB-231 cells already reached their limits in regard to their migratory and proliferative activities so that hMSCs are not able to further enhance them. In contrast, the metastatic potential of MDA-MB-231 cells may not be fully exploited and, hence, can be further increased by MSCs via CCL5.

MSCs also affect other types of cancer. Yu et al. showed that MSCs isolated from adipose tissues stimulated tumor growth when injected together with the lung cancer cell line H460 or the human glioblastoma-astrocytoma cell line U87MG in nude mice [81]. In tissue culture experiments, hMSCs stimulated the proliferation of H460 or U87MG cells suggesting that the effect of hMSCs on tumor growth was direct. Also indirect effects of MSCs on tumor expansion has been described. Djouad et al. showed that B16 melanoma cells, that were able to form tumors in immunocompetent syngeneic mice, failed to do so in allogeneic mice [82]. Tumor growth by B16 cells could be rescued in allogeneic mice, if MSCs were co-injected along with the B16 cancer cells. It is thought that, in the allogenic mice, the immunosuppressive activity of the MSCs prevented clearance of the tumor cells by the host immune system. Djouad and co-workers also demonstrated that Renca adenocarcinoma cells grew faster in mice when co-injected with MSCs [83], although, *in vitro* co-culture experiments, MSCs failed to affect the growth rate of Renca cells. Again it is believed that MSCs stimulated tumor growth *in vivo* by inhibiting the immune response.

Some studies show that MSCs can also act inhibitory on tumor growth. When Maestroni et al. compared the ability of Lewis lung carcinoma or B16 melanoma to form tumors in mice in the presence vs. absence of MSCs they found that, in the presence of bone marrow stroma, tumor formation was attenuated [84]. Similarly, when rat colon carcinoma cells entrapped in a gelatin matrix were implanted into rats, the extent of tumor outgrowth was reduced when MSCs were present [85]. Also the growth of gliomas in Fisher 344 rats was reported to be negatively modulated by MSCs [69].

Another study showed that hMSCs intravenously injected into athymic nude mice bearing Kaposi sarcomas entered the tumors and inhibited their growth [86]. This growth-inhibitory effect of hMSCs was accompanied by a decrease in the activity of AKT in the tumor cells suggesting that hMSCs induced an inhibition of the PI3K/AKT pathway. In support of this notion, overexpression of a constitutively active form of AKT rendered the Kaposi sarcoma cells resistent to hMSCs. The hMSC effect on the Kaposi sarcoma cells seems to be mediated by direct cell-cell contact as antibodies against E-cadherin prevented hMSC from modulating the tumor cell activity. Qiao et al found that, when hMSCs were injected together with H7402 or HepG2 hepatoma cells into SCID mice, the onset of tumor formation was delayed [87]. The anti-tumor effect of hMSCs was confirmed by tissue culture experiments demonstrating that hMSCs decreased proliferation and increased apoptosis by reducing the expression of pro-apoptotic proteins.

Cancer cells have also been shown to act back on MSCs. MDA-MB-231 and to a lesser extent MCF-7 breast cancer cells were found to stimulate the migratory activity of hMSCs in the Boyden chamber [76]. This effect could be mimicked by conditioned medium derived from these breast cancer cell lines. In addition, hMSCs were found to move towards and enter MCF-7 spheroids. Three MDA-MB-231 derived factors, the chemokine MCP-1 (CCL-2), cyclophilin B and hepatoma-derived growth factor (HDGF), have been shown to be able to stimulate hMSC migration [88,89]. Of these, MCP-1 are also secreted by the T47D breast cancer cell line as well as by primary breast cancer-derived stromal and epithelial cells [89]. Hence, breast cancer cells in general may be able to enhance the migratory activity of hMSCs. Also conditioned medium (CM) from B85 human colorectal cancer cells stimulated the migration of hMSCs [90]. Comparative cDNA microarray analyses of the hMSC exposed to CM from B85 cells and bone marrow revealed that the expression of 104 genes were upregulated in response to B85-CM. These genes included a number of genes coding for chemokines, such as SDF-1 (CXCL-12) and MCP-1. Interestingly, knock-down of SDF-1 in hMSCs abrogated the stimulatory effect of B85-CM. This suggests that factor(s) secreted by B85 colorectal cancer cells stimulated an SDF-1 dependent autocrine loop in hMSCs causing these cells to move faster.

Conclusion

There is striking evidence that MSCs are attracted to wounds and facilitate wound healing by downregulating the inflammatory response and by differentiating to those cell types that are required to restore the function of the injured tissue. Given their imazing plasticity MSCs may generally function as "repair cells" that quickly adopt to the needs of the tissue to which they have been recruited. In terms of cancer, this need may be the recruitment of cells that promote proliferation and migration and inhibit apoptosis. In fact, exposed to tumor-conditioned medium, MSCs have been found to differentiate to carcinoma-associated fibroblasts (CAFs) that are known to be involved in cancer progression [91]. Cancer may also "use" MSCs as a shield against the attack by the immune system. And, since exposure of cancer to anti-cancer drugs have been shown to result in an increase of a population of cells that express stem cell markers [92], MSCs may also help cancer cells to survive drug attacks as MSCs are drug-resistant [93]. The similarity of MSCs with cancer stem cells (CSCs) has even led to the discussion of whether, in certain cancers, CSCs are MSCs [94]. On the other hand, their tropism for cancers makes MSCs an ideal tool for delivering anti-cancer drugs to many types of cancers and may help to develop more specific strategies for cancer treatment.

REFERENCES

[1] Friedenstein, A. J., Piatetzky, S., II & Petrakova, K. V. (1966) Osteogenesis in transplants of bone marrow cells. *J Embryol Exp Morphol, 16*, 381-390.

[2] Friedenstein, A. & Kuralesova, A. I. (1971) Osteogenic precursor cells of bone marrow in radiation chimeras. *Transplantation, 12*, 99-108.

[3] Caplan, A. I. (1991) Mesenchymal stem cells. *J Orthop Res., 9*, 641-650.

[4] Friedenstein, A. J., Chailakhyan, R. K., Latsinik, N. V., Panasyuk, A. F. & Keiliss-Borok, I. V. (1974) Stromal cells responsible for transferring the microenvironment of the hemopoietic tissues. Cloning in vitro and retransplantation in vivo. *Transplantation, 17*, 331-340.

[5] Wexler, S. A., Donaldson, C., Denning-Kendall, P., Rice, C., Bradley, B. & Hows, J. M. (2003) Adult bone marrow is a rich source of human mesenchymal 'stem' cells but umbilical cord and mobilized adult blood are not. *Br J Haematol, 121*, 368-374.

[6] Phinney, D. G. (2002) Building a consensus regarding the nature and origin of mesenchymal stem cells. *J Cell Biochem Suppl, 38*, 7-12.

[7] Dominici, M., Le Blanc, K., Mueller, I., Slaper-Cortenbach, I., Marini, F., Krause, D., Deans, R., Keating, A., Prockop, D. & Horwitz, E. (2006) Minimal criteria for defining multipotent mesenchymal stromal cells. The International Society for Cellular Therapy position statement. *Cytotherapy, 8*, 315-317.

[8] Beyer Nardi, N. & da Silva Meirelles, L. (2006) Mesenchymal stem cells: isolation, in vitro expansion and characterization. *Handb Exp Pharmacol*, 249-282.

[9] Zuk, P. A., Zhu, M., Mizuno, H., Huang, J., Futrell, J. W., Katz, A. J., Benhaim, P., Lorenz, H. P. & Hedrick, M. H. (2001) Multilineage cells from human adipose tissue: implications for cell-based therapies. *Tissue Eng, 7*, 211-228.

[10] Crisan, M., Yap, S., Casteilla, L., Chen, C. W., Corselli, M., Park, T. S., Andriolo, G., Sun, B., Zheng, B., Zhang, L., Norotte, C., Teng, P. N., Traas, J., Schugar, R., Deasy, B. M., Badylak, S., Buhring, H. J., Giacobino, J. P., Lazzari, L., Huard, J. & Peault, B. (2008) A perivascular origin for mesenchymal stem cells in multiple human organs. *Cell Stem Cell, 3*, 301-313.

[11] Uccelli, A., Moretta, L. & Pistoia, V. (2008) Mesenchymal stem cells in health and disease. *Nat Rev Immunol, 8*, 726-736.

[12] Jiang, X. X., Zhang, Y., Liu, B., Zhang, S. X., Wu, Y., Yu, X. D. & Mao, N. (2005) Human mesenchymal stem cells inhibit differentiation and function of monocyte-derived dendritic cells. *Blood, 105*, 4120-4126.

[13] Ramasamy, R., Fazekasova, H., Lam, E. W., Soeiro, I., Lombardi, G. & Dazzi, F. (2007) Mesenchymal stem cells inhibit dendritic cell differentiation and function by preventing entry into the cell cycle. *Transplantation, 83*, 71-76.

[14] Aggarwal, S. & Pittenger, M. F. (2005) Human mesenchymal stem cells modulate allogeneic immune cell responses. *Blood, 105*, 1815-1822.

[15] Beyth, S., Borovsky, Z., Mevorach, D., Liebergall, M., Gazit, Z., Aslan, H., Galun, E. & Rachmilewitz, J. (2005) Human mesenchymal stem cells alter antigen-presenting cell maturation and induce T-cell unresponsiveness. *Blood, 105*, 2214-2219.

[16] Bartholomew, A., Sturgeon, C., Siatskas, M., Ferrer, K., McIntosh, K., Patil, S., Hardy, W., Devine, S., Ucker, D., Deans, R., Moseley, A. & Hoffman, R. (2002) Mesenchymal stem cells suppress lymphocyte proliferation in vitro and prolong skin graft survival in vivo. *Exp Hematol, 30*, 42-48.

[17] Di Nicola, M., Carlo-Stella, C., Magni, M., Milanesi, M., Longoni, P. D., Matteucci, P., Grisanti, S. & Gianni, A. M. (2002) Human bone marrow stromal cells suppress T-lymphocyte proliferation induced by cellular or nonspecific mitogenic stimuli. *Blood, 99*, 3838-3843.

[18] Rasmusson, I., Ringden, O., Sundberg, B. & Le Blanc, K. (2005) Mesenchymal stem cells inhibit lymphocyte proliferation by mitogens and alloantigens by different mechanisms. *Exp Cell Res, 305*, 33-41.

[19] Krampera, M., Glennie, S., Dyson, J., Scott, D., Laylor, R., Simpson, E. & Dazzi, F. (2003) Bone marrow mesenchymal stem cells inhibit the response of naive and memory antigen-specific T cells to their cognate peptide. *Blood, 1*01, 3722-3729.

[20] Glennie, S., Soeiro, I., Dyson, P. J., Lam, E. W. & Dazzi, F. (2005) Bone marrow mesenchymal stem cells induce division arrest anergy of activated T cells. *Blood, 105*, 2821-2827.

[21] Selmani, Z., Naji, A., Zidi, I., Favier, B., Gaiffe, E., Obert, L., Borg, C., Saas, P., Tiberghien, P., Rouas-Freiss, N., Carosella, E. D. & Deschaseaux, F. (2008) Human leukocyte antigen-G5 secretion by human mesenchymal stem cells is required to suppress T lymphocyte and natural killer function and to induce CD4+CD25highFOXP3+ regulatory T cells. *Stem Cells, 26*, 212-222.

[22] Rasmusson, I., Ringden, O., Sundberg, B. & Le Blanc, K. (2003) Mesenchymal stem cells inhibit the formation of cytotoxic T lymphocytes, but not activated cytotoxic T lymphocytes or natural killer cells. *Transplantation, 76*, 1208-1213.

[23] Spaggiari, G. M., Capobianco, A., Abdelrazik, H., Becchetti, F., Mingari, M. C. & Moretta, L. (2008) Mesenchymal stem cells inhibit natural killer-cell proliferation, cytotoxicity, and cytokine production: role of indoleamine 2,3-dioxygenase and prostaglandin E2. *Blood, 111*, 1327-1333.

[24] Sotiropoulou, P. A., Perez, S. A., Gritzapis, A. D., Baxevanis, C. N. & Papamichail, M. (2006) Interactions between human mesenchymal stem cells and natural killer cells. *Stem Cells, 24*, 74-85.

[25] Spaggiari, G. M., Capobianco, A., Becchetti, S., Mingari, M. C. & Moretta, L. (2006) Mesenchymal stem cell-natural killer cell interactions: evidence that activated NK cells

are capable of killing MSCs, whereas MSCs can inhibit IL-2-induced NK-cell proliferation. *Blood, 107*, 1484-1490.

[26] Raffaghello, L., Bianchi, G., Bertolotto, M., Montecucco, F., Busca, A., Dallegri, F., Ottonello, L. & Pistoia, V. (2008) Human mesenchymal stem cells inhibit neutrophil apoptosis: a model for neutrophil preservation in the bone marrow niche. *Stem Cells, 26*, 151-162.

[27] Campioni, D., Lanza, F., Moretti, S., Ferrari, L. & Cuneo, A. (2008) Loss of Thy-1 (CD90) antigen expression on mesenchymal stromal cells from hematologic malignancies is induced by in vitro angiogenic stimuli and is associated with peculiar functional and phenotypic characteristics. *Cytotherapy, 10*, 69-82.

[28] Campioni, D., Rizzo, R., Stignani, M., Melchiorri, L., Ferrari, L., Moretti, S., Russo, A., Bagnara, G. P., Bonsi, L., Alviano, F., Lanzoni, G., Cuneo, A., Baricordi, O. R. & Lanza, F. (2009) A decreased positivity for CD90 on human mesenchymal stromal cells (MSCs) is associated with a loss of immunosuppressive activity by MSCs. *Cytometry B Clin Cytom, 76*, 225-230.

[29] Corcione, A., Benvenuto, F., Ferretti, E., Giunti, D., Cappiello, V., Cazzanti, F., Risso, M., Gualandi, F., Mancardi, G. L., Pistoia, V. & Uccelli, A. (2006) Human mesenchymal stem cells modulate B-cell functions. *Blood, 107*, 367-372.

[30] Traggiai, E., Volpi, S., Schena, F., Gattorno, M., Ferlito, F., Moretta, L. & Martini, A. (2008) Bone marrow-derived mesenchymal stem cells induce both polyclonal expansion and differentiation of B cells isolated from healthy donors and systemic lupus erythematosus patients. *Stem Cells, 26*, 562-569.

[31] Brooke, G., Cook, M., Blair, C., Han, R., Heazlewood, C., Jones, B., Kambouris, M., Kollar, K., McTaggart, S., Pelekanos, R., Rice, A., Rossetti, T. & Atkinson, K. (2007) Therapeutic applications of mesenchymal stromal cells. *Semin Cell Dev Biol, 18*, 846-858.

[32] Rojas, M., Xu, J., Woods, C. R., Mora, A. L., Spears, W., Roman, J. & Brigham, K. L. (2005) Bone marrow-derived mesenchymal stem cells in repair of the injured lung. *Am J Respir Cell Mol Biol, 33*, 145-152.

[33] Natsu, K., Ochi, M., Mochizuki, Y., Hachisuka, H., Yanada, S. & Yasunaga, Y. (2004) Allogeneic bone marrow-derived mesenchymal stromal cells promote the regeneration of injured skeletal muscle without differentiation into myofibers. *Tissue Eng, 10*, 1093-1112.

[34] Kurozumi, K., Nakamura, K., Tamiya, T., Kawano, Y., Kobune, M., Hirai, S., Uchida, H., Sasaki, K., Ito, Y., Kato, K., Honmou, O., Houkin, K., Date, I. & Hamada, H. (2004) BDNF gene-modified mesenchymal stem cells promote functional recovery and reduce infarct size in the rat middle cerebral artery occlusion model. *Mol Ther, 9*, 189-197.

[35] Barbash, I. M., Chouraqui, P., Baron, J., Feinberg, M. S., Etzion, S., Tessone, A., Miller, L., Guetta, E., Zipori, D., Kedes, L. H., Kloner, R. A. & Leor, J. (2003) Systemic delivery of bone marrow-derived mesenchymal stem cells to the infarcted myocardium: feasibility, cell migration, and body distribution. *Circulation, 108*, 863-868.

[36] Mahmood, A., Lu, D., Lu, M. & Chopp, M. (2003) Treatment of traumatic brain injury in adult rats with intravenous administration of human bone marrow stromal cells. *Neurosurgery, 53*, 697-702.

[37] Wu, G. D., Nolta, J. A., Jin, Y. S., Barr, M. L., Yu, H., Starnes, V. A. & Cramer, D. V. (2003) Migration of mesenchymal stem cells to heart allografts during chronic rejection. *Transplantation, 75*, 679-685.

[38] Kidd, S., Spaeth, E., Dembinski, J. L., Dietrich, M., Watson, K., Klopp, A., Battula, V. L., Weil, M., Andreeff, M. & Marini, F. C. (2009) Direct evidence of mesenchymal stem cell tropism for tumor and wounding microenvironments using in vivo bioluminescent imaging. *Stem Cells, 27*, 2614-2623.

[39] Ortiz, L. A., Gambelli, F., McBride, C., Gaupp, D., Baddoo, M., Kaminski, N. & Phinney, D. G. (2003) Mesenchymal stem cell engraftment in lung is enhanced in response to bleomycin exposure and ameliorates its fibrotic effects. *Proc Natl Acad Sci USA, 100*, 8407-8411.

[40] Chen, J., Li, Y., Wang, L., Zhang, Z., Lu, D., Lu, M. & Chopp, M. (2001) Therapeutic benefit of intravenous administration of bone marrow stromal cells after cerebral ischemia in rats. *Stroke, 32*, 1005-1011.

[41] Park, K. S., Jung, K. H., Kim, S. H., Kim, K. S., Choi, M. R., Kim, Y. & Chai, Y. G. (2007) Functional expression of ion channels in mesenchymal stem cells derived from umbilical cord vein. *Stem Cells, 25*, 2044-2052.

[42] Li, G. R., Sun, H., Deng, X. & Lau, C. P. (2005) Characterization of ionic currents in human mesenchymal stem cells from bone marrow. *Stem Cells, 23*, 371-38.

[43] Tondreau, T., Lagneaux, L., Dejeneffe, M., Massy, M., Mortier, C., Delforge, A. & Bron, D. (2004) Bone marrow-derived mesenchymal stem cells already express specific neural proteins before any differentiation. *Differentiation, 72*, 319-326.

[44] Krabbe, C., Zimmer, J. & Meyer, M. (2005) Neural transdifferentiation of mesenchymal stem cells--a critical review. *Apmis, 113*, 831-844.

[45] Wislet-Gendebien, S., Hans, G., Leprince, P., Rigo, J. M., Moonen, G. & Rogister, B. (2005) Plasticity of cultured mesenchymal stem cells: switch from nestin-positive to excitable neuron-like phenotype. *Stem Cells, 23*, 392-402.

[46] Toma, C., Pittenger, M. F., Cahill, K. S., Byrne, B. J. & Kessler, P. D. (2002) Human mesenchymal stem cells differentiate to a cardiomyocyte phenotype in the adult murine heart. *Circulation, 1*05, 93-98.

[47] Wang, J. S., Shum-Tim, D., Chedrawy, E. & Chiu, R. C. (2001) The coronary delivery of marrow stromal cells for myocardial regeneration: pathophysiologic and therapeutic implications. *J Thorac Cardiovasc Surg, 122*, 699-705.

[48] Ito, T., Suzuki, A., Imai, E., Okabe, M. & Hori, M. (2001) Bone marrow is a reservoir of repopulating mesangial cells during glomerular remodeling. *J Am Soc Nephrol,* 12, 2625-2635.

[49] Lin, F., Cordes, K., Li, L., Hood, L., Couser, W. G., Shankland, S. J. & Igarashi, P. (2003) Hematopoietic stem cells contribute to the regeneration of renal tubules after renal ischemia-reperfusion injury in mice. *J Am Soc Nephrol, 14*, 1188-1199.

[50] Kale, S., Karihaloo, A., Clark, P. R., Kashgarian, M., Krause, D. S. & Cantley, L. G. (2003) Bone marrow stem cells contribute to repair of the ischemically injured renal tubule. *J Clin Invest, 112*, 42-49.

[51] Lee, R. H., Seo, M. J., Reger, R. L., Spees, J. L., Pulin, A. A., Olson, S. D. & Prockop, D. J. (2006) Multipotent stromal cells from human marrow home to and promote repair of pancreatic islets and renal glomeruli in diabetic NOD/scid mice. *Proc Natl Acad Sci USA, 103*, 17438-17443.

[52] Hess, D., Li, L., Martin, M., Sakano, S., Hill, D., Strutt, B., Thyssen, S., Gray, D. A. & Bhatia, M. (2003) Bone marrow-derived stem cells initiate pancreatic regeneration. *Nat Biotechnol, 21*, 763-770.

[53] Phinney, D. G. & Isakova, I. (2005) Plasticity and therapeutic potential of mesenchymal stem cells in the nervous system. *Curr Pharm Des, 11*, 1255-1265.

[54] Amado, L. C., Saliaris, A. P., Schuleri, K. H., St John, M., Xie, J. S., Cattaneo, S., Durand, D. J., Fitton, T., Kuang, J. Q., Stewart, G., Lehrke, S., Baumgartner, W. W., Martin, B. J., Heldman, A. W. & Hare, J. M. (2005) Cardiac repair with intramyocardial injection of allogeneic mesenchymal stem cells after myocardial infarction. *Proc Natl Acad Sci USA, 102*, 11474-11479.

[55] Itescu, S., Schuster, M. D. & Kocher, A. A. (2003) New directions in strategies using cell therapy for heart disease. *J Mol Med, 81*, 288-296.

[56] Xu, J., Lu, Y., Ding, F., Zhan, X., Zhu, M. & Wang, Z. (2007) Reversal of diabetes in mice by intrahepatic injection of bone-derived GFP-murine mesenchymal stem cells infected with the recombinant retrovirus-carrying human insulin gene. *World J Surg, 31*, 1872-1882.

[57] Rosland, G. V., Svendsen, A., Torsvik, A., Sobala, E., McCormack, E., Immervoll, H., Mysliwietz, J., Tonn, J. C., Goldbrunner, R., Lonning, P. E., Bjerkvig, R. & Schichor, C. (2009) Long-term cultures of bone marrow-derived human mesenchymal stem cells frequently undergo spontaneous malignant transformation. *Cancer Res, 69*, 5331-5339.

[58] Burns, J. S., Abdallah, B. M., Schroder, H. D. & Kassem, M. (2008) The histopathology of a human mesenchymal stem cell experimental tumor model: support for an hMSC origin for Ewing's sarcoma? *Histol Histopathol, 23*, 1229-1240.

[59] Li, N., Yang, R., Zhang, W., Dorfman, H., Rao, P. & Gorlick, R. (2009) Genetically transforming human mesenchymal stem cells to sarcomas: changes in cellular phenotype and multilineage differentiation potential. *Cancer, 115*, 4795-4806.

[60] Riggi, N., Suva, M. L., Suva, D., Cironi, L., Provero, P., Tercier, S., Joseph, J. M., Stehle, J. C., Baumer, K., Kindler, V. & Stamenkovic, I. (2008) EWS-FLI-1 expression triggers a Ewing's sarcoma initiation program in primary human mesenchymal stem cells. *Cancer Res, 68*, 2176-2185.

[61] Studeny, M., Marini, F. C., Champlin, R. E., Zompetta, C., Fidler, I. J. & Andreeff, M. (2002) Bone marrow-derived mesenchymal stem cells as vehicles for interferon-beta delivery into tumors. *Cancer Res, 62*, 3603-3608.

[62] Xin, H., Kanehira, M., Mizuguchi, H., Hayakawa, T., Kikuchi, T., Nukiwa, T. & Saijo, Y. (2007) Targeted delivery of CX3CL1 to multiple lung tumors by mesenchymal stem cells. *Stem Cells, 25*, 1618-1626.

[63] Dvorak, H. F. (1986) Tumors: wounds that do not heal. Similarities between tumor stroma generation and wound healing. *N Engl J Med, 315*, 1650-1659.

[64] Kidd, S., Spaeth, E., Klopp, A., Andreeff, M., Hall, B. & Marini, F. C. (2008) The (in) auspicious role of mesenchymal stromal cells in cancer: be it friend or foe. *Cytotherapy, 10*, 657-667.

[65] Ishii, G., Sangai, T., Oda, T., Aoyagi, Y., Hasebe, T., Kanomata, N., Endoh, Y., Okumura, C., Okuhara, Y., Magae, J., Emura, M., Ochiya, T. & Ochiai, A. (2003) Bone-marrow-derived myofibroblasts contribute to the cancer-induced stromal reaction. *Biochem Biophys Res Commun, 309*, 232-240.

[66] Direkze, N. C., Hodivala-Dilke, K., Jeffery, R., Hunt, T., Poulsom, R., Oukrif, D., Alison, M. R. & Wright, N. A. (2004) Bone marrow contribution to tumor-associated myofibroblasts and fibroblasts. *Cancer Res, 64*, 8492-8495.

[67] Luetzkendorf, J., Mueller, L. P., Mueller, T., Caysa, H., Nerger, K. & Schmoll, H. J. (2009) Growth-inhibition of colorectal carcinoma by lentiviral TRAIL-transgenic human mesenchymal stem cells requires their substantial intratumoral presence. *J Cell Mol Med*, Epub ahead of print.

[68] Menon, L. G., Kelly, K., Yang, H. W., Kim, S. K., Black, P. M. & Carroll, R. S. (2009) Human bone marrow-derived mesenchymal stromal cells expressing S-TRAIL as a cellular delivery vehicle for human glioma therapy. *Stem Cells, 27*, 2320-2330.

[69] Nakamura, K., Ito, Y., Kawano, Y., Kurozumi, K., Kobune, M., Tsuda, H., Bizen, A., Honmou, O., Niitsu, Y. & Hamada, H. (2004) Antitumor effect of genetically engineered mesenchymal stem cells in a rat glioma model. *Gene Ther, 11*, 1155-1164.

[70] Fritz, V., Noel, D., Bouquet, C., Opolon, P., Voide, R., Apparailly, F., Louis-Plence, P., Bouffi, C., Drissi, H., Xie, C., Perricaudet, M., Muller, R., Schwarz, E. & Jorgensen, C. (2008) Antitumoral activity and osteogenic potential of mesenchymal stem cells expressing the urokinase-type plasminogen antagonist amino-terminal fragment in a murine model of osteolytic tumor. *Stem Cells, 26*, 2981-2990.

[71] Yong, R. L., Shinojima, N., Fueyo, J., Gumin, J., Vecil, G. G., Marini, F. C., Bogler, O., Andreeff, M. & Lang, F. F. (2009) Human bone marrow-derived mesenchymal stem cells for intravascular delivery of oncolytic adenovirus Delta24-RGD to human gliomas. *Cancer Res, 69*, 8932-8940.

[72] Sonabend, A. M., Ulasov, I. V., Tyler, M. A., Rivera, A. A., Mathis, J. M. & Lesniak, M. S. (2008) Mesenchymal stem cells effectively deliver an oncolytic adenovirus to intracranial glioma. *Stem Cells, 26*, 831-841.

[73] You, M. H., Kim, W. J., Shim, W., Lee, S. R., Lee, G., Choi, S., Kim, D. Y., Kim, Y. M., Kim, H. & Han, S. U. (2009) Cytosine deaminase-producing human mesenchymal stem cells mediate an antitumor effect in a mouse xenograft model. *J Gastroenterol Hepatol, 24*, 1393-1400.

[74] Parekkadan, B., van Poll, D., Suganuma, K., Carter, E. A., Berthiaume, F., Tilles, A. W. & Yarmush, M. L. (2007) Mesenchymal stem cell-derived molecules reverse fulminant hepatic failure. *PLoS On., 2*, e941.

[75] Karnoub, A. E., Dash, A. B., Vo, A. P., Sullivan, A., Brooks, M. W., Bell, G. W., Richardson, A. L., Polyak, K., Tubo, R. & Weinberg, R. A. (2007) Mesenchymal stem cells within tumour stroma promote breast cancer metastasis. *Nature, 449*, 557-563.

[76] Dittmer, A., Hohlfeld, K., Lutzkendorf, J., Muller, L. P. & Dittmer, J. (2009) Human mesenchymal stem cells induce E-cadherin degradation in breast carcinoma spheroids by activating ADAM10. *Cell Mol Life Sci, 66*, 3053-3065.

[77] Hombauer, H. & Minguell, J. J. (2000). Selective interactions between epithelial tumour cells and bone marrow mesenchymal stem cells. *Br J Cancer, 82*, 1290-1296.

[78] Fierro, F. A., Sierralta, W. D., Epunan, M. J. & Minguell, J. J. (2004) Marrow-derived mesenchymal stem cells: role in epithelial tumor cell determination. *Clin Exp Metastasis, 21*, 313-319.

[79] Rhodes, L. V., Muir, S. E., Elliott, S., Guillot, L. M., Antoon, J. W., Penfornis, P., Tilghman, S. L., Salvo, V. A., Fonseca, J. P., Lacey, M. R., Beckman, B. S., McLachlan, J. A., Rowan, B. G., Pochampally, R. & Burow, M. E. (2009) Adult

human mesenchymal stem cells enhance breast tumorigenesis and promote hormone independence. *Breast Cancer Res Treat*, Epub ahead of print.

[80] Sasser, A. K., Mundy, B. L., Smith, K. M., Studebaker, A. W., Axel, A. E., Haidet, A. M., Fernandez, S. A. & Hall, B. M. (2007) Human bone marrow stromal cells enhance breast cancer cell growth rates in a cell line-dependent manner when evaluated in 3D tumor environments. *Cancer Lett, 254*, 255-264.

[81] Yu, J. M., Jun, E. S., Bae, Y. C. & Jung, J. S. (2008) Mesenchymal stem cells derived from human adipose tissues favor tumor cell growth in vivo. Stem Cells De., 17, 463-473.

[82] Djouad, F., Plence, P., Bony, C., Tropel, P., Apparailly, F., Sany, J., Noel, D. & Jorgensen, C. (2003) Immunosuppressive effect of mesenchymal stem cells favors tumor growth in allogeneic animals. *Blood, 102*, 3837-3844.

[83] Djouad, F., Bony, C., Apparailly, F., Louis-Plence, P., Jorgensen, C. & Noel, D. (2006) Earlier onset of syngeneic tumors in the presence of mesenchymal stem cells. *Transplantation, 82*, 1060-1066.

[84] Maestroni, G. J., Hertens, E. & Galli, P. (1999) Factor(s) from nonmacrophage bone marrow stromal cells inhibit Lewis lung carcinoma and B16 melanoma growth in mice. *Cell Mol Life Sci, 55*, 663-667.

[85] Ohlsson, L. B., Varas, L., Kjellman, C., Edvardsen, K. & Lindvall, M. (2003) Mesenchymal progenitor cell-mediated inhibition of tumor growth in vivo and in vitro in gelatin matrix. *Exp Mol Pathol, 75*, 248-255.

[86] Khakoo, A. Y., Pati, S., Anderson, S. A., Reid, W., Elshal, M. F., Rovira, II, Nguyen, A. T., Malide, D., Combs, C. A., Hall, G., Zhang, J., Raffeld, M., Rogers, T. B., Stetler-Stevenson, W., Frank, J. A., Reitz, M. & Finkel, T. (2006) Human mesenchymal stem cells exert potent antitumorigenic effects in a model of Kaposi's sarcoma. *J Exp Med, 203*, 1235-1247

[87] Qiao, L., Xu, Z., Zhao, T., Zhao, Z., Shi, M., Zhao, R. C., Ye, L. & Zhang, X. (2008) Suppression of tumorigenesis by human mesenchymal stem cells in a hepatoma model. *Cell Res, 18*, 500-507.

[88] Lin, S. Y., Yang, J., Everett, A. D., Clevenger, C. V., Koneru, M., Mishra, P. J., Kamen, B., Banerjee, D. & Glod, J. (2008) The isolation of novel mesenchymal stromal cell chemotactic factors from the conditioned medium of tumor cells. *Exp Cell Res, 314*, 3107-3117.

[89] Dwyer, R. M., Potter-Beirne, S. M., Harrington, K. A., Lowery, A. J., Hennessy, E., Murphy, J. M., Barry, F. P., O'Brien, T. & Kerin, M. J. (2007) Monocyte chemotactic protein-1 secreted by primary breast tumors stimulates migration of mesenchymal stem cells. *Clin Cancer Res, 13*, 5020-5027.

[90] Menon, L. G., Picinich, S., Koneru, R., Gao, H., Lin, S. Y., Koneru, M., Mayer-Kuckuk, P., Glod, J. & Banerjee, D. (2007) Differential gene expression associated with migration of mesenchymal stem cells to conditioned medium from tumor cells or bone marrow cells. *Stem Cells, 25*, 520-528.

[91] Mishra, P. J., Humeniuk, R., Medina, D. J., Alexe, G., Mesirov, J. P., Ganesan, S., Glod, J. W. & Banerjee, D. (2008) Carcinoma-associated fibroblast-like differentiation of human mesenchymal stem cells. *Cancer Res, 68*, 4331-4339.

[92] Levina, V., Marrangoni, A. M., DeMarco, R., Gorelik, E. & Lokshin, A. E. (2008) Drug-selected human lung cancer stem cells: cytokine network, tumorigenic and metastatic properties. *PLoS One, 3*, e3077.

[93] Mueller, L. P., Luetzkendorf, J., Mueller, T., Reichelt, K., Simon, H. & Schmoll, H. J. (2006) Presence of mesenchymal stem cells in human bone marrow after exposure to chemotherapy: evidence of resistance to apoptosis induction. *Stem Cell, 24*, 2753-2765.

[94] Jorgensen, C. (2009) Link between cancer stem cells and adult mesenchymal stromal cells: implications for cancer therapy. *Regen Med, 4*, 149-152.

In: Stem Cell Research: New Developments
Editors: Hiroshi Tanaka and Michael C. F. Chang
ISBN: 978-1-61942-081-6

Chapter 12

Cancer Stem Cells and Metastasis

Benjamin Tiede and Yibin Kang*
Princeton University, Princeton, NJ, US

Abstract

Recent insights regarding the function of cancer stem cells are particularly intriguing when considered in the context of the metastatic cascade. As evidence for the direct involvement of cancer stem cells in initiating the growth of metastatic lesions is scant, this chapter will focus on known events in malignant transformation that are likely to involve or affect cancer stem cells, which may give rise to primary tumors of varying degrees of malignancy and metastatic potentials. The role of cancer stem cells in the later steps of the metastasis cascade will also be discussed. Finally, this chapter will explore potential characteristics vulnerabilities of cancer stem cells involved in metastasis, and speculate on how these weaknesses may be exploited to generate novel therapeutic and diagnostic approaches.

Introduction

The cancer stem cell (CSC) hypothesis, although proposed many years ago, has undergone a renaissance in the past few years as evident by the isolation and characterization of CSCs responsible for initiating tumorigenesis of a variety of solid and hematopoietic malignancies [1]. Part of the excitement surrounding this field has hinged on the fact that CSCs have been shown to be responsible for driving the recurrence of chemoresistant tumors [2]. As such, research into CSC function has sought to identify critical CSC vulnerabilities in order to improve cancer treatment. Ironically though, most CSC studies have focused on the role of CSCs during primary tumorigenesis, but not metastasis, which is responsible for 90% of cancer related fatalities [3]. Therefore, the primary goals of this chapter are to speculate on

* Correspondence concerning this article should be addressed to: Dr. Yibin Kang, Ph.D. Department of Molecular Biology, Princeton University, Princeton, NJ 08544, USA, Phone: +1 609 258 8834; Fax: +1 609 258 2340; ykang@princeton.edu.

what portions of the metastatic cascade are mediated by CSCs, identify critical research needed to validate these claims, and finally discuss how cancer treatment can shift to focus on the role of CSCs in metastasis.

Before proceeding with investigating the role of CSCs in metastasis, it is important to operationally define two different types of CSCs that play a role in two distinct steps in the tumorigenesis/metastasis cascade. The first population of CSCs (herein referred to as primary tumor CSCs, or pCSCs) are those that have been extensively studied for their role in primary tumorigenesis, and may give rise to highly or lowly metastatic tumors depending on early oncogenic events that drive their formation. The other population of CSCs (dubbed metastatic CSCs or mCSCs) are tumor cells that break off from the primary tumor, travel to the distant sites of metastasis and are responsible for the initiation and the propagation of metastatic lesions.

Poor Prognosis, Primary Tumors and pCSCs

For many years, tumor progression was believed to be the end result of a series of Darwinian natural selections that repeatedly enriched for cells that were fit to survive in the primary tumor microenvironment. While this idea undoubtedly holds a great deal of credence, it did leave one conceptual gap unanswered; how could metastatic cells that are adapted to travel through the circulation and survive at foreign tissues or organs be selected for at the site of the primary tumor? It would seem to be the case that mutations that favor metastasis but do not confer an advantage in primary tumor growth would not be enriched for in the primary tumor. One possible reconciliation to this puzzle is that metastasis potential is actually endowed early during tumorigenesis whereby initial oncogenic events produce distinct classes of tumors with distinct degrees of malignancy [4]. This speculation is likely to hold true when evaluating tumors which consist of subtypes that have a high degree of cellular and molecular heterogeneity (such as breast cancer and leukemia), compared to more homogeneous tumors such as colon and pancreatic cancers [5]. As such, this chapter will primarily focus on evidence from breast cancer and leukemia.

The early predetermination of malignancy hypothesis is supported by numerous studies which provided evidence that different prognoses, including risk of recurrence and distant metastasis, can be detected by profiling the bulk of the primary tumor. The fact that these phenotypes are shared by many of the primary tumor cells suggests that these cells share a common ancestor that was transformed and then expanded into the bulk of the tumor, rather than the entire tumor undergoing the same deregulation independently. For example, genomic analysis of breast tumors indicated at least five different subtypes for breast cancer based on their distinct gene expression profiles: a basal epithelial-like group, an ERBB2-overexpressing group, a normal breast-like group, a luminal A and a luminal B group [6,7]. Survival analyses showed significantly different outcomes for the patients belonging to the various groups, including a poor prognosis for the basal-like, $ERBB2^+$ and luminal B subtypes [6]. Furthermore, it has been shown that expression profiling of primary tumor masses can identify poor prognosis signatures which can effectively predict metastasis formation [8,9,10,11]. Finally, expression profiling of a range of mouse breast cancer models revealed both a common tumorigenesis signature shared by all tumor types, and unique signatures that depended on the initial oncogenic events that correlated with subsequent tumor malignancy phenotypes [12].

The fact that the bulk of the tumor mass expresses a gene signature that can predict metastasis behavior suggests that metastasis potential is endowed early in tumorigenesis so that most cells express the poor prognosis signature, rather than later in tumorigenesis where a few highly metastatic variants would break off from the primary tumor. However, it should be kept in mind that these possibilities are not mutually exclusive; proof that poor prognosis signatures exist in certain tumors does not rule out the possibility for rare metastasis variants to arise late in tumorigenesis. Genomic profiling of primary tumors or metastases by nature will not be able to detect rare, metastatic variants which would not be populous enough to influence total tumor RNA levels [13]. Nevertheless, identifying the precise origin and characterizing the early activity of pCSCs remains a critical avenue of research to be explored to help explain tumor progression and metastasis.

pCSC Origins and Metastasis

Connecting the observations about tumor poor prognosis signatures with the CSC theory of carcinogenesis, a number of questions arise concerning how the origin and propagation of pCSCs could possibly account for the tumor-wide poor prognosis signatures that are observed. For instance, it is unknown whether the same pCSC population can give rise to tumors of varying degrees of malignancy if challenged by different transformation events (see Figure 1). Factors such as genomic instability, oncogenic stress, and microenvironment interactions could potentially alter the same pCSC population to produce tumors of different phenotypes. Early evidence in a leukemia model indicates this is the case as pre-pCSCs from a dendritic cell like leukemia can differentiate into both benign and malignant cell types depending on a variety of factors including the injection site and the immune background of the host [14]. Future studies should seek to expand these observations by testing different oncogenic stresses on the same population of pCSCs or pre-pCSCs to determine the precise role of early oncogenic events, before the majority of the tumor is formed, in predisposing tumors to metastasize.

It is also feasible that similar oncogenic stresses challenging two distinct cell populations, for instance a normal adult stem cell and a committed progenitor, could produce tumors of varying degrees of malignancy (see Figure 2). Preliminary evidence supporting this notion has come from studies which have sought to define the origin of pCSCs, where it has been suggested that both normal stem cells and committed progenitors could serve as the target for transformation. It is believed that normal stem cells or committed progenitors, rather than mature cell types, are the target for transformation because many mutational events rely on DNA replication and cell division: events which are restricted to stem/progenitor cells [5,15].

The inherent self-renewal capacity and long lifespan of normal adult stem cells presumably allows for a greater window of opportunity for their transformation by oncogenic events that may occur over a long period of time. The fact that normal adult stem cells often share surface marker expression profiles with their cancerous counterparts suggests, but does not prove, that normal stem cells may be the origin of pCSCs [1]. For instance, it could be the case that transformed progenitors re-adopt a stem cell surface profile as part of their oncogenesis (there is a precedent for normal epithelial cells to re-adopt a stem cell phenotype in a Wnt-dependent fashion in the hair follicle [16]). Additionally, there is a ~6 fold expansion of mammary stem cells in pre-neoplastic mouse mammary glands in a breast cancer model [17], but again, this does not prove that the normal stem cells are the origin of pCSCs. What has been lacking in the field is the observation or induction of transformation of adult stem cells into pCSCs as opposed to retrospective analyses. Part of the reason why this has been difficult lies in the fact that outside of the hematopoietic system true, adult tissue-specific stem cells have been difficult to identify and isolate. In contrast, it has been much easier to identify committed progenitors because of the less stringent criteria needed to characterize and isolate them, and their relative abundance compared to tissue-specific stem cells.

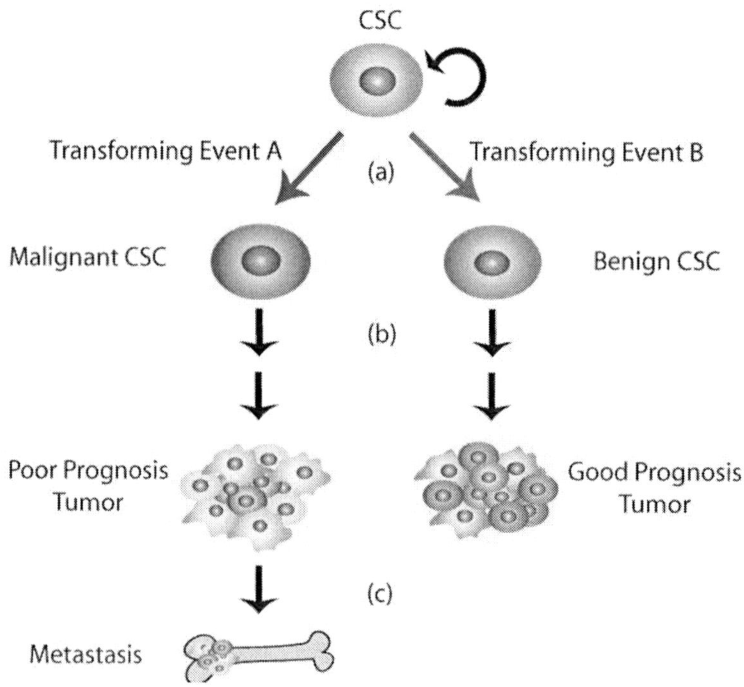

Figure 1. Single origin model of tumorigenesis. In this model, tumors of varying degrees of malignancy are the product of the same cellular origin because of different transformation events (a). These stresses result in the formation of distinct pCSCs (b) that divide and expand into good or poor prognosis tumors (c) that have a differential metastasis capacity.

The fact that committed progenitors are much more abundant than stem cells also suggests, based on probability, that they are more likely to be the target of oncogenic transformation. Given that committed progenitors are easier to isolate than true adult stem cells, it is not surprising that there is better evidence for committed progenitors serving as the origin of CSCs. For instance, committed myeloid progenitors have been shown to initiate leukemia development in mice when they are forced to overexpress Bcl-2 and BCR/ABL [18]. Furthermore, the 15:17 chromosome translocation associated with human acute promyelocytic leukemia (APL) is only found in committed progenitors, and not in hematopoietic stem cells [19]. Granulocyte-macrophage progenitors have also been shown to induce leukemia development, either when activating a self-renewal program through the upregulation of the Wnt/β-catenin pathway [20] or by the forced expression of the MLL-AF9 fusion protein [21]. Interestingly, expression profiling of the MLL-AF9 expressing cells revealed that they retained a progenitor gene expression profile, and not a hematopoietic stem cell profile. Similar evidence has also indicated that neural progenitors are likely to be the target of oncogenic transformations [22].

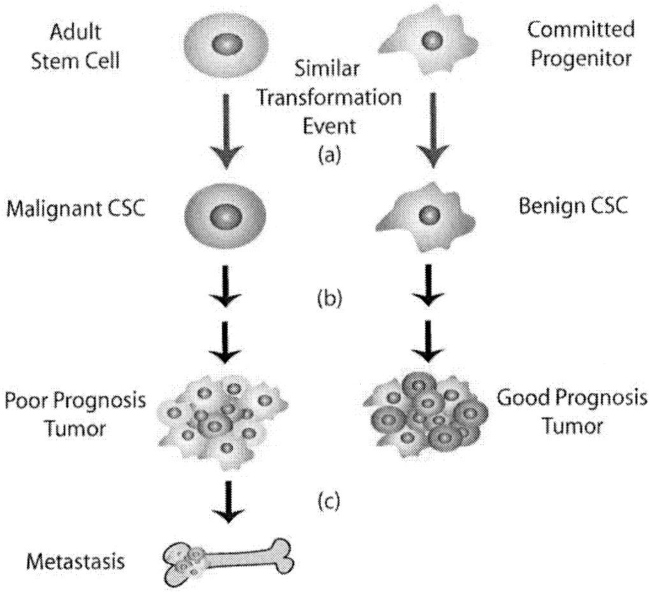

Figure 2. Multiple origin model of tumorigenesis. As opposed to Figure 1, in this scenario, differential metastasis ability is the result of a similar transformation event happening in different target populations (a, b). It is hypothesized, but not proven, that stresses initiated in normal adult stem cells will produce tumors that will metastasize more (c), because of their cellular plasticity and enhanced mobility.

Given that there is evidence for both normal adult stem cells and committed progenitors to serve as the origin of CSCs, and knowing that there are many different paths to tumorigenesis, it is likely to be the case that both stem cells and committed progenitors can serve as the targets for transformation. In fact, it has been shown that EGFR activation, combined with the loss of Arf and Ink4a is sufficient to drive the formation of high grade malignant gliomas in both transformed astrocytes and neural stem cells [23]. What is not clear however is if CSCs derived from different cell types can produce tumors with varying degrees of malignancy. Preliminary evidence has indicated that the same oncogenic stress can induce the formation of tumors with differential metastasis ability if induced in different starting populations. Forced expression of SV-40 large T antigen, hTERT and H-ras-v12 in two distinct human mammary epithelial cell types, derived from the same origin but cultured in different conditions, resulted in tumors with completely different metastasis capacity [24].

Further characterization of the initial oncogenic events that drive CSC formation, particularly with respect to endowing the pCSCs with the ability to metastasize may help to identify clinically relevant prognostic indicators for future tumor malignancy. For instance, it may be possible to isolate pCSCs from a given tumor and determine if they express a unique signature, the figurative "root" of the poor prognosis signature, which would provide stronger prognostic value over sampling of the entire tumor. It also should be kept in mind that most experimental manipulations to decipher the origin of pCSCs typically (by design) test one experimental variable at a time (i.e. whether the challenging stem cells and progenitors with an oncogenic stress results in tumor formation). While this aids in analysis of data, it unfortunately leads to oversimplification of complex *in vivo* interactions.

For instance, it may be the case that an initial transformation event *in vivo* may happen in a stem cell population which results in a pre-neoplastic cell that after differentiating into a progenitor is subject to a second transformation event that leads to typical tumor growth. There is strong observational evidence in leukemia and comparatively weaker evidence from breast cancer studies to suggest this progressive tumorigenesis model happens *in vivo*. Hallmark fusion proteins associated with chronic myelogenous leukemia (CML) as well as acute myelogenous leukemia (AML) (BCR-ABL and AML1-ETO, respectively) can be detected in human hematopoietic stem cells, however these cells are not tumorigenic [20,25]. Instead, further mutations that are only seen in downstream progeny are required to fully initiate tumorigenesis. In breast cancer, it has been shown that tumorigenic $CD44^+$ CSCs are clonally related to and share many genomic alterations with $CD24^+$ cells, but that $CD24^+$ cells express unique mutations [26]. This observation was interpreted to mean that $CD24^+$ cells are the progeny of $CD44^+$ cells that have undergone and initial transformation event. Experimentally testing scenarios such as these (and not just making retroactive conclusions based on tumor heterogeneity) will require a new wave of innovative research design strategies.

METASTATIC CANCER STEM CELLS

In addition to playing significant roles early during the tumorigenesis process that ultimately affect metastasis propensity, CSCs also play a significant role after tumor formation, during the formation of the actual metastatic lesion. Just as pCSCs are required for the initiation of the primary tumor, mCSCs are likely to be required for the formation of metastatic lesions. It has been known that a single cell is capable of initiating metastasis [27]. Thus, given the high number of cells found circulating in the blood of cancer patients and the comparatively low metastasis incidence, it seems likely that only rare CSCs could initiate metastatic lesions. These CSCs, termed metastatic CSCs or mCSCs, are a distinct entity from the pCSCs that gave rise to the primary tumor (although they may share many of the same properties, such as expression of critical tumor propagation factors). mCSCs must also express proteins that endow them with the ability to survive in the blood or lymphatic system as well to adapt to the different environments at the future site of metastasis. For instance, it has been shown that pancreatic mCSCs are a contained in a subset of $CD133^+$ CSCs that also express CXCR4 [28], which is known to be important in homing/anchorage of metastatic cells. Just as pCSCs are rare within a primary tumor, and are the only cells that can induce formation of a new tumor, mCSCs may be the only cells that can break off from the primary tumor and form a metastatic lesion. This could explain the observation that many cancer cells can be detected in the blood of patients with primary tumors, but they all do not form metastasis [29]. Only when a mCSC colonizes a foreign tissue or organ will a metastatic lesion form.

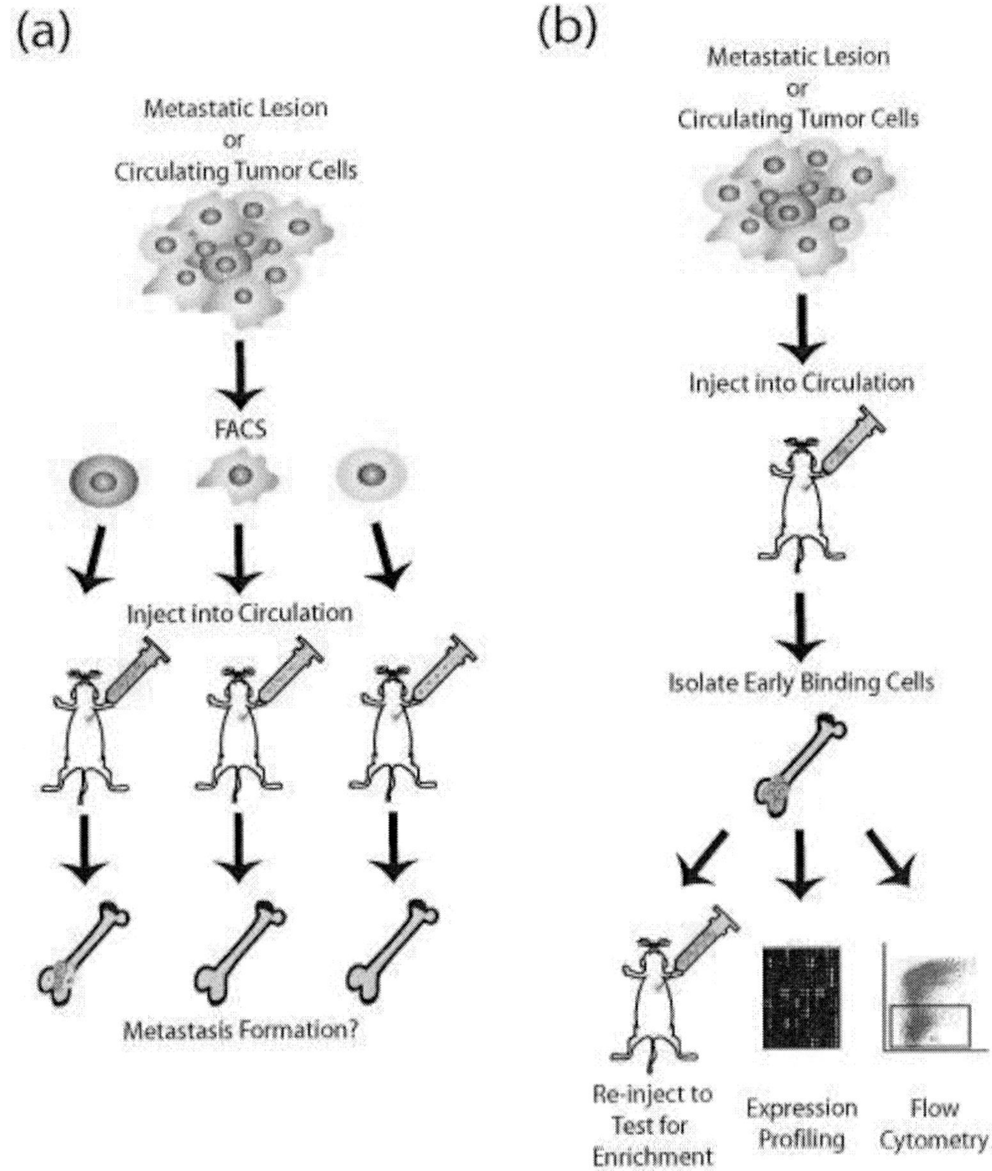

Figure 3. Two different strategies to prospectively identify mCSCs *in vivo*. In (a), a metastatic lesion or cancer cells isolated from the circulation of affected individuals are fractionated using FACS and then injected directly into the circulation of recipient mice. This allows for the direct determination of which cells are able to extravasate, colonize, and expand into a metastatic lesion, but requires the use of previously identified surface markers. As a complementary approach, (b) involves isolating similar tumor cells and injecting them directly into the circulation without fractionating them using FACS (labeling tumor cells with a drug selection marker or GFP would likely be critical before injecting). Soon after injection (~12hr to 2 days later), the cells which initially colonize the metastatic site are selected for, expanded in culture if needed, and reinjected to test for enriched tumorigenicity. These cells could be analyzed by expression profiling or flow cytometry to identify markers to enrich for these cells from other metastatic lesions to enable in further identification and characterization.

Despite speculation of their existence, the direct identification of mCSCs has only been accomplished in one experimental system [28], but could be done by similar xenograft transplantation assays that are used to identify pCSCs. Instead of fractioning a primary tumor and testing different cell populations for their ability to form primary tumors in subcutaneous or orthotopic transplantation models, metastatic lesions or tumor cells collected from the circulation of tumor bearing subjects need to be collected, fractionated based on different cell surface profiles, and tested *in vivo* using experimental metastasis assays (see Figure 3a). These assays directly test the ability of cells to colonize the lung, bone, brain and other organs by injection into the blood circulation. If tumor cells were injected subcutaneously or orthotopically primary tumorigenesis would be a prerequisite of the cells in question, which may not be a property that mCSCs are endowed with. This approach understandably bypasses the initial intravasation step required for circulating tumor cells, but given the high numbers of circulating tumor cells that can be detected, this omission may not be a detrimental one. A complementary approach would involve isolating cells that initially lodge in the bone, lung or any metastatic site soon after injection in an experimental metastasis assay and testing to see if they have an enriched metastatic ability compared to the parental population that was initially injected (see Figure 3b). If this was the case, expression profiling could be used to identify relevant surface proteins that could be used to enrich for the mCSCs in the parental population which could then be characterized in subsequent testing.

It is interesting to note that in the identification of breast pCSCs, the majority of the tumor samples that were used to test pCSC function were pleural effusions, rather than primary tumors [30]. This could be the reason why the expression profiling of these cells identified a unique "invasiveness gene signature" that negatively correlated with metastasis free survival in breast and other cancer types [31]. Furthermore, cells with the breast CSC phenotype $CD44^{+}CD24^{-}$ [30] have been shown to be highly invasive *in vitro* [32], to overexpress motility and chemotaxis gene signatures [26], to be some of the first cells to metastasize to the bone in breast cancer patients [33], and when present in high numbers at the primary tumor to correlate clinically with distant metastasis [34]. These cells are also shown to contain a minority "side population", a group of cells known to have stem cell phenotypes and be chemoresistant [35]. These observations all suggest that breast pCSCs, in addition to forming primary tumors, may actually function as mCSCs as well.

Although the exact identity of mCSCs remains unknown, it is possible to study critical parts of the metastatic cascade that would affect their growth. For example, it has been shown that $CD133^{+}$ glioma CSCs are more adept at inducing angiogenesis, a critical early step in metastasis progression, during tumor formation compared to $CD133^{-}$ cells [36]. While this is clearly indicative of a role for CSCs in the early parts of the metastasis cascade, metastasis research relevant to the function of CSCs typically focuses on later steps in metastasis (i.e., determining tissue specificity, colonization and expansion).

Just as pCSCs are thought to share properties with normal stem cells, so too is the case with mCSCs. Connecting these stipulations, one of the most relevant avenues of research related to mCSCs concerns the role of the supportive niche, or microenvironment that metastatic cells reside in.

THE (PRE)-METASTATIC NICHE AND MCSCS

From drosophila through vertebrates, the protection, growth, and differentiation of normal adults stem cells have been shown in a variety of systems to be regulated by nearby niche cells that provide both a physical location for stem cells to reside in as well as secreting molecules to regulate stem cell function (reviewed in [37]). Interestingly, signaling molecules, such as Wnts and TGFβ, found to be secreted at normal stem cell niches are factors known to be important in tumor growth and metastasis [38]. Additionally, if mCSCs are similar to normal stem cells in that they have a high degree of cellular plasticity, they are likely to be better then other tumor cells at surviving in a foreign niche that is different than the microenvironment at the site of the primary tumor. It is possible that when mCSCs engraft in a tissue they may kick out resident stem cells from their niche. For instance, it is known that osteolytic bone metastasis results in the activation of endosteal osteoclasts [39] which can promote the mobilization of endosteal hematopoietic progenitor cells in the bone marrow [40]. In addition to invading already established niches, metastatic cells have also been shown to induce niche formation prior to leaving the primary tumor site.

In a seminal report in 2005, it was shown that metastatic lung and melanoma cells secrete factors including vascular endothelial growth factor (VEGF) and placental growth factor (PlGF) which induce the recruitment of bone marrow derived cells to the future sites of metastasis (dubbed the pre-metastasis niche) [41]. Blocking these factors was sufficient to reduce tumor metastasis, and interestingly, treating mice with conditioned media from one tumor type was sufficient to redirect the tissue tropisms of the other type. This suggested that once the pre-metastasis niche was initiated, factors were secreted by cells in the niche back to the primary tumor to help recruit metastatic cells. Two possible candidates to mediate this effect are the S100 cytokines S100A8 and S100A9. These cytokines, expressed by myeloid cells, were shown to be upregulated in the pre-metastatic lungs of tumor bearing mice, and when blocked reduced metastasis to the lung [42]. The molecular basis of this effect seems to be the induction of the p38 Map kinase pathway which enhanced tumor cell migration and invasion [42]. Once located in the niche, it is speculated that mCSCs may enter a period of dormancy, similar to that of normal adult stem cells, whereby some re-activation signal may trigger their expansion into a full blown metastatic lesion (see Figure 4) [1]. However, at this point, this idea remains purely speculation and lacks experimental validation.

Other microenvironment factors known to be important during tumorigenesis and metastasis may specifically be important in the regulation of mCSC growth and expansion. For example, when secreted by stromal cells, growth regulators such as Bmp and its inhibitor GREMLIN-1, which are known to regulate normal stem cell proliferation, have been shown to regulate basal cell carcinoma primary tumor growth [43]. Whether this is true in metastasis, and specifically in the regulation of mCSC behavior, remains to be determined. A number of other heterotypic examples between tumor cells and their microenvironment known to play a role in metastasis, such as hypoxia and immune surveillance (reviewed in [44,45]), may also specifically affect mCSCs. However, without their precise identity known, direct studies to characterize these interactions remain far off. Once identified, tests could be designed to determine whether or not circulating cancer cells from a patient contain a population of mCSCs which would predict future metastasis.

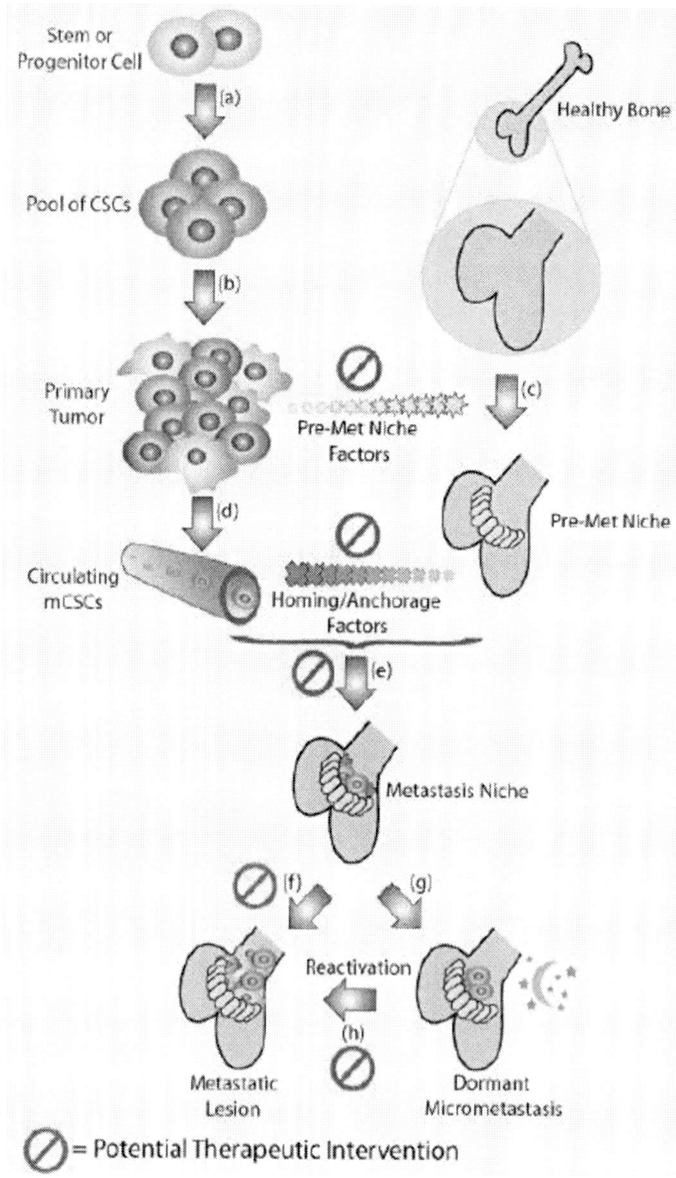

Figure 4. Critical stem cell-niche interactions in regulating metastasis (from [1]). Regardless of how it is derived (a), a pool of malignant pCSCs is formed which expands into a primary tumor (b). This primary tumor is capable of secreting pre-metastasis niche factors such as VEGF and PLGF (c) that induces the expression of homing and anchorage factors such as the S100 cytokines which guide circulating mCSCs (d). Once these mCSCs lodge in the niche (e), they can either proliferate into a metastatic lesion immediately (f) or enter into a period of dormancy (g) whereby reactivation signals induce their expansion (h). Ø = potential steps to target by therapeutic intervention.

As the mCSC population that initially lodges in a metastatic niche is likely very small, profiling the aforementioned niche responses to tumor metastasis may provide an easier means to detect early metastatic lesions. Further research into mCSC behavior, both reliant and independent of niche interactions hopefully will lead to the development of the most clinically effective cancer therapeutics to date.

Metastasis, CSCs and Chemotherapy

Much of the hype surrounding the CSC field has centered on the idea that by treating a small, typically chemoresistant population of cells responsible for initiating tumors, cancer treatment might finally deplete tumors of their lifeblood. However, the idea that these therapies might be designed to specifically ablate mCSCs has usually been little more than an afterthought. This fact should not be taken lightly as even if a CSC based therapy depletes all the tumor initiating cells from the primary tumor, mCSCs that have left the primary tumor and potentially have different molecular profiles than their primary tumor counterparts could be resistant to these therapies. It is also worth noting that many of these proposed therapies speculate on what the critical vulnerabilities of CSCs are, often times based on the known behavior of normal adult stem cells. However, before proceeding to discuss these approaches, it is important to think about the means of validating potential therapeutics, and about potential side effects of CSC based therapeutics.

The traditional standard of evaluating the effectiveness of a given anti-cancer drug is to determine the amount the drug can halt or shrink tumor growth. This is potentially problematic when considering CSC based therapeutics, since these cells are a minority population within a tumor. Treatment with CSC targeting agents in conjunction with traditional therapeutics may only result in a modest, if any, shrinking of the primary tumor compared to traditional drugs alone, but could have significant benefits when evaluating the recurrence- or metastasis-free survival. With respect to the potential side effects of CSC based therapy, there has been concern that if CSCs share properties with normal stem cells, then CSC based therapy may have deleterious side effects on these crucial cell types. This may not be much of a problem for breast cancer, where mastectomy is already an established acceptable treatment option but could be very serious for leukemia, where the normal stem cell and progenitor counterparts are essential for immune function. However, the increased proliferative potential of CSCs may provide a therapeutic window that could be exploited. This seems to be the case as leukemia initiating cells and normal hematopoietic stem cells have a differential dependence on the tumor suppressor PTEN [46].

Self-Renewal and Differentiation

Normal stem cells are known to possess the unique ability to self-renew to maintain a stem-cell pool and to differentiate into more committed progenitors. It is believed that either blocking CSC self-renewal ability or inducing differentiation may deplete these cells from the body. There are a variety of studies indicating this is the case in brain cancer. Treating glioblastoma derived neurospheres (cells dependent on stem cell function) with cyclopamine to block the Hedgehog pathway eliminated their ability to form new neurospheres. Additionally after cyclopamine treatment, glioblastoma cells were no longer able to form tumors *in vivo* [47]. Similar studies have demonstrated that using retinoic acid, a useful differentiation inducer in acute promyelocytic leukemia, also induces differentiation of glioblastoma cells [48]. Alternatively, using a γ-secretase inhibitor to block the Notch pathway resulted in differentiation of medulloblastoma cell lines, and a loss of colony- and tumor-forming ability. This effect appears to be due to a specific depletion of $CD133^+$ CSCs

[49]. Despite these significant findings, it remains to be determined whether mCSCS can be targeted by similar strategies or if they require unique therapeutic targeting.

Metastasis Niche

One therapeutic strategy unique to mCSCs involves targeting the critical mCSC/niche interactions that affect homing, engraftment and growth of tumor cells. It has been shown that blocking the pre-metastasis niche initiation using VEGF or PlGF antibodies was sufficient to reduce metastasis [41]. However, after the niche is initiated, other factors may be useful drug targets in blocking the binding of mCSCs to the niche. One possible factor is CXCR4, which is critical for leukemia cells binding to their niche [50], is important in breast cancer metastasis [51], and has been shown to enrich for mCSCs in pancreatic cancer [28]. Another factor is CD44, which positively selects for breast pCSCs. Blocking CD44 in a acute myelogenous leukemia model resulted in a significant deficiency in engraftment, even when the leukemia CSCs were injected directly into the bone marrow, indicating a specific defect in binding not homing [52]. Similar conclusions were also drawn regarding the essential nature of CD44 in chronic myelogenous leukemia [53]. Once mCSCs are identified and characterized extensively, it will be interesting to note determine what other factors are supplied by the niche to maintain their growth, and if these are potential therapeutic targets.

Reactivation

It is speculated, but remains to be proven, that mCSCs reside in niches in a state of dormancy before expanding into a full blow metastatic lesion. If this is the case, identifying the critical reactivation factors will certainly be of great interest. These potential therapies could have an advantage over drugs that target the homing or seeding of mCSCs because by the time of tumor diagnosis, mCSCs may have already left the primary tumor, migrated and lodged in metastatic niches. However, developing these therapeutics will not happen in the near future since the dormancy model first needs to be validated and characterized before creating drugs.

CSC Clearance

Cell surface marker profiling of CSCs may be useful beyond teasing out tumor initiating populations from the bulk of the tumor mass; the markers identified may be useful in creating cell specific clearance therapies, such as DNA vaccines or oncolytic viruses. When $CD44^{+}CD24^{-/low}$ pleural effusion cells are infected with capsid modified oncolytic adenoviruses, their tumor initiating capacity is abrogated [35]. Furthermore, these viruses when administered after tumor formation were able to significantly deplete the $CD44^{+}/CD24^{-/low}$ population within tumors. Since the surface markers used to identify CSCs are also shared by normal, non tumor cells, specific targeting of the viruses to the CSC population is likely to be a major hurdle to overcome in this line of research.

Conclusion

The unprecedented excitement surrounding the CSC field is certainly grounded in significant theoretical and experimental evidence. This excitement is particularly warranted when considering the role of CSCs in metastasis, since metastasis is responsible for the overwhelming majority of cancer deaths coupled with the fact that CSCs have been shown to be chemoresistant [2,3]. Characterizing the role of CSCs in metastasis involves two distinct portions of the metastatic cascade. First, the role of initial oncogenic events is important in deriving pCSCs that eventually produce tumors of varying degrees of malignancy. Understanding these events is likely to provide more prognostic, rather than therapeutic value. On the contrary, profiling the function of mCSCs, which are important for actually initiating and perpetuating metastatic lesion growth, may lead to novel therapeutic strategies. However, prudence dictates that scientists should acknowledge that while CSCs are a particularly intriguing line of research, at this juncture, we yet don't know if we will be successful in developing any new safe and effective therapeutics. Nevertheless, the future is filled with interesting avenues of research in the CSC field, many of which should shift to focus on the role of CSCs in metastasis and not just tumorigenesis. These studies may result in the development of the most powerful tools in prognostic and therapeutic oncology.

References

[1] Li F, Tiede B, Massague J, Kang Y (2006) Beyond tumorigenesis: cancer stem cells in metastasis. *Cell Res.*

[2] Bao S, Wu Q, McLendon RE, Hao Y, Shi Q, et al. (2006) Glioma stem cells promote radioresistance by preferential activation of the DNA damage response. *Nature 444*: 756-760.

[3] Jemal A, Siegel R, Ward E, Murray T, Xu J, et al. (2007) Cancer statistics, 2007. CA *Cancer J. Clin. 57*: 43-66.

[4] Bernards R, Weinberg RA (2002) A progression puzzle. *Nature 418*: 823.

[5] Stingl J, Caldas C (2007) Molecular heterogeneity of breast carcinomas and the cancer stem cell hypothesis. *Nat. Rev. Cancer.*

[6] Sorlie T, Perou CM, Tibshirani R, Aas T, Geisler S, et al. (2001) Gene expression patterns of breast carcinomas distinguish tumor subclasses with clinical implications. *Proc. Natl. Acad. Sci. USA 98*: 10869-10874.

[7] Perou CM, Jeffrey SS, van de Rijn M, Rees CA, Eisen MB, et al. (1999) Distinctive gene expression patterns in human mammary epithelial cells and breast cancers. *Proc. Natl. Acad. Sci. USA 96*: 9212-9217.

[8] van de Vijver MJ, He YD, van't Veer LJ, Dai H, Hart AA, et al. (2002) A gene-expression signature as a predictor of survival in breast cancer. *N. Engl. J. Med. 347*: 1999-2009.

[9] van 't Veer LJ, Dai H, van de Vijver MJ, He YD, Hart AA, et al. (2002) Gene expression profiling predicts clinical outcome of breast cancer. *Nature 415*: 530-536.

[10] Wang Y, Klijn JG, Zhang Y, Sieuwerts AM, Look MP, et al. (2005) Gene-expression profiles to predict distant metastasis of lymph-node-negative primary breast cancer. *Lancet 365*: 671-679.

[11] Ramaswamy S, Ross KN, Lander ES, Golub TR (2003) A molecular signature of metastasis in primary solid tumors. *Nat. Genet. 33*: 49-54.

[12] Desai KV, Xiao N, Wang W, Gangi L, Greene J, et al. (2002) Initiating oncogenic event determines gene-expression patterns of human breast cancer models. *Proc. Natl. Acad. Sci. USA 99*: 6967-6972.

[13] Hynes RO (2003) Metastatic potential: generic predisposition of the primary tumor or rare, metastatic variants-or both? *Cell 113*: 821-823.

[14] Chen L, Shen R, Ye Y, Pu XA, Liu X, et al. (2007) Precancerous stem cells have the potential for both benign and malignant differentiation. *PLoS ONE 2*: e293.

[15] Cairns J (2002) Somatic stem cells and the kinetics of mutagenesis and carcinogenesis. *Proc. Natl. Acad. Sci. USA 99*: 10567-10570.

[16] Ito M, Yang Z, Andl T, Cui C, Kim N, et al. (2007) Wnt-dependent de novo hair follicle regeneration in adult mouse skin after wounding. *Nature 447*: 316-320.

[17] Shackleton M, Vaillant F, Simpson KJ, Stingl J, Smyth GK, et al. (2006) Generation of a functional mammary gland from a single stem cell. *Nature 439*: 84-88.

[18] Jaiswal S, Traver D, Miyamoto T, Akashi K, Lagasse E, et al. (2003) Expression of BCR/ABL and BCL-2 in myeloid progenitors leads to myeloid leukemias. *Proc. Natl. Acad. Sci. USA 100*: 10002-10007.

[19] Turhan AG, Lemoine FM, Debert C, Bonnet ML, Baillou C, et al. (1995) Highly purified primitive hematopoietic stem cells are PML-RARA negative and generate nonclonal progenitors in acute promyelocytic leukemia. *Blood 85*: 2154-2161.

[20] Jamieson CH, Ailles LE, Dylla SJ, Muijtjens M, Jones C, et al. (2004) Granulocyte-macrophage progenitors as candidate leukemic stem cells in blast-crisis CML. *N. Engl. J. Med. 351*: 657-667.

[21] Krivtsov AV, Twomey D, Feng Z, Stubbs MC, Wang Y, et al. (2006) Transformation from committed progenitor to leukaemia stem cell initiated by MLL-AF9. *Nature.*

[22] Vescovi AL, Galli R, Reynolds BA (2006) Brain tumour stem cells. *Nat. Rev. Cancer 6*: 425-436.

[23] Bachoo RM, Maher EA, Ligon KL, Sharpless NE, Chan SS, et al. (2002) Epidermal growth factor receptor and Ink4a/Arf: convergent mechanisms governing terminal differentiation and transformation along the neural stem cell to astrocyte axis. *Cancer Cell 1*: 269-277.

[24] Ince TA, Richardson AL, Bell GW, Saitoh M, Godar S, et al. (2007) Transformation of Different Human Breast Epithelial Cell Types Leads to Distinct Tumor Phenotypes. *Cancer Cell 12*: 160-170.

[25] Blair A, Hogge DE, Ailles LE, Lansdorp PM, Sutherland HJ (1997) Lack of expression of Thy-1 (CD90) on acute myeloid leukemia cells with long-term proliferative ability in vitro and in vivo. *Blood 89*: 3104-3112.

[26] Shipitsin M, Campbell LL, Argani P, Weremowicz S, Bloushtain-Qimron N, et al. (2007) Molecular definition of breast tumor heterogeneity. *Cancer Cell 11*: 259-273.

[27] Fidler IJ, Talmadge JE (1986) Evidence that intravenously derived murine pulmonary melanoma metastases can originate from the expansion of a single tumor cell. *Cancer Res. 46*: 5167-5171.

[28] Hermann P, Huber S, Herrler T, Aicher A, Ellwart J, et al. (2007) Distinct Populations of Cancer Stem Cells Determine Tumor Growth and Metastatic Activity in Human Pancreatic Cancer. *Cell Stem Cell 1*: 313-323.

[29] Fidler IJ (2003) The pathogenesis of cancer metastasis: the 'seed and soil' hypothesis revisited. *Nat. Rev. Cancer 3*: 453-458.

[30] Al-Hajj M, Wicha MS, Benito-Hernandez A, Morrison SJ, Clarke MF (2003) Prospective identification of tumorigenic breast cancer cells. *Proc. Natl. Acad. Sci. USA 100*: 3983-3988.

[31] Liu R, Wang X, Chen GY, Dalerba P, Gurney A, et al. (2007) The prognostic role of a gene signature from tumorigenic breast-cancer cells. *N. Engl. J. Med. 356*: 217-226.

[32] Sheridan C, Kishimoto H, Fuchs RK, Mehrotra S, Bhat-Nakshatri P, et al. (2006) CD44+/CD24- breast cancer cells exhibit enhanced invasive properties: an early step necessary for metastasis. *Breast Cancer Res. 8*: R59.

[33] Balic M, Lin H, Young L, Hawes D, Giuliano A, et al. (2006) Most early disseminated cancer cells detected in bone marrow of breast cancer patients have a putative breast cancer stem cell phenotype. *Clin. Cancer Res. 12*: 5615-5621.

[34] Abraham BK, Fritz P, McClellan M, Hauptvogel P, Athelogou M, et al. (2005) Prevalence of CD44+/CD24-/low cells in breast cancer may not be associated with clinical outcome but may favor distant metastasis. *Clin. Cancer Res. 11*: 1154-1159.

[35] Eriksson M, Guse K, Bauerschmitz G, Virkkunen P, Tarkkanen M, et al. (2007) Oncolytic Adenoviruses Kill Breast Cancer Initiating CD44(+)CD24(-/Low) Cells. *Mol. Ther.*

[36] Bao S, Wu Q, Sathornsumetee S, Hao Y, Li Z, et al. (2006) Stem Cell-like Glioma Cells Promote Tumor Angiogenesis through Vascular Endothelial Growth Factor. *Cancer Res. 66*: 7843-7848.

[37] Moore KA, Lemischka IR (2006) Stem cells and their niches. Science 311: 1880-1885.

[38] Li L, Neaves WB (2006) Normal stem cells and cancer stem cells: the niche matters. *Cancer Res. 66*: 4553-4557.

[39] Guise TA, Mohammad KS, Clines G, Stebbins EG, Wong DH, et al. (2006) Basic mechanisms responsible for osteolytic and osteoblastic bone metastases. *Clin. Cancer Res. 12*: 6213s-6216s.

[40] Kollet O, Dar A, Shivtiel S, Kalinkovich A, Lapid K, et al. (2006) Osteoclasts degrade endosteal components and promote mobilization of hematopoietic progenitor cells. *Nat. Med. 12*: 657-664.

[41] Kaplan RN, Riba RD, Zacharoulis S, Bramley AH, Vincent L, et al. (2005) VEGFR1-positive haematopoietic bone marrow progenitors initiate the pre-metastatic niche. *Nature 438*: 820-827.

[42] Hiratsuka S, Watanabe A, Aburatani H, Maru Y (2006) Tumour-mediated upregulation of chemoattractants and recruitment of myeloid cells predetermines lung metastasis. *Nat. Cell Biol. 8*: 1369-1375.

[43] Sneddon JB, Zhen HH, Montgomery K, van de Rijn M, Tward AD, et al. (2006) Bone morphogenetic protein antagonist gremlin 1 is widely expressed by cancer-associated stromal cells and can promote tumor cell proliferation. *Proc. Natl. Acad. Sci. USA 103*: 14842-14847.

[44] Barnhart BC, Simon MC (2007) Metastasis and stem cell pathways. *Cancer Metastasis Rev. 26*: 261-271.

[45] Gupta GP, Massague J (2006) Cancer metastasis: building a framework. *Cell 127*: 679-695.

[46] Yilmaz OH, Valdez R, Theisen BK, Guo W, Ferguson DO, et al. (2006) Pten dependence distinguishes haematopoietic stem cells from leukaemia-initiating cells. *Nature 441*: 475-482.

[47] Bar EE, Chaudhry A, Lin A, Fan X, Schreck K, et al. (2007) Cyclopamine-Mediated Hedgehog Pathway Inhibition Depletes Stem-Like Cancer Cells in Glioblastoma. *Stem Cells*.

[48] Park DM, Li J, Okamoto H, Akeju O, Kim SH, et al. (2007) N-CoR pathway targeting induces glioblastoma derived cancer stem cell differentiation. *Cell Cycle 6:* 467-470.

[49] Fan X, Matsui W, Khaki L, Stearns D, Chun J, et al. (2006) Notch pathway inhibition depletes stem-like cells and blocks engraftment in embryonal brain tumors. *Cancer Res. 66*: 7445-7452.

[50] Tavor S, Petit I, Porozov S, Avigdor A, Dar A, et al. (2004) CXCR4 regulates migration and development of human acute myelogenous leukemia stem cells in transplanted NOD/SCID mice. *Cancer Res. 64*: 2817-2824.

[51] Kang Y, Siegel PM, Shu W, Drobnjak M, Kakonen SM, et al. (2003) A multigenic program mediating breast cancer metastasis to bone. *Cancer Cell 3*: 537-549.

[52] Jin L, Hope KJ, Zhai Q, Smadja-Joffe F, Dick JE (2006) Targeting of CD44 eradicates human acute myeloid leukemic stem cells. *Nat. Med. 12*: 1167-1174.

[53] Krause DS, Lazarides K, von Andrian UH, Van Etten RA (2006) Requirement for CD44 in homing and engraftment of BCR-ABL-expressing leukemic stem cells. *Nat. Med. 12*: 1175-1180.

In: Stem Cell Research: New Developments
Editors: Hiroshi Tanaka and Michael C. F. Chang
ISBN: 978-1-61942-081-6

Chapter 13

Human Adult Stem Cells as Targets for Cancer Stem Cells: Evolution; Oct-4 Gene and Cell-to-Cell Communication

James E. Trosko*
Michigan State University, East Lansing, Michigan, US

Abstract

To examine the factors involving human carcinogenesis in order to design new strategies for prevention and treatment, a new approach from the current reductionalistic molecular oncological view will have to be made. In addition, this view must take into account both biological and cultural evolutionary factors that interact with the biology of the pathogenesis of cancer. An integrated hypothesist that links many incomplete hypotheses, such as the stem cell or de-differentiation theories of cancer, the multi-stage, multi-mechanism or "initiation/promotion/progression" theory, the mutation and epigenetic theories of carcinogenesis, and the "cancer stem cells" hypothesis, has been outlined. The emergence of somatic and germ-line stem cells during the biological evolution of the multi-cellular organism created new functions to regulate, homeostatically, phenotypes, such as growth control, differentiation, apoptosis, senescence and adaptive functions of terminally differentiated cells. The evidence supporting the stem cells as target cells for the initiation process was reviewed. The biological consequence of the initiation of an adult stem cell appears to be the inhibition of asymmetric cell division, or the blockage of "mortalization" of a normal "immortal" stem cell, not the "immortalization" of a normal, "mortal" cell. Promotion, functionally, is the clonal expansion of initiated stem cells by both mitogenesis and the inhibition of apoptosis. These promoting conditions occur during wound healing, compensatory hyperplasia after cell death, chronic inflammation, growth factors and by many dietary and environmental, non-mutagenic chemicals. All of these promoting conditions inhibit cell-cell communication, either by disruption of gap junctions in progenitor cells or by

* Correspondence concerning this article should be addressed to: James E. Trosko, E-Mail: james.trosko@ht.msu.edu.

interfering with secreted negative growth regulator-receptor signalling in cells not having functional gap junctions, thereby releasing initiated stem cells from mitotic inhibition. Tumor promoters are characterized by threshold levels, exposing the initiated cells for regular and long periods of time in the absence of anti-promoters and having species, gender, cell-type specificities. The normal stem cell appears to give rise to the initiated stem cell which ultimately can accrue all the phenotypes of an invasive, metastatic "cancer stem cell". As the tumor grows, some of these cancer stem cells can partially differentiate to become cancer "non-stem cells". Finally, to understand how cultural evolution affects the human cancer patterns, domestication of certain animals helped to change dietary habits which can influence the carcinogenic process. These dietary factors can influence the adult stem cells, in utero and postnatally, so as to either increase or decrease the risk to cancer by altering the stem cell pools and by increasing or decreasing the promotion of the initiated stem cells. This might provide a mechanistic basis for the "Barker hypothesis".

"Nothing in biology makes sense except in the light of evolution."
T. Dobzansky [1]

Introduction: The Complexicity of a Complicated Disease; The Interaction of Biological and Cultural Evolutionary Factors

The use of this quote by Theodosius Dobzhansky was done with a specific intent, namely, that in any attempt to understand carcinogenesis in human beings, outside the process of both biological and cultural evolution, will always come up with incomplete explanations. This review will attempt to provide some newer insights to this extremely complex disease. It should also be stated up front that "cancer" is not a single disease but multiple diseases that share several phenotypes or "hallmarks of cancer" [2]. Indeed, each cancer will be characterized by different phenotypes and genotypes within the tumor itself, due to alterations in the tumor micro-environment, causing both genetic and epigenetic instability as the tumor progresses.

Given this reality, one might wonder if any meaningful prevention and treatment strategies can be developed, not only for specific types of cancer (e.g., lung, prostate, colon), but, also, for different individuals with the same diagnosed cancer that shares the same 6 "hallmarks of cancer". This brings to mind a story of Albert Einstein's remark to a reporter who heard him gave a public lecture on his new theory of relativity. After his talk, this young reporter asked, "Professor Einstein, now that you physicists understand the workings of the universe, don't you think it's *complicated?* Einstein looked at the reporter and responded by saying, "Young man, if you *know nothing* of the universe, it is, indeed, *very complicated!* However, when you *begin to understand* it, it is *merely complex!*"

The goal of this overview *Commentary* is to try to integrate a number of well-known hypotheses of carcinogenesis (e.g., the stem cell versus the de-differentiation hypotheses, the multi-stage, multi-mechanism or "initiation, promotion, progression hypothesis; mutation versus epigenetic theories; and the oncogene- tumor suppression gene hypothesis of carcinogenesis). The attempt will, hopefully, demonstrate that this complicated carcinogenic process is "merely" complex. However, even with this incomplete understanding, new improved strategies can be made to prevent and treat the various cancers. Hopefully, unlike the old Indian fable of the six blind men who tried to describe the whole elephant, from which they only touched one part, medical science will at least try to integrate the different parts from various individual views in order to get a more realistic view of carcinogenesis.

No One Appendage Describes an Elephant, Nor Does Only One Thing Cause Cancer!

From early Greek observations to *Percival Pott's* observation on the relationship of soot to scrotal cancers in chimney sweepers and to the recent "discovery" of "cancer stem cells" [3], fundamental observations for hundreds of years have been made that give some insight into the factors influencing this whole animal/human biological process. However, the embryologists, pathologists, physiologists, biochemists, and molecular biologists saw cancers within the prisms of their reductionalistic training. The explosion of reductionalistic data being produced today, unfortunately, has no integrated framework on to which these data can be meaningfully interpreted. Because of the "success" of modern molecular oncology, with the discovery of oncogenes and tumor suppressor genes, many of the old observations and insights concerning the whole animal process of carcinogenesis have been ignored. The very idea that understanding the sequence of the human DNA will give us the "answer" to why we get cancer and how we can "cure" it, sounds much like the old fable of the 6 blind man.

In the field of embryology, Markert saw cancer as some developmental process that had been interfered with ("Cancer as a disease of differentiation") [4]. The following quote from one of his papers describes, beautifully, his perspective that has much relevance to our current understanding [5].

> "Cells interact and communicate during embryonic development and through inductive stimuli mutually direct the divergent courses of their differentiation. Very little cell differentiation is truly autonomous in vertebrate organisms. The myriad cell phenotypes present in mammals, for example, must reflect a corresponding complexity in the timing, nature, and amount of inductive interactions. Whatever the nature of inductive stimuli may be, they emerge as a consequence of specific sequential interactions of cells during embryonic development.
>
> The first embryonic cells, blastomeres, of mice and other mammals are all totipotent. During cleavage and early morphologenesis these cells come to occupy different positions in the three-dimensional embryo. Some cells are on the outside, some inside. The different environments of these cells cause the cells to express different patterns of metabolism in accordance with their own developing programs of gene function. These patterns of metabolism create new chemical environments for nearby cells and these changed environments induce yet new programs of gene function in responding cells. Thus a progressive series of reciprocal interactions is established between the cellular environment and the genome of each cell. These interactions drive the cell along a specific path of differentiation until a stable equilibrium is reached in the adult. Thereafter little change occurs in the specialized cells and they become remarkably refractory to changes in the environment. They seem stably locked into the terminal patterns of gene function characteristic of adult

> cells. The genome seems no longer responsible to the signals that were effective earlier in development.
>
> Of course, changes can occur in adult cells that lead to renewed cell proliferation and altered differentiation as seen in neoplasms, both benign and malignant, but such changes are very rare indeed when one considers the number of cells potentially available for neoplastic transformation. Possibly, mutations in regulatory DNA of dividing adult cells can occasionally lead to new and highly effective programs gene function that we recognize as neoplastic or malignant. However, most genetic changes in adult cells can probably lead to cell death since random changes in patterns of gene activity are not likely to be beneficial."

Pierce, also, saw carcinogenesis as a defect in the differentiation of stem cells ("Cancer as a stem cell disease") [6]. After examining many hundreds of Morris hepatomas, Van R. Potter proposed the concept of "oncogeny as partially blocked ontogeny" [7]. It should be noted that while these scientists did not have individual stem cells on which to study the process of carcinogenesis, the concept of stem cells was sufficient to explain both the processes of development and carcinogenesis. It should be noted that the operational definition of an embryonic stem cell of today is that they will form teratomas when placed back into an adult animal. Ironically, both embryologists and stem cell researchers use this observation of the cancer field as a criterion of stemness.

When it was shown that all the cells within a tumor were clonally- derived, it provided even more experimental evidence of the role of stem cells and differentiation in carcinogenesis. It might seem a bit conflicting that, while all the cells within a tumor are genotyically and phenotypically unique [8], they were all derivatives of a single stem cell. The concept of genomic and epigenomic instability of the carcinogenic process was created to explain this apparent dilemma [9,10]. It must be pointed out, however, the idea that genomic and epigenomic stability is the "cause" of cancer has to be tempered with the possibility that these might be the consequence of a cell becoming a cancer cell, rather that the instability being the "cause" of cancer. Regardless of the ultimate resolution of this academic problem, this heterogeneity has been, and will continue to be, a major problem for prevention and treatment of cancer. That this is the case, for each tumor and each cell within that tumor, a different intracellular physiology, generated by different gene expressions and genetic abnormalities, poses a problem for treatment strategies.

From Single Cell Organisms to Multi-Cellular Organisms: Cancer as the "Faustian Bargain" we Paid for our Survival

Until relatively recently, both the public and scientists wondered why the germ theory could not explain cancer as a disease. Even though clues that environmental agents, such as chimney soot, were associated with scrotal cancers by Percival Pott, it was difficult to put together a meaningful scientific hypothesis at that time. Although the clue that genetic factors might play a role came when Boveri [11] noticed abnormalities in chromosomes in cancer cells, until more direct evidence, such as the lack of the ability to repair ultraviolet light-induced DNA lesions in a cancer prone skin cancer syndrome, xeroderma pigmentosum [12], did a new perspective emerge. The role of the inability to repair UV-induced DNA lesions was associated with the production of mutations [13,14] and the molecular basis of specific

UV mutations in the p53 tumor suppressor gene of skin cancer cells [15]. The new paradigm was generated, "cancers as mutagen" [16], that took hold and from that time until just recently, carcinogenesis research became very reductionalistic with the new focus on the specific genes in cells, when mutated, "proto-oncogenes" and "tumor suppressor" were thought to provide the ultimate understanding of the carcinogenic process.

There is no doubt today, that the production of mutations does play a role in the complex carcinogenic process, as evidenced by (a) the inherited germ line mutations that led to cancer predispositions, such as the xeroderma pigmentosum, retinoblastoma, Down's, Fanconi's anemia, etc [17]; (b) agents associated with the induction of cancer inducing mutations in various short term in vitro assays; (c) mutations found in the oncogenes or tumor suppressor genes of cancer cells; and (d) DNA lesions found in cells of the cancer prone organs treated with various carcinogens. However, as will be discussed later, this view was too narrow, for it now has been shown that epigenetic alterations in the nuclear genome (defined here as the alteration in the expression of the genome at the transcriptional, translational or posttranslational levels) could also give rise to a component of the carcinogenic process.

However, to continue the focus on the role of evolution and cancer, one must realize that without mutations (as well as epigenetic changes) in the genome, that first living single cell organism would not have survived as a species. Clearly, if that early organism did not form any new genetic sequences, when the environment changes, as it inevitably has changed, and will continue to change, the genes that coded for those proteins and enzymes would be useless in the new challenging environment. The species could not survive in new harsh environments. Therefore, without the ability to protect DNA from having DNA lesions and from repairing, perfectly, the DNA lesions being formed by the errors of DNA repair or by errors of DNA replication, mutations could be generated in a population. In such cases, possibly one of those mutations could code for a protein that allows the organism to survive and reproduce, and, thus, saving the species. However, we must view the two extremes in mutation production. No mutations clearly lead to species failure in a changing environment. Too many mutations would also complicate survival. This is especially true in a multi-cellular organism.

Therefore, obviously, during the course of evolution, a balance was made between (a) protecting the DNA from any external damage that might lead to mutations and the perfect repair and replicating of DNA (which would lead to the extinction of the species) and (b) the lack of excessive DNA protection and the excessive production of errors of DNA repair and replication (which would also lead to the extinction of the species). While single cell organisms survive by unrestricted or immortalized ability to reproduce, in a population that is large enough, the population will have a few individuals that had accrued a mutation that allowed it to survive and reproduce when its sibs could not. Only temperature, nutrient depletion, pH changes, gravity and radiation would have environmental limiting influence on these single cell organisms' ability to proliferate.

When during the course of biological evolution that the first multi-cellular organism appeared, several new phenotypes had to accompany this new society of cells. Clearly, the aggregation of cells into a closed system would not have survived environmental changes had there not been some evolutionary advantage. One advantage would have been the appearance of specialized cells within the closed system that would enhance the survivability of the group as a whole. The appearance of the ability to form these specialized cells or *to differentiate* from a very primitive state to a very high "differentiated" cell, which could perform "higher order" functions, such as touch, sight, thermal regulation, muscle movement, etc., added to the single cell organism's ability to proliferate in, basically, an uncontrolled manner.

However, if a social colony of cells, which could form cooperating, but specialized functions, had no growth control, the colony would, in effect, become a tumor. Therefore, a second new phenotype had to be a new form of *growth control* in a closed system. In a society of single cell organisms, there are methods of "communicating" with each other via secreted factors. During the transition from the single cell to the multi-cell organism, this communication mechanism was not lost, but it was supplemented by the appearance of the gap junction, a membrane-associated protein channel that allows direct transfer of ions and small regulatory substrates to be transferred between the coupled cells [18]. Today, twenty connexin genes, those coding the proteins that are assembled into hexamers that comprise the hemi-channel of the cell which couples with the neighboring hemi-channel, are evolutionarily conserved, thus implying their importance in the survival of the metazoan [19]. These different connexin genes appear to serve the function of providing differential signalling mechanisms to regulate various cellular functions, including allowing for differential differentiation within an organism [20]. Equally important, these new means of communication between neighboring cells in direct contact with each other seem to be involved in growth control via "contact inhibition" [21].

Another new phenotype also appeared during this transition in evolution. It was the function of *programmed cell death* or *apoptosis*. If, in fact, a multi-cellular organism was to be successful in maintaining its species, it could also "improve" its ability to survive by changing its phenotype to add new survival functions, such as the transition from an insect larva to a flying butterfly. However to make this extraordinary advance, those specialized cells of the larva had to give way to new cells that would be needed for pigmentation, flight muscles, wings and other new sensory organs. This could only happen if whole battery of genes in those cells, needed for the larval function, is replaced with new differentiated cells having new battery of genes expressed for the new functions of a flying butterfly. The original fertilized egg of that butterfly had both sets of genes but they were expressed only when needed for that particular stage of development.

Equally important during this transition of the single to multi-cell organism was the "Faustian" bargain. That is, in return for higher order functions that differentiation of highly specials cells could give to the species' survival, was the "mortality" or senescence of the whole organism. Clearly, if *all* the cells of the multi-cellular organism senesced or became mortal, the species would not survive. With the appearance of the ability to form specialized *"immortal" germ cells,* the "Faustian" bargain, then, excluded the germ cells from the curse of "mortality". Moreover, if the multi-cell organ was to have additional adaptive functions, such as continued growth of the non-germ line cells, tissue replacement of damaged or diseased tissue, and for extended life span, not only was the germ-line cells privileged with the characteristic of "immortality", but also, some somatic or non-germ cells were selected that had this feature. These germ line and somatic "immortal cells" are the so-called adult "stem" cells.

If we now view these new phenotypes that emerged during multi-cellular development, and if we view what happens in a multi- celled organism when it has a cancer, we note that cancers (a) no longer have growth control; (b) can not terminally differentiate; (c) do not apoptose normally; and (d) have the ability to be immortal. In effect, they have "de-evolved" to a single-cell organism-like state. It is interesting to note that the appearance of the connexin gene appeared early in the evolution of the multi-cellular organism [22]. It is also interesting that cancer cells have no functional gap junctional intercellular communication [23], either because the connexin genes were never expressed or that they were expressed but rendered non-functional by activated oncogenes or mutations [24]. Whether this association of the loss of function of the gap junction with the loss of growth control, differentiation, abnormal apoptosis and the appearance of immortality in the cancer cell was just coincidence or causal, has to be resolved.

STEM CELLS, CELL COMMUNICATION AND DEVELOPMENT

During the development of a human being from a single fertilized egg, the zygote or "toti-potent" stem cell, approximately 100 trillion cells are produced. In order that development of the embryo, fetus, neonate, adolescent, mature and geriatric individual be normal, a very delicate orchestration of communication processes (extra-, intra, and gap junctional inter-cellular communication mechanisms) must be integrated, in order that the hierarchy of different cell types (embryonic, pluri-potent, multi-potent, bi-polar stem cells; progenitor stems, and terminally-differentiated cells) be done in a sequential, concatenated manner to allow the total genome to be specifically regulated in each cell type (Figure 1).

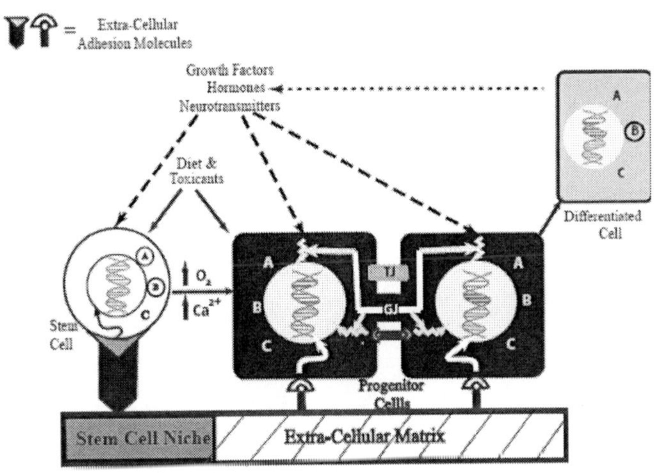

Figure 1. Gap junctions in cellular homeostasis. Extracellular signals, such as growth factors, toxicants, extra-cellular matrices and cell adhesion molecules that vary for each cell type (adult stem cell, progenitor and terminally-differentiated), interact with membrane receptors, which then activate intracellular signal transduction pathways that induce the transcription of genes (A,B,C) through activated transcription factors. These specific intracellular pathways operate under cascading systems that cross communicate with each other in controlling the expression of genes that direct the proliferation, differentiation and apoptosis of cells within a tissue. These multiple intracellular signalling check points are further modulated by intercellular signals traversing gap junctions, thereby maintaining the homeostatic state of a tissue. Abnormal interruption of these integrated signalling pathways by food-related and environmental toxicants results in diseased states, such as the tumor promotion phase of carcinogenesis, teratogenesis during early development, atherogenesis, immunotoxicity, reproductive- and neuro-toxicities.

Genes for "stemness", such as Oct-4, nanog, Sox-2 [25], must be expressed in the embryonic and adult stem cells (multi-potent, bi-polar). Other genes must be expressed in order that specific differentiation genes might be regulated during development, growth and in cell replacement in tissues, and during wound-healing. Gap junctions genes, the 20 connexin genes [19], do seem to be required for the specific differentiation of cells within and between tissues of different organs [20]. Temporal expressions of genes are needed for the normal process of apoptosis or programmed cell death and even for removal of damaged cells [26]. For cells in solid tissues, gap junction function seems to be required for apoptosis to occur [27].

This extremely complex communication between the adult stem cells in their niches [28], their committed progenitor or "transit" cells [29], and the terminally- differentiated daughter cells must exist. Since it seems that the early blastocyte cells do not have function gap junctions [30], and that several adult human stem cells also do not express their connexin genes or have functional gap junctional intercellular communication (GJIC) [31], communication between the stem cells and the surrounding committed progenitor cells, that do seem to have gap junctions, and the terminally differentiated cells, that might or might not have gap junctions during their whole life time, must be mediated by secreted factors [32-33]. The progenitor cells, both epithelial, endothelial, and fibroblasts, do have contact-inhibitory means to regulate proliferation [34]. Gap junctions have been associated with growth control [35], differentiation [36] and apoptosis [27].

The stem cell is defined as a cell that has the ability to divide either symmetrically to form two identical daughter stem cells (if it divides to commit both daughter to terminal differentiation, that would be the end of that stem cell's contribution to the organism's life) or asymmetrically to form one daughter cell (a progenitor) that is now committed to form a lineage of differentiated cells and one daughter that remains capable of self-renewal or stemness. To view stem cells, in this light, is to realize that a stem cell is naturally an "immortal" cell and it becomes "mortal" when it is induced to form a terminally-differentiated or "mortal" cell. Therefore, this decision point in a multi-cellular organism's evolutionary advance over single cell organism, namely, the control of symmetric versus asymmetric cell division will be of critical importance during normal development and during carcinogenesis.

Exactly how a stem cell determines whether it should divide symmetrically or asymmetrically is not currently known. However, from a conceptual standpoint, the stem cell must receive a number of signalling mechanisms. The first is signalling the stem cell receives from its anchored niche-substrate extra-cellular molecules. In the case of non-anchored stem cells, extra-cellular secreted signalling ions and molecules probably provide the same signal. Together with the secreted factors such as a hormone, growth factor, cytokine, chemokine, or ions, such as calcium, that might trigger some specific intra-cellular signalling, the net-effect of these signals would be result of the "cross-talk" of these extra- cellar signalling triggered intra-cellular signal pathways. Together with an important environmental factor, oxygen [37], the net effect of the interactive signals determine which genes are going to be transcribed and which existing proteins will be posttranslationally-modified for activity, inaction or ubquitization. That will lead to the molecular decision mechanism for symmetric or asymmetric cell division.

Conceptually, one model that might help to explain how the role of gap junctions might come into play in this process of symmetric and asymmetrical stem cell division. In Figure 2, it is speculated that, depending on the mix of signals a stem cell gets in its niche, the stem cell anchored to the niche extra-cellar matrix might form a mitotic division plane that is parallel to the plane of the stem cell niche extra-cellular matrix. In this case, the new daughter that is still attached to the niche extra-cellular matrix will continue to receive the same signal as did its stem cell mother.

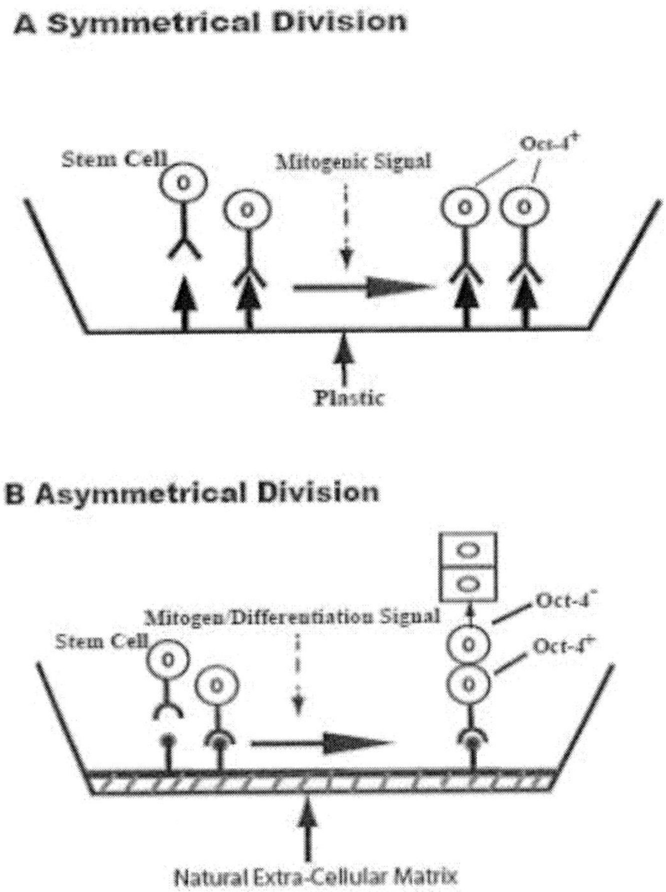

Figure 2. These diagrams illustrate two possible means by which stem cells (Oct-4+) decide to divide by symmetrical or asymmetrical division. In panel A, if a stem cell binds to a specific extracellular matrix, as symbolized by attaching to a coated plastic dish, the signal received combines with signals in the medium (growth factors, Ca++, nutrients, oxygen, etc.) to stimulate genes and gene products to bring about the division plane to be perpendicular to the attachment plane. As a result, both daughter cells continue to have identical signalling as did the maternal stem cell (symmerical cell division or expansion of the stem cell population). In panel B, the stem cell binds to a different substrate molecule, as represented by a natural extra-cellular molecule, such as laminin or collagen type 4. In this case, the signal this substrate molecule induces a different intracellular signal that interacts with the same signals from the medium, Ca++, oxygen, etc. to stimulate different genes and gene products to cause a division plane within the stem cell to be formed parallel to the attachment plane. In this case, the daughter cell on the bottom will mimic the same intracellular signalling as its maternal stem cell. Important to note that if these stem cells do not have functional gap junctional intercellular communication, then these signals are not transmitted to the other daughter cell because that daughter cell does not interact with the substrate signal. As a result, these daughter cells receive a different set of combined signals that trigger a commitment to become a progenitor and ultimately terminally differentiated progeny.

On the other hand, because the other daughter is not attached to the extra-cellular niche matrix and does not communicate directly via gap junctions to its sister cell (a stem cell), its new mix of signals coul d induce the expression of connexin genes and form functional gap junctions. This cell is now a progenitor cell and is growth inhibited every time it is stimulated to proliferate by these gap junctions and it can differentiate via these gap junctions.

On the other hand, if the mix of signals the anchored stem cell gets triggers genes that cause the mitotic division plane to be vertical to the stem cell niche plane, then both new daughter cells would still be anchored to the same extra-cellular matrix molecule that helped to determine stemness. Since neither sister stem cell has gap junctions, they do not differentiate.

The Stem Cell or De-differentiation Hypothesis of Carcinogenesis

One of the oldest theories of cancer is that a cancer cell started as a stem cell but was blocked in its ability to terminally differentiate or to become "mortal". That is the essence of Markert's quote and led to his view that cancer was a disease of differentiation [4]. In addition, the views of Pierce ("Cancer as a stem cell disease") [6], Potter's concept of "oncogeny as partially blocked ontogeny" [7], together with the experimental demonstrations of the clonal origin of all the cells within a tumor [37-38] and the immortally of tumor cells, contribute to a hypothesis that the normal immortal stem cell was the target cell for the ultimate cancer cell.

Yet this hypothesis has not gone unchallenged, as there are those who feel any cell, save those terminally-differentiated cells with no nuclei (red blood cells or lens cells), can de-differentiate to the "embryonic-stem" cell state and then progress to the carcinogenic process. In more modern terms, this "de-differentiation" might be re-named, "re-programmed" [39]. In deed, with some evidence being presented, adult differentiated mouse fibroblasts have been interpreted to be re-programmed after being genetically modified to over express copies of the Oct-4 gene [40-42]. Yet, these data also can be challenged in that the original adult mouse skin fibroblast culture probably contained some normal adult skin stem cells expressing Oct-4. The transfected recovered cells might have been a transfected normal skin adult stem cell. More experiments will be needed to resolve this possibility.

The de-differentiation hypothesis does challenge the basic tenet in science, namely, *Ocham's Razor*. Whenever multiple hypotheses are offered to explain an observation, one should first stick with the simplest explanation for it is the easiest to disprove. In the case of the de-differentiation hypothesis, one needs to re-program the genome, such that, at least those genes that limited the life span of the progenitor or terminally differentiate cell would need to be repressed and the stemness or Oct.4 gene be expressed. Basically, while in principle, this is logical, it does add another step in an otherwise, already complex carcinogenic process.

Probably another concept that has to be considered, in the context of the stem cell theory, is the current paradigm in the cancer field, namely, that the first step in the carcinogenic process must be the induction of "immortalization" in a normal, "mortal" cell [43]. In this paradigm, cancer is thought to arise from a normal, mortal cell, such as a primary culture of mammalian tissue. Since these primary cells, primarily fibroblasts, were characterized as having a finite life span in vitro, the "Hayflick limit" [44], any induced neoplastic cell derived from this population was assumed to be "mortal". Therefore, the first step in the carcinogenic process was to induce "immortality" in a mortal, normal cell. This allowed the immortalized cell to live long enough to accrue additional genetic and epigenetic changes needed for complete neoplastic transformation. However, if the target cell for carcinogenesis is the stem cell, then one can see the current paradigm is exactly backwards. If the stem cell, which is naturally "immortal" until it is induced to differentiate or to become "mortal", is the stem cell, then the new paradigm should be that the first step in the carcinogenetic process must be to block "mortalization" of an immortal normal stem cell. This now sets up the discussion of the next hypothesis of carcinogenesis.

Stem Cells, the Multi-Step, Multi-Mechanism Carcinogenic Process of Initiation, Promotion and Progression

With the possible exception of the formation of teratomas, all other cancers appear to require multiple distinct events from each other, in order that a single, normal cell becomes an invasive, metastatic cancer cell, having all those "Hallmarks" associated with all cancer cells. With the early demonstration using mouse skin and rabbit ears [45,46], it was shown that a one" hit" hypothesis of carcinogenesis was inappropriate to explain the multiple treatments an organism must get in order that a tumor appear.

Even with later studies on human genetic predisposing cancer syndromes, such as retinoblastoma [47], it was clearly evident that, just because all the cells of a person's body contained the cancer-predisposing gene, only a very few gave rise to a cancer.

In these early animal experiments, the concepts of "initiation", "promotion" and "progression" were coined, as "operation" terms.

Initiation was the event that occurred in only a few cells of organism, was basically *irreversible.* If the initiator was known to be associated with the induction of the target organ when given at high concentrations or doses, then at a low, non-cancer- inducing concentration or dose, the animal will not form any tumors. However, if followed by the next step (promotion), one can surmise that an irreversible event had occurred in a few cells of that organism. In the case of the mouse skin or rat liver, the initiated cell could remain quiescent in the animal for months, only to be stimulated later to start the carcinogenic process. The initiated cell did not die or was not "restored" to the normal state during this period. *Operationally,* initiation is only the production of a stable cell that can not terminally differentiate or apoptose easily. Consequently, initiation is that fundamental event that affects a stem cell's ability to divide, asymmetrically. This is probably the most accurate operational definition of initiation. While few studies have given us an insight as to what might be the gene or genes involved in this critical biological process of stem cells, Ko and associates have identified a gene, CoAA, that could be involved in this process [48]. A conceptual manner of viewing this initiation process in an adult stem cell is seen in Figure 4.

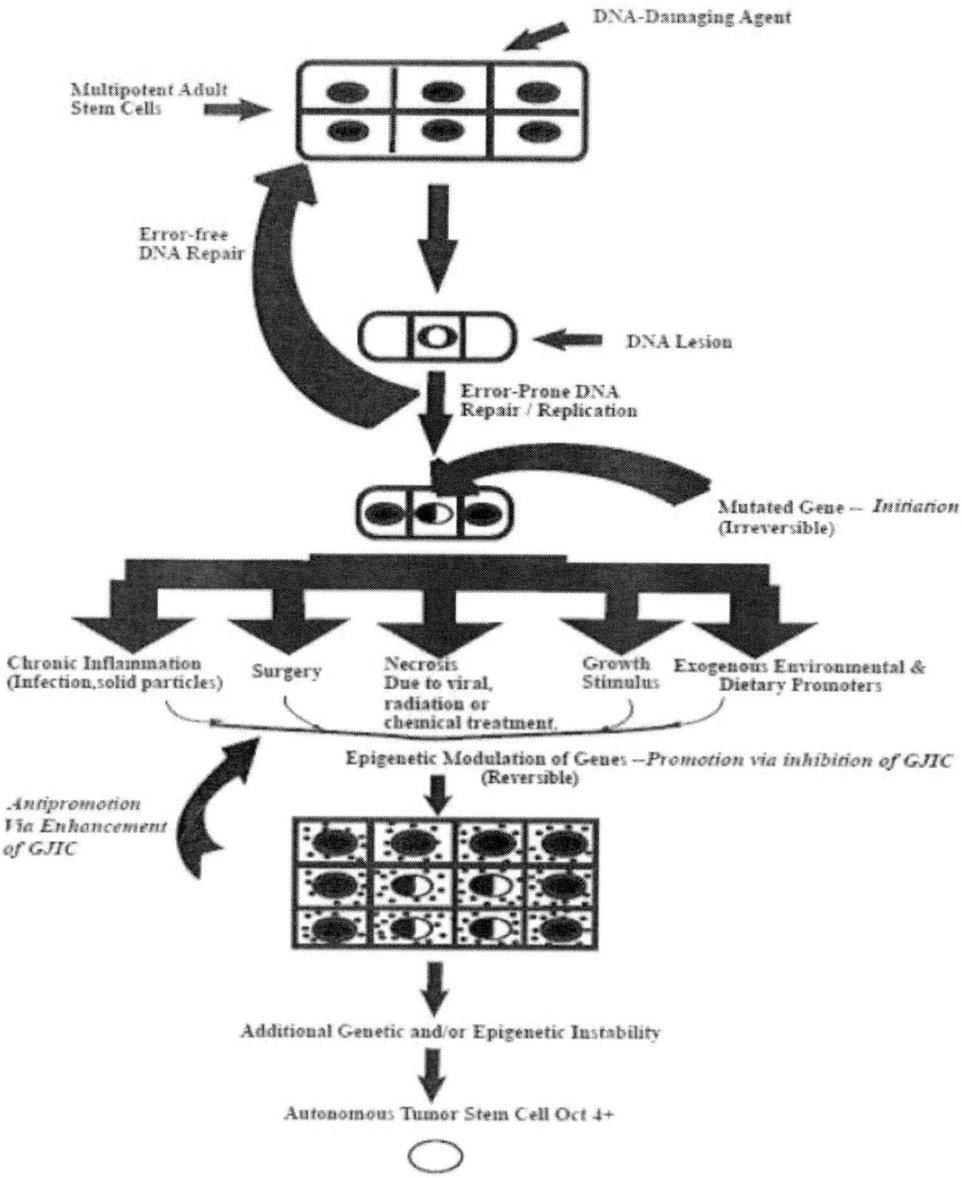

Figure 3. A diagrammatic heuristic scheme to depict the postulated mechanisms of the initiation and promotion phase of carcinogenesis. DNA lesions, induced by physical mutagens or by errors in DNA replication, are substrates in adult stem cells (Oct-4+) that can be fixed if they are not removed in an error-free manner prior to DNA replication. Promotion includes those conditions (i.e., chronic inflammation induced by infectious agents, solid particles; surgery or wounding; necrotic cell death; normal growth stimuli caused by growth factors, hormones; and exogenous epigenetic natural and synthethic epigenetic molecules), in which a pluripotent, but surviving, initiated adult stem cell (Oct-4+), can escape the nonproliferative state. The build up of initiated cells allows them to "resist" the anti-mitotic influence of neighboring non-initiated cells. In addition, the changing micro-environment within the growing benign tumor will cause some of the initiated adult stem cells to partially differentiate into cancer non-stem cells. This, together with either addition mutations or stable epigenetic changes, might allow a given initiated adult stem cell to have autonomous, invasive properties of a malignant cell.

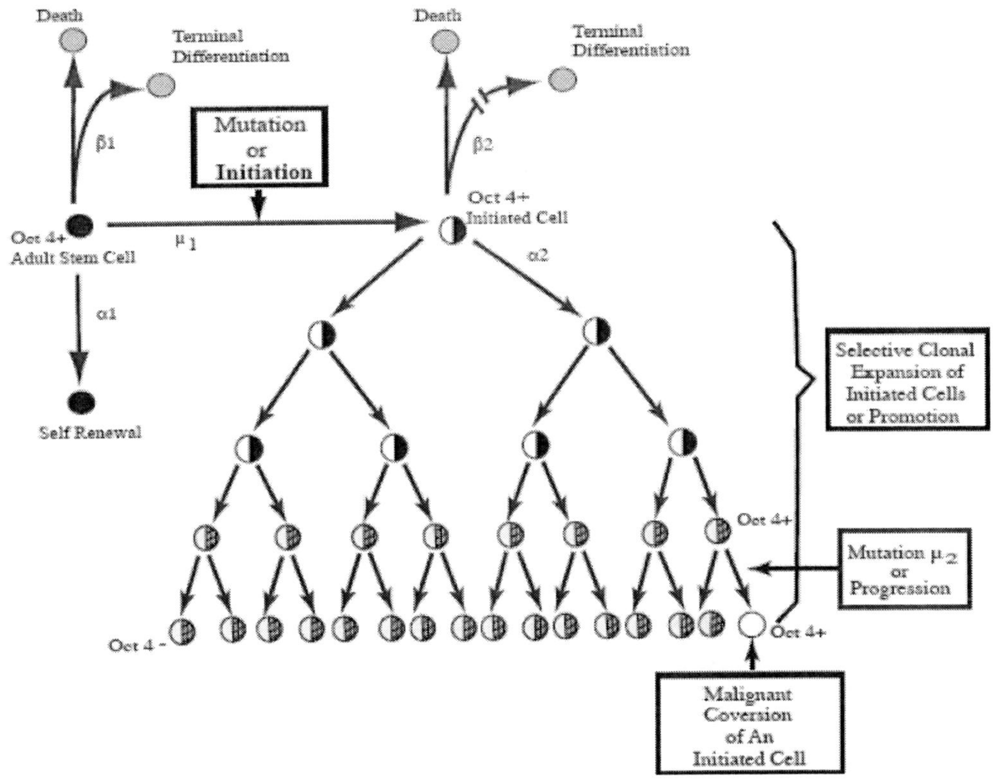

Figure 4. In this diagram, a normal adult stem cell is shown dividing asymmetrically to form one daughter that is committed to ultimately terminally differentiate. The other daughter is designated to be identical to its mother adult stem cell (Oct-4+). If that adult stem cell is exposed to some condition that prevents asymmetrical cell division, but does not suppress the Oct-4 expression, it is operationally an initiated cell. That is, if mitotically stimulated to divide, it divides symmetrically to form two initiated, non-terminally differentiated cell. Initiation is, then, defined as the process that prevents an "immortal" normal adult stem cell to terminally differentiate or become "mortal". These adult initiated stem cells are still Oct-4 positive or benign cancer stem cells. As these initiated Oct-4+ cells are stimulated to proliferate and resist apoptosis, the growing benign tumor micro-environment changes, some of these initiated Oct-4 + cells can partially differentiate into "cancer non-stem cells"[Oct-4 negative]. Evening, additional stable mutational or epigenetic events occur, providing the benign Oct-4+ cancer stem cells to become invasive, metastatic "cancer stem cells".

Promotion, on the other hand, was that process that occurred only after the animal was initiated (or as will be seen later, it could also occur on cells that were "spontaneously" initiated). In fact, especially in the case of a long-lived species, such as the human being, all individuals have spontaneously-initiated cells, and the longer one lives, the greater that number of initiated stem cells. The process of tumor promotion is when the initiated animal is exposed on a regular basis, for a long period of time, at threshold and above concentrations and in the absence of "anti-promoters", causing the single initiated cell to form a tumor. In the absence of this promotion process, no tumors appear [49]. Clearly, if the promotion process is stopped or interrupted, or given together with anti-promoters, then no initiated cell can accrue the necessary characteristics needed to have all the "hallmarks" of cancer. *Operationally,* the promotion process, one that is interruptible or even reversible [50], is one where the single "initiated" cell can be clonally expanded to reach a mass of cells, in which one cell can now acquire an addition stable change to give it a more selective advance to acquire more changes. It was also noted that promotion, which leads to the expansion of initiated cells, also involves the acquisition of a resistance to apoptosis. Therefore, the increased accumulation of initiated cells by promotion could be the result of mitogenesis and an inhibition of apoptosis.

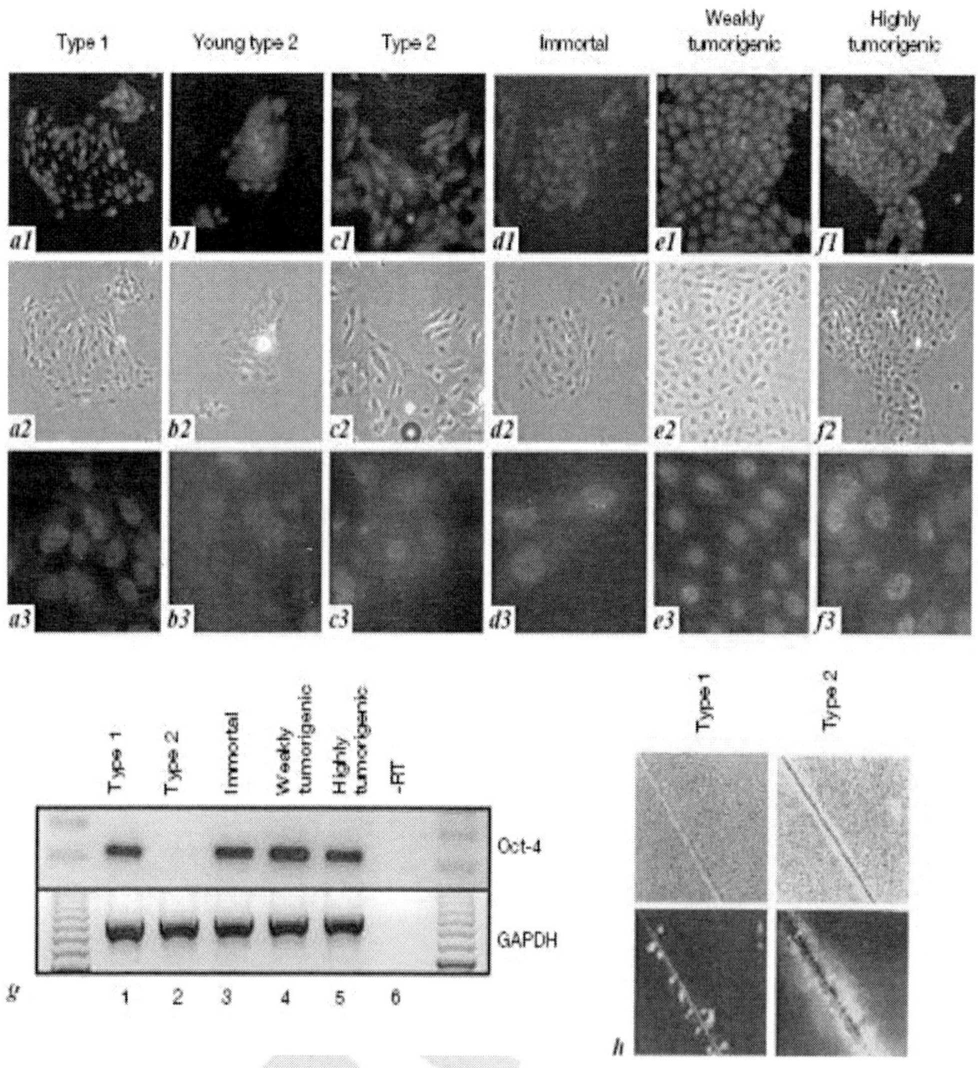

Figure 5. The composite of these three figures illustrated that (a) the clonally-derived normal human adult breast stem cells expressed Oct-4 (Figure 5.A panel) via immunohistochemical use of fluorescent antibodies to Oct-4 in the normal breast stem cells, but not in the differentiated breast cells (Figure 5.C panel), still expressed in SV40 "immortalized" normal breast stem cells which were not tumorigenic (Figure 5.D panel), still expressed in the irradiated and weakly tumorigenic breast stem cells (Figure 5.E panel) and expressed in the neu/ErB-2 highly transformed clone (Figure 5.F panel). In Figure 5.G, the RT-PCR data correlated with the immunohistochemical data of Oct-4 in this series of human breast adult stem cells. In Figure 5.H, the data clearly show that the normal breast adult stem cells have no functional gap junctional intercellular communication as measured by the fluorescent.

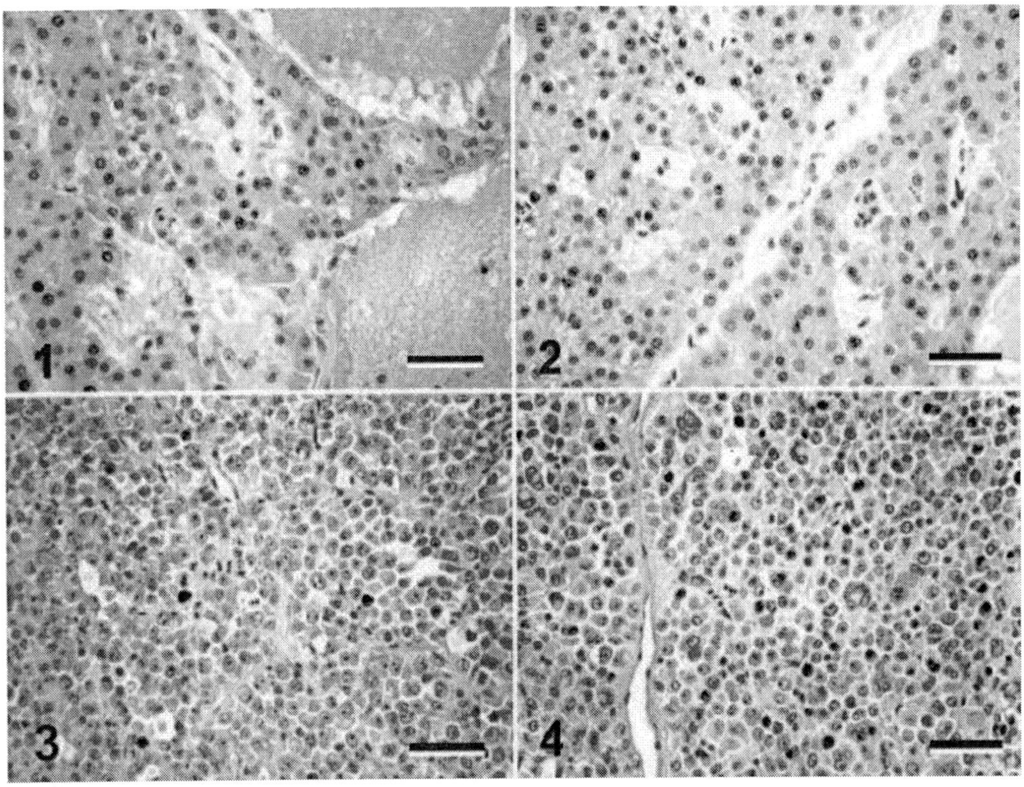

Figure 6. These photographs of Oct4 expression in spontaneous canine tumors reflect the intertumor and intratumor variation. Low (Figures 1, 3) and High (Figures 2, 4) frequencies of Oct-4 expressing cells in canine hepatocellular carcinomas (Figures 1, 2) and seminomas (Figures 3, 4 , respectively. Variation in the relative proportion of the Oct-4 –positive cells (brown nuclear precipitate) was seen in both between and within different types of spontaneous canine tumors. Immunohistochemical staining with mouse anti-human Oct-4 monoclonal antibody was visualized with the substrate 3,3'-diaminobenzidine with hematoxylin counterstain. Bar= 80 μm. Permission granted by American Society of Veterinary Pathology, Allen Press, Lawrence, Kansas, USA.

Promotion appears to be able to allow an initiated cell to escape mitotic suppression by surrounding normal cells. The literature has shown that (a) wound healing after removal of tissue by surgery, (b) chronic inflammation, (c) cell death due to burns, viruses, or non-genotoxic toxicants, such as alcohol or carbon tetrachloride, (d) growth factors and hormones, and (e) exogenous non-genotoxic chemicals, such as Phenobarbital or polybrominated biphenols, can be tumor promoters. Promotion has been shown to be induced in initiated rodent skin, ears, mammary tissue, bladder, and liver. Physical agents, such as asbestos fibers, carbon particles, and solid metal objects, such as nanoparticles, can induce chronic inflammation to act as promoters [51]. There are species and strain specific promoters [52].

Although it was postulated in 1979 that tumor promoters worked, mechanistically, by inhibiting gap junctional intercellular communication [53], it still has not been integrated into the cancer field, as evidenced by the lack of references to this insight by the molecular oncologists. Most, if not all, chemical tumor promoters have been shown to inhibit, reversibly, GJIC at threshold and above concentrations which are non-cytotoxic [54]. In fact, the role of gap junctions has further been strengthened by the fact that many chemopreventive and anti-carcinogenic agents, such as green tea, [55], resveratrol [56,57], caffeic acid phenylester [58], or chemotherapeutic agents, such as lovastatin [59], kaempherol [60], SAHA [61], and beta-sitosterol [62], restore GJIC in cancer cells, Even various oncogenes, such as ras, src, neu, mos, have been shown to inhibit, stably, GJIC [63]. Genetic transfection of connexin genes in non-GJIC functioning cancer cells restores GJIC and normal cell growth with reduced tumorigenicity [63]. On the other hand, anti-sense connexin genes in normal cells triggered the tumorigenic phenotype of these cells [63]. Collectively, the role of GJIC must play some role, as Lowenstein and Kanno predicted in 1966 [64], in the carcinogenic process.

Progression is the final complex step (probably involving multi-events) that, *operationally*, converts one single initiated cell in the heterogeneous clone produced by promotion (e.g., a skin papilloma, liver enzyme foci, a colon polyp or a nodule in the breast). This step, also, appears to be irreversible and leads, ultimately, to an invasive, metastatic cell with all the "hallmarks of cancer".

To try to integrate the stem cell theory into this "initiation/ promotion/progression" hypothesis, it should be obvious that, if initiation occurs in an adult normal immortal stem cell, the initiation event must be the process that inhibits asymmetric cell division, but not the symmetric cell division of an immortal adult stem cell. This could, then, induce signalling in some of the "pre-cancer stem cells" so that they "partially" differentiate into " cancer non-stem cells", cancer cells which are no longer able to sustain the growth of the tumor.

THE MUTATION OR EPIGENETIC THEORIES OF CARCINOGENESIS

Since inherited genes that predispose cancer in patients, such as xeroderma pigmentosum or retinoblastoma, carry a germ line mutation. In the case of cells of the skin-cancer predisposed xeroderma pigmentosum, which do not repair their DNA after ultraviolet light-induced DNA damage [65], their cells have a higher mutation frequency than their normal counterparts [13,14]. From this, it is clear that mutations must play some role in carcinogenesis. In deed, when one examines oncogenes and tumor suppressor genes in various tumor cells, one frequently finds mutations in these genes. Especially, in the case of the mutations of the p53 gene in skin cancer patients, the mutations found correspond to that expected type if formed from unrepaired UV lesions of these cells [15]. Even in the cancer prone multi-cancer syndrome, Bloom's syndrome, the spontaneous mutation rates were found to be higher than from cells of normal patients [66].

These kinds of examples provide strong evidence that mutations, being basically an irreversible event, could be the mechanistic basis for the "initiation" event that starts the multi-stage process. This assumption has been carried over to the prominent paradigm of today's cancer research field, namely, "carcinogen as mutagen" [67]. However, the uncritical interpretation of results from in vitro studies to test if "carcinogens" are mutagens, as well as from ill-design bioassays on rodents [68], has brought massive confusion to the cancer-risk assessment field, as well as to practice assessment of new drugs and chemicals. While this does not imply that mutations do not play a role in carcinogenesis, it does question if *chemicals* (not radiation) cause mutations found in the oncogenes and tumor suppressor genes of the tumors associated with that exposure. With the demonstration that the mutation spectrum of an oncogene found in tumor cells of cigarette smokers being essentially the same as the spectrum for mutations found in the oncogenes of lung tumors of non-smokers [69], the question is raised whether the chemicals in cigarette smoke acted as promoters, rather than as initiators [68]. Animal experiments, as well as epidemiological evidence from smokers who quit smoking, suggest, strongly, that these chemicals acted more like promoters than initiators. Stopping smoking acted as stopping phorbol esters or phenobarbital on the interruption of promotion of skin and liver cancers, respectively. Must recently, Upham and co-workers [70-72] showed that the predominant chemicals in cigarette smoke performed, mechanistically, like tumor promoters, at non-cytotoxic concentrations. Promoters, by blocking intercellular communication, either by interfering with secreted growth inhibitors or their receptor-signaling, or by reversibly blocking GJIC, could block the cellular functions of "contact-inhibition", differentiation, or apoptosis. All three of these cellular phenotypes are affected by the carcinogenic process.

The important point to be made here, in trying to resolve the issue of finding DNA lesions in cells after an animal or cells in culture are exposed to chemicals associated with the appearance of tumors or neoplastic transformed cells, is that there are two sources of DNA which could be targets for DNA damage caused by electrophiles or free radicals. The first is the mitochondrial DNA where oxidative metabolism is occurring and the second is the nuclear DNA, which is sequestered away from oxidative damaging free radicals and electrophiles (except during ionizing radiation). In addition, there are three types of cells in which these two DNA targets are found, the few stem cells, the many progenitor cells with a limited life span and the terminally differentiated cells, which do not proliferate or give rise to cancers. Since very few of the studies demonstrating the existence of DNA lesions after chemical exposures separate the two sources of DNA before analysis, one can not rigorously state these lesions are those that led to mutations found in the oncogenes of tumor cells found after the chemical exposure. If one does find these DNA lesions in the nuclear DNA then, in all likelihood, the cell would have died from such massive production of electrophiles and free radicals that exceeded the cellular defence mechanisms, and traversed from the cytoplasm to the nuclear membrane. Under those conditions, the plasma membrane would be destroyed and the cell would die by necrosis. The death of these cells (usually the terminal differentiated cells, which express large amounts of metabolizing enzymes) could act as "indirect" tumor promoters by stimulating the stem cells to proliferate. If the stem cell was previously initiated by errors in replication or by UV radiation induced mutations, then the chemical could give the appearance of causing the DNA damage and mutations. In brief, while a statement suggesting that chemicals do not induce mutations that cause cancer is clearly heretical, the evidence suggesting otherwise is yet to be rigorously demonstrated. These so-called "mutagenic carcinogens" are more likely tumor promoters rather than initiators. These cancer-associated chemicals selectively promote spontaneously initiated stem cells [68].

If mutations might be the mechanistic basis for the initiation and the progression stages, one should not ignore the possibility that a stable epigenetic event could also bring about an initiation event. In the case of teratomas, it has been shown that a metastatic teratocarcinoma cell, when placed back into a blastocyst of a genetically-marked mouse, could participate in the normal development of a mosaic mouse, whereby, the teracarcimoa cells helped to generate normal tissues [73]. This could not have happened if the original teratocarcinoma cell was generated by an irreversible mutational event. The example also re-enforces the stem cell theory of cancer. The normal definition of an embryonic stem cell is that it forms a teratoma when injected into an adult animal. That implies the embryonic stem cell, when placed in a strange micro-environment, will modulate its gene expression patterns in bizarre ways, so as to differentiate but in an unorganized fashion. If a mutated cancer cell is transplanted into an adult host, it might partially differentiate or even partly apoptose, but will continue to form a tumor.

Oncogenes, Tumor Suppressor Genes and Cancer Cells

The success of modern molecular oncology, with the discovery of oncogenes and tumor suppressor genes, easily diverted the cancer community from the classic whole animal studies to that of mutated DNA sequences in certain genes associated with a cell becoming a cancer. The emergence of the Human Genome project, with its promise to cure human diseases, such as cancer, simply by comparing sequences of cancer and non cancer patients, as well as providing new strategies for prevention or “cures”, turns out not to be able to deliver on many of those promises. In fact, the insights, gained by the classic studies on carcinogenesis, as well as some of the ignored “hallmarks” of cancer [74], have already provided new insights without the need for all that Human Genomic information.

Harris has reviewed hundreds of studies on the most common tumor suppressor gene found in human cancers (but it should be noted, not all human cancers), the p53 gene [75]. Multiple oncogenes have been identified and are still being reported [48]. In brief, the functional roles, albeit each works by different molecular/biochemical mechanisms, of these two classes of cancer-related genes is to stimulate the growth of pre-malignant (initiated) and malignant cells and to inhibit the growth of these pre-malignant cells, respectively. *Operationally*, stimulation of the increase of initiated cells can occur by either or both inhibiting “contact-inhibition” and apoptosis and by stimulating mitogenesis. In addition, this includes the fact that initiation, operationally, *prevents asymmetric cell division of the initiated adult stem cell under normal conditions*, the oncogene or tumor suppressor genes might affect the regulation of symmetric and asymmetric cell division. Few in the cancer field have addressed this as a fundamental problem to be solved. Since oncogene and tumor suppression genes affect cell proliferation and cell cycle regulation of the single cell, the molecular oncologists have ignored the fact that cell proliferation also involves cell-cell interactions, either heterogeneous, such as stromal- epithelial interactions [76,77] by secreted factors (extra-cellular communication) or by gap junctional intercellular communication between heterologous and homologous cells within a tissue [78]. In other words, there are other genes working at a higher systems level, which transcends the reductionalists’ thinking that predominates the cancer field today.

The fact that gap junction genes have been shown to be tumor suppressor genes, and the function of the these connexin genes is to affect intercellular regulation of single cell’s cycle cycle control, to differentiate by receiving signals from without the cell or to apoptose by reaching signals from outside the cell, a different manner of viewing carcinogens must be gained than just from molecular or in vitro studies. As the late V.R. Potter had stated [79]:

"The cancer problem is not merely a cell problem; it is a problem of cell interaction, not only within tissues, but also with distal cells in other tissues. But in stressing the whole organism, we must also remember that the integration of normal cells with the welfare of the whole organism is brought about by molecular messages acting on molecular receptors."

ADULT STEM CELLS AS THE TARGETS FOR CARCINOGENIC INITIATION

Given the previous experiments that demonstrated cancer cells were "immortal", that they resisted terminal differentiation but could partially differentiate under certain conditions, that they were monoclonally derived and that they could invade and metastasize, as well as induce angiogenesis, one is struck by the similarities of these "hallmarks" of cancer with the normal properties of stem cells. Two "hallmarks" that were not identified were the stem-like nature of the cancer cell and the lack of functional cell-cell communication [74].

Conceptually, however, the initiation/promotion/progression hypothesis seems, best, to support the idea that the single cell that is initiated is a normal adult stem cell. In the case of teratomas, the single cell might be an embryonic stem cell. However, in adult cancers, since stem cells do exists for most, if not all, organs, these cells, being either multi-potent or bi-potent, could after initiation, depending on the genes affected and the micro-environment, in which the cell finds itself, cause partially differentiation of the initiated stem cell into the identifiable tumor types of that particular organ (e.g., hepatocellular carcinomas or cholangiocellular carcinomas in the liver). In other words, for some initiated adult stem cells, these new changes in the micro-environment can induced these cells to have asymmetric cell division in order to partially differentiate.

Initiation is that operational step to cause a cell, presumably an adult stem cell, to start the complex evolutionary process for all tumors. If this cell is a normal, immortal adult stem cell, and if it is assumed that the initiation process is one that inhibits the stem cell to asymmetrically divide (i.e., it cannot normally terminally differentiate), then, "Are initiated stem cells those that give rise to the so-called newly discovered *"cancer stem cells*" which have the potential to perpetuate the growth of a tumor?" [80]. Clearly, in a tumor, there are *"cancer non-stem cells",* those that appear to be partially differentiated and can not perpetuate the growth of the tumor [81]. Of course, it has not been rigorously ruled out that some differentiated progenitor cell could be "re-programmed" to de-differentiate to become "immortal" again and then start the carcinogenic process. In this case, the "initiation" step would be the so-called "immortalization" of a normal, mortal progenitor cell as the prevailing hypothesis would suggest [43].

However, there are times when "Ocham's Razor" comes in handy in trying to resolve multiple scientific interpretations of observations. In the case of the "de-differentiation" or "re-programming" hypothesis of the origin of cancer cells, if an adult or somatic differentiated cell is "initiated", it must involve at least one additional step before it can utilize its new-found "immortality", compared to the normal adult step cell which is naturally immortal" at the time of initiation. Recent claims that an adult mouse skin fibroblast cell could be "re-programmed" when genetically transfected with "stemness" genes, such as oct-4, nanog, etc, would seem, at least, to keep open the possibility that "initiation" of an adult differentiated cell might happen [40-42]. However, in this case, "initiation" is operationally very different than "initiation" of a normal immortal adult stem cell. It must include two steps; one to reprogram whole sets of genes that determine the differentiation of a mature, differentiated skin fibroblast cell, which had its Oct-4 (and other "stemness" genes) transcriptionally suppressed and its senescence genes transcriptionally, operational. It, then, had to start where the normal adult get was when it was "initiated", namely already immortal but now blocked in its ability to divide asymmetrically under normal conditions.

However, there is another interpretation of these results of "re-programming" of an adult somatic, differentiated skin fibroblast cell. That is, if the original rescued genetically-engineered cell, done with a drug-resistance gene that presumably turned on the stemness genes, was originally a normal adult stem cell with it's already expressed Oct-4 and other stemness genes, then, in fact, those rescued cells were hardly highly differentiated somatic differentiated skin fibroblasts. The point being made is that adult stem cells do exist in most, if not all, adult organs, especially the skin. Many adult stem cells have been isolated from adult tissues that express Oct4 and did not express the connexin genes or have functional gap junctions [82-88]. These are real multi-potential stem or bi-potential stem cells. They are not simply pluri-potential embryonic stem cells migrating throughout the body of adult organisms.

Since adult stem cells have been isolated for many years, "Is there evidence that these adult stem cells can give rise to cancer?" The answer is "yes". When human adult breast stem cells were isolated and reported in 1995 [83], it was, then, subsequently shown that SV40 could block their ability to terminally differentiate (an operational definition of initiation) [89]. These cells were unable to form tumors in an appropriated animal model. While SV40 and other viruses (i.e. human papilloma virus) have been termed, "immortalizing viruses", it appears that this might be a major misnomer. It is well known that when primary human cell cultures are infected with these viruses, the majority of the cells eventually go through "crises", while a few rare cells survive and are characterized as "immortal". The idea is that either some rare insertional mutational event had occurred in these few surviving cells or that the virus genome somehow affected the senescence genes to be re-programmed" and the immortalization process started. There is a simpler explanation, supported by the experiments with human adult breast stem cells [31]. That is, the infecting SV40 or papilloma viruses, while infecting all the cells of the primary culture, only affected the few adult stem cells of that culture. These viruses did not induce "immortalization" but, in fact, blocked "mortalization" of an already normal, immortal adult stem cell. Chang and associates showed that these cells were able to perpetuate themselves in vitro and, upon, radiation and oncogene transfection become tumorigenic, whereas, no normal, differentiated human adult breast epithelial cell became "immortal" or neoplastically transformed [89].

It's important to discuss how the original adult human kidney stem cell was isolated and reported in 1987 [82]. The idea that stem cells might be the target cell for initiating the carcinogenic process came from studies to determine the extreme variability of inducing neoplastic transformed Syrian hamster cells in vitro. Nakano and T'so were trying to discern why cultures of Syrian hamster embryo cells could be exposed to some carcinogen on one day in the lab and formed many neoplastic transformed clones, but in the same cultures, on another day or in another lab, no transformants were induced [90]. To make a long story short, they noticed that, only in those cultures with "contact-insensitive" populations of cells, could one obtain neoplastic transformed clones. Our lab speculated these "contact insensitive", normal embryonic cells in these cultures might be stem cells. We further reasoned that their "contact-insensitivity" was the result of not expressing connexin genes or having functional gap junctional intercellular communication. We, therefore, assumed, in all adult tissues, there existed a few adult stem cells that did not have functional GJIC. By designing an in vitro assay with lethally-irradiated human fibroblast cells, which have functional GJIC, we disassociated normal kidney tissue into single cells. This mixture of normal kidney cells contained the many progenitor cells, which have functional GJIC, the terminally differentiated cells which can not proliferate and the few adult stem cells, which we assumed had no functional GJIC. After putting these cells on the lethally irradiated monolayer of human fibroblasts, we obtained a few clones of cells, which were later shown to be the adult stem cells of the human kidney (They expressed no connexin genes or had functional GJIC but they expressed Oct-4). As controls in this experiment, 8 human carcinoma cell lines, which had no GJIC, also could be recovered on this assay system. The rationale for the selection system was that if a normal cell had functional GJIC, it would couple with the dying x ray lethally-irradiated cells and die. Only those cells with no functional GJIC would proliferate on this monolayer. All of the human adult stem cells that have been reported appear not to express any connexion genes or have functional GJIC [82-88].

The reality is that in an adult animal, including the human being, adult committed stem cells exists normally for tissue replacement and growth. These stem cells are not merely pluripotent or multi-potent stem cells floating around only to differentiate when needed in particular micro-environments. Each tissue contains these stem cells. It is these adult organ-specific stem cells that are the suspected targets for the initiation of the carcinogenic process.

Cancer Stem Cells: A Re-Discovery of an Old Idea

One of the recent paradigm-changing observations that has occurred in the cancer field happened when Al Hajj et al [80] reported that they identified a presumptive unique class of breast cancer cells within the breast tumor that had the ability to perpetuate the growth of the tumor, i.e., a breast *"cancer stem cell",* whereas the other cancer cells within that tumor did not have this ability. These might be referred to as *cancer non-stem cells*. They are partially differentiated and ultimately senesce or apoptose. Later, Ponti et al [91] were able to show that these breast cancer stem cells to perpetuate the growth of the tumor. However, much earlier, Chang and his associates had already identified and partially characterized the normal human breast stem cell and showed that these stem cells could be "initiated" and neoplastically transformed [92]. In effect, he produced, in vitro, the human breast cancer stem cell that gave rise to a tumor when the cells were placed into an immune-compromised mouse.

Historically, when it was shown that the embryonic stem cell expressed a few unique "embryonic stem cell markers" (e.g., Oct-4, Sox 2, nanog genes) [93], Oct-4 seemed to have been correctly identified, early in the characterization of expressed genes in embryonic stem cells, as a critical "stemness-determining gene" [94]. Later, observations showed that when these cells differentiated, the oct-4 gene was transcriptionally suppressed [95]. There were others that claimed that no Oct-4 expression could be found in normal differentiated tissues.

Then, when a few reports saw Oct-4 expression in a few cells of some types of tumors [96,97], it was suggested that Oct-4 must have been re-expressed or re-programmed during the neoplastic transformation process. It has been used to confirm the accepted paradigm [43] that the normal differentiated progenitor cells do not express immortalizing potential that the Oct-4 gene seems to possess.

Because our group, believers in the stem cell theory of cancer, knew the adult differentiated tissues must have a few adult stem cells, which were probably overlooked in these previous reports, we decided to examine the many isolated human adult stem cells we had in our lab (kidney, breast, liver, pancreas, mesenchyme) for the expression of Oct-4. We also assumed that these few normal adult stem cells were the target cells for the cancers seen in human organs. In addition to testing for Oct-4, we also tested for the expression of the major connexins and for functional GJIC which is required for these stem cells to differentiate. In brief, we showed that all of these normal adult stem cells expressed Oct-4 and when the stem cells differentiated, Oct-4 was repressed.

In a classic set of experiments, Dr. Chang's group obtained a series of clonally-derived cells from the normal adult breast stem cells which (a) could be differentiated into normal epithelial cells (no expression of Oct-4, but they expressed Cx43 and had functional GJIC); (b) were SV-40 transfected but non-tumorigenic and unable to terminally differentiate, had Oct-4 expressed but no GJIC; (c) after x-rayed irradiated produced a weakly tumorigenic clone with Oct-4 expressed; and (d) which, after a neu/Erb2 transfection, a highly tumorigenic derivative of the weakly tumorigenic clone was obtained, which still expressed Oct-4 [98]. In essence, we showed that Oct-4 was expressed in the normal adult stem cell, stayed expressed when SV40 prevented asymmetric cell division, remained expressed during the induction of tumorigenesis by X rays and oncogene transfection. It was transcriptionally suppressed only during differentiation of the normal adult stem cells [98]. These differentiated breast epithelial cells were unable to re-program the Oct-4 gene or become immortal or tumorigenic under the conditions where the normal adult stem cell was easily blocked from differentiating and neoplastically transformed. These experiments clearly support the stem cell theory and are harder to explain using the "de-differentiation" or "re-programming" hypothesis of carcinogenesis.

It is important to note that these normal breast adult stem cells expressed the estrogen receptor, a marker found in a majority of human breast cancers. In addition, since the commonly used human breast carcinoma cell line in breast cancer studies, MCF-7, expresses the estrogen receptor, but not the connexin43 gene [99], but does express the Oct-4 in vitro [98], one might speculate that MCF-7 was originally derived from a normal adult breast stem cell similar to our normal human isolated adult breast stem cell.

It is also important to note that MCF-7 is not a homogeneous cell population [98]. It is an immortal cell line because it contains some "cancer stem cells" that help to perpetuate the cell line indefinitely. *In vitro, as in vivo, the cells create different micro-environments for these cancer stem cells, causing some of them to partially differentiate into cancer non-stem cells or to regain some asymmetric cell division potential.* The implication from these observations is that, all tumors during their growth will be a mixture of cancer stem cells and cancer non-stem cells. The ratio of these two types of cancer cells is probably influenced by some stromal-epithelial interactions, as has been demonstrated in vivo and in vitro [76,77,100].

To illustrate this, we were the first to detect in vivo that 100% of 83 canine tumors from 21 different organ sites expressed Oct-4 in the tumors (the "cancer stem cells", but the ratio of the cancer stem cell to the cancer non-stem cells varied from tumor to tumor. [81] Later it was shown that 34/35 human bladder tumors expressed Oct-4, and the ratio of the two types varied widely between tumors [101]. At this point, one can only speculate that the differences in the ratio of the two types of cancer cells might be due to genetic, environmental or dietary factors that influences symmetric and asymmetric cell division of the cancer stem cell.

In a recent cautionary note, it was stated that "tumor growth need not be driven by rare cancer stem cells" [102]. The authors drew their conclusion, based on showing that isolated primary pre-B7B lymphoma cells from 3 independent Eu-myc transgenic mice could give rise to tumors in congenic mice, independent of the cells injected. Their conclusion, based on everyone's assumption was that, in all tumors, the "cancer stem cells" were "rare". In the study on canine tumors, and on human bladders [81,101], the numbers of Oct-4 "cancer stem cells" varied widely. Therefore, this cautionary note might be very misleading.

The excitement seen after the reports of the existence of various "cancer stem cells" has given new insights to the reasons why past cancer therapies have failed, i.e., they failed to target the "cancer stem cells" in the tumors. In addition, one of the explanations why these various therapeutic treatments failed was because the treatments, themselves, induced drug resistance genes that allowed these drug resistant cells to re-emerge. It now seems that a more plausible explanation exists for "induced drug resistance". The normal adult stem cell and its derived "cancer stem cell" might be naturally resistant to toxic chemotherapeutic agents. Again, the quote, "Nothing in biology makes sense except in the light of evolution", seems appropriate here.

From an evolutionary standpoint, if, during the emergence of the multi-cellular organism and the development of both germ line stem cells and adult somatic stem cells, both the stem cells and their differentiate lineage progeny were equally sensitive to environmental toxicant, the individual, hence, species, would never have survived. Therefore, it was imperative that the stem cells evolved with some mechanism(s) to protect itself from the exposure to these toxic agents. One means was to develop mechanisms to pump out foreign chemicals before they could damage the cell. Therefore, if an organism is exposed to some toxic agent, the differentiated cells might die; however, if the adult stem cell survived, it could replace the dead, specialized, differentiated cells and the organism and species would survive.

Evidence has been reported that, when tumor cells are exposure to some toxic fluorescent agent and then passed through a cell sorter, two populations of cells are recovered. One that contains the fluorescent compound and the other, the "side population", cells are non-fluorescent. It is these "side population" cells that seem to have stem-like properties, in that they can differentiate into the cell-lineage from which the tumor is derived [103]. One of these factors that rendered these cells to be drug resistant is because they naturally expressed various drug resistant genes, such as ABCG-2 [104].

In brief, drug resistance was not induced by the cancer chemotherapy, but it was the result of "cancer stem cells", which are naturally, expressing drug resistance genes, were selected from the mixed population of cancer cells.

A new perspective for cancer prevention and therapy is now obvious. The real target cell for prevention and treatment should be the "cancer stem cells". Oct-4 expression appears to by a critical gene to maintain "stemness" of both the normal stem cell and "cancer stem" cell. The ultimate goal in cancer prevention and therapy will be to render, transcriptionally or posttranslationally, the Oct-4 gene inoperative.

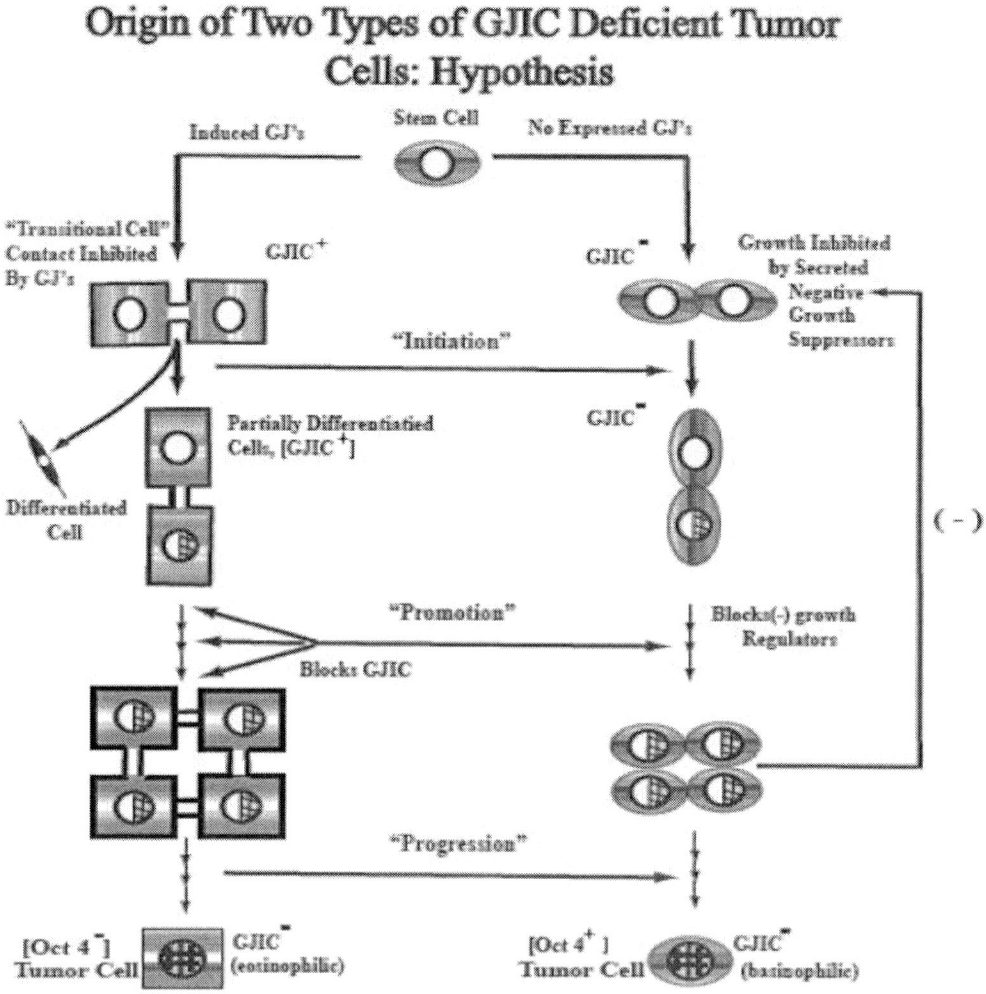

Figure 7. This figure illustrates a hypothesis to explain the existence of two types of cancer cells, namely, those that lack GJIC communication because (a) the connexin genes were never transcribed, as in HeLa or MCF-7 cancer cell lines, or (b) the expressed connexion genes could not form functional gap junctions due to oncogenes or mutations that render the connexin proteins forming functional gap junction, as in ras, raf, neu, src or mos-activated oncogene-transformed cancer cells. In other words, all cancer cells seem to be dysfunctional with regard to having GJIC, either because the connexin genes were never transcribed or if the transcribed proteins were not functional. There are several possible explanations, one being that the original stem cell, lacking expressed connexins, got initiated and subsequently promoted by agents that inhibited secreted negative growth regulators of stem cells. These might be the origin of the "cancer stem" cells. Now the cancer cells with activated oncogenes might inactivate functional GJIC by modifying, posttranslationally, the connexin proteins and gap junctions. There could be at least two explanations for this. One is that if the very early committed progenitor cells of the adult stem cell was initiated while it still expressed Oct-4 and telomerase, then its growth inhibition via gap junctions had to be inhibited by promoters that reversibly blocked GJIC, until late in promotion, when activated oncogenes stably and irreversibly inhibited gap junction proteins, such as via hyper-phosphorylation of connexins by ras, src and neu. Alternatively, these non-functional GJIC tumor cells might be derived from "cancer stem cells" but which were partially differentiated by the developing and changing microenvironments of all tumors to become "cancer non-stem cells".

This goal still has the same current intractable problem that has been plaguing the old therapeutic approaches. Since Oct-4 is expressed in both the normal and cancer stem cells, one must be able to target only the cancer stem cell, in order from preventing the therapy from reducing the normal stem cell pool. In addition, since the tumor contains both the cancer stem and cancer non-stem cells, which could inhibit the therapy designed to target the cancer stem cells, a dual approach might be implemented.

First, apply some therapy that can "easily" remove these cancer non-stem cells. After these are reduced, if the cancer stem cells, which express oct-4 and drug resistance genes, inhibiting the pump activity at the functional or enzymatic level, then treating with a toxic chemical, used to kill the cancer non-stem cells, would render these cancer stem cells to behave as functional cancer non-stem cells.

This approach has been tried in the past without our current knowledge of the cancer stem cell concept. Another strategy would be to target the Oct-4 gene with transcriptionally-modifying potential to block its expression, using targeting strategies that identify the organ markers for the adult stem cells, such as the estrogen receptor for adult human breast cancer stem cells and some other "cancer stem cell" marker not expressed in the normal adult stem cell.

Dietary Modulation of Normal and Cancer Stem Cell Pools: A View of How Diet, Systems View of Cell Biology, and the Risk to Cancer Interact

It is well known that genetic predispositions, gender, developmental state, caloric balance (gluttony or caloric restriction), exercise, life style, cultural, environmental, medical, or pharmacological treatments can influence the multi-stage, multi-mechanism process of carcinogenesis. What is clearly emerging is the powerful role that dietary factors play in experimental, as well as epidemiological studies, to either increase or decrease one's risk to various cancers. What has not been clearly demonstrated is, the interaction of these dietary factors and the adult normal and cancer stem cells. In fact, a new view is emerging that takes us away from only thinking, reductionalistically, about what might happen in a single adult stem cell that eventually could give rise to an initiated cancer stem cell, but how diet can involve the stem cell pool to affect the risk to increase or decrease the risk to cancer from a *systems* vantage point. In deed, this new view also will take our attention away from only viewing the cancer stem cell role as only a biological problem, but one that involves many cultural evolutionary changes.

Because of cultural evolution, which affects our dietary intake of the quantity and quality of food much more rapidly than the biological evolution needed to adapt to these changes, the long biological evolutionary adaptive balance with the diet of early humanoids, the new dietary behaviours are creating many new health problems [105-109]. Transmigration studies of humans have shown in several cases that the patterns of cancer frequencies of various ethnic groups conform to the new cultural (presumably) dietary behaviour compared to their country of origin.

Because of modern methods of altering native cultural diets to global diets, cancer patterns are changing. In fact, for a number of reasons, these new dietary habits are shaped by economic costs, availability of certain foods (depletion of tuna for sushi and sashimi), substitution of red meats for fish, agricultural genetic breeding of foods that sell or are needed for "fast food industries", and the psychological selling via mass marketing. The complexity of "diets" (calories, vitamins, nutrients, food components, processing and preparation of foods, etc.) makes epidemiological studies difficult to interpret since these studies are but a small snapshot in a dynamic time and place experience in an ever-changing dietary climate probably within every 20 years. These studies are now compounded in complexity by increasing uses of food supplements, pharmaceutical drugs, changing life styles and individual behaviours. The World Health Organization's estimation that there might be more over weight individuals than under weight in the world today suggests that global chronic (as well as acute) diseases are being affected by, on one hand, too many calories (not necessarily too many nutrients) or too few calories and nutrients [110]. Therefore, the next question has to be asked: "Which of the three stages of carcinogenesis seem to be most affected by diet modification?"

One can speculate that, since the initiation stage must take place in a single cell in a limited number of critical cancer-related genes, either by a mutational or stable epigenetic event, it will be impossible to reduce the risk to zero in the body of 100 trillion cells, most of which are not the target or adult stem cells. Initiation can occur when DNA damage is not repaired correctly (errors in DNA repair), such as in the xeroderma pigmentosum example. We can, of course, prevent the risk from being higher, such as not exposing ourselves to too much sunlight. In addition, we must recognize that mutations can be produced every time a cell replicates (errors in replication). We can never prevent this source of mutations that might initiate an adult stem cell. Cells are replicating day and night, 7 days a week and for our whole lives. Therefore, it is would seem that we will never reduce to zero the initiating event. *In fact, this source of spontaneously-originating errors in replication of DNA in stem cells might be the main source of initiated cells of the body, except for the UV-light induced initiation of skin stem cells.*

Promotion, on the other hand, takes decades, in most cases (except in children), to reach the progression stage. From a practical standpoint of designing an intervention chemoprevention strategy that would be the most efficacious, to decrease the risk to carcinogenesis, at least from the view that we, as individuals, might have some control of this process, the promotion phase would be a *life-long* process. Since the progression phase appears to occur in a single promoted initiated cell (a "pre-cancer stem cell"), that requires the phenotypes needed for invasion, metastasis and induction of angiogenesis, it might also be impossible to modify, appreciably, this phase of carcinogenesis because one might not know when to intervene. *By intervening during the promotion phase (during one's adult lifespan), diet can make a difference on the progression, hence carcinogenic transition.*

There is no question, that using the initiation, promotion and progression models of carcinogenesis, one can increase or decrease the cancer frequencies. Even using surrogate in vitro models, (transformation assays; gap junction modulation assays, etc.), one can identify dietary, as well as environmental factors, that can either increase or decrease endpoints in these models that correspond to the experimental or epidemiological evidence [111]. Of course, while there hasn't been perfect correspondence of the in vitro assay results with the experimental or epidemiological data, it should not be surprising, given the shortcomings of in vitro and in vivo animal data [68], let alone epidemiological data [112]. Most of these studies are lacking the mechanistic basis of either the assays used or the understanding of the biology of the carcinogenic process in the design or interpretation of the epidemiological studies.. The failure of the CARET study is a perfect example of this point [113]. The original design ignored previous studies on the mechanism of action of this class of natural chemicals on GJIC [114]. In addition, studies have shown that anti-oxidants can become pro-oxidants [115]. It has even been shown that some of the same class of molecules could become tumor promoters [116]. By the same interesting challenge to our understanding, many tumor promoters have been shown to be anti- carcinogens [117-119]. The conflicting and non-reproducible epidemiological studies are also not surprising, because human populations can not be controlled like rats in a laboratory. Genetic differences, exposures to unreported factors that might be additive, antagonistic or even synergistic to the factor that is under study, critical threshold concentrations, anti-oxidant proficiencies or deficiencies of the individuals, time and duration of exposures, etc., can modify the results of one study compared to another.

The critical importance of understanding the underlying mechanisms of promotion and the role of stem cells in carcinogenesis have not yet entered the cancer prevention or treatment area. A case in point is the recent TASK FORCE REPORT to suggest new approaches to identify potential cancer chemo-preventive compounds [120]. No mention was made of the mechanistically-based in vitro (and in vivo) assay, based on the prevention of tumor promoting agents from down-regulating gap junctional intercellular communication. Many agents that can, reversibly, down regulate GJIC have been shown to be potential tumor promoters by various biochemical mechanisms [121]. The consequence of inhibiting GJIC by any biochemical mechanism in normal tissues is dis-regulation of homeostasis of cell proliferation and differentiation of stem cells, progenitor and differentiated cells. Classic tumor promoters, such as phorbol esters and phenobarbital, have shown correspondence of the in vitro results with the in vivo results [52]. In deed, even the opposite case to support the role of GJIC in chemoprevention, and even chemotherapy, has been made in vitro, as well as in vivo., with a large number of dietary factors, such as green tea [55], resveratrol [56,57], caffeic acid ethyl ester [58], beta-sitosterol [62]and lovastatin [59], SAHA [61].

Why Dogs and Cows Caused Human Prostate and Breast Cancers: The Interaction of Biological and Cultural Evolution, Diet, Adult Stem Cells and Cancer

To bring this *Commentary* to full circle, the quote made by D. Coffey should serve to provide a "systems view" of the human cancer problem. In his article comparing the similarities of breast and prostate cancers, he stated:

> "Certainly, looking for simple relation will not be sufficient, but delineating the exact mechanisms of cell cycle control and stem cell development in prostate cancer should be helpful in understanding these early preneoplastic lesions and their relations to diet." [122].

Up until now, the focus for trying to understand the complex carcinogenic process has been through the "light of biological evolution". The formation of a multi-cellular organism created a need to coordinate cell proliferation, differentiation, apoptosis, senescence and adaptive responses of adult stem cells, progenitor and terminally-differentiated cells. The need to have both somatic and germ-line stem cells served both the individual and species The fact that the DNA is not immune to DNA damage, errors in repair or in DNA replication was selected for a the production of mutations at a rate that would ensure survival of the species in an ever changing physical environment, yet not so high as to jeopardize either the individual or species' survival. Neither the somatic adult stem cells nor the germ-line stem cells were immune to these mutations.

In the case of the human species, the individual was served by these somatic adult stem cells to provide growth, differentiation of highly specialized cells, and wound-healing. These were needed to allow the individual to live long enough to reach sexual maturation, to leave offspring, and to take care of the offspring until they were able to repeat this process. This ensured the survival of the species. After that period of life span (approximately mid-fourties), the individual's contribution to evolution was essentially finished. At which time, sufficient mutations had occurred in both the germ line and somatic stem cells. The geriatric individual, save for some accumulated experiences ("wisdom"), was basically a drain on limited resources for the survival of the young. As pointed out above, the adult stem cell is most likely the target cell for cancer. However, the multi-stage, multi-mechanism carcinogenic process, probably played little role as a negative selection factor for evolution, as most cancers would appear long after the median life span of most individuals in early pre- and real human biological evolutionary history.

Clues to the roles of both biological and cultural evolution, diet and breast and prostate cancers have been noted before [122,123]. Unlike the roles that biological evolution, changing physical environment and diets of non-human animals played in their evolution, human's brought with them the emergence of 4 critical new phenotypes [to consciously create symbols; to communicate with those symbols; to create new technologies using those symbols and communication skills; and to value or make choices on which technology to use or not use [124]. Unlike non-human animals, their "detritus" disappears in short time. However, as it has been stated by a philosopher, "Men build walls and walls build men". The point being that what we do to our physical and cultural environments has lasting and major impacts on future generations of both the non-human animal and the human animal.

Human beings have created a cultural environment which, among many other things, shapes both our physical environment and our diet. As noted in the subtitle of this section, early humans learned a few things that helped to rescue them from hunting and gathering and a "feast-fast"- type of dietary behaviour that shaped our biological evolution. That is, we had to have those molecular, cellular and physiological adaptive features, stored in the genome of our germ and somatic stem cells, that allowed us to survive under these "feast and fast"-conditions. We inherited these from our pre-human and non-human animal ancestors. With the domestication of the cow, which provided work, food, and clothing, and of the dog, which aided human's hunting abilities; we find clues as to how these cultural evolutionary facts have impacted on human stem cells and cancer. In both of these cases, these two animals have helped to "cause" breast, colon and prostate cancers in humans. In the case of the bovine, one might note there seems not to be any significant mammary cancers associated with its existence, so why is there a link to human breast cancer? In the case of the canine, this animal seems to have a significant prostate cancer problem similar to human beings [122,123]. Can comparative oncology provide some answers or will a simple "systems" view do?

To first view how diet might affect the multi-stage, multi-mechanism process of carcinogenesis, we need to view the shared general concepts of the aforementioned integrated hypothesis, and how prostate and breast carcinogenesis might have a "higher order" or cultural component in their dietary risk factors.

When one views the current studies on the cancers found in the atomic bomb survivals of Hiroshima and Nagasaki, breast cancers seem to be one of the highest solid tumors to which could be attributed to the exposures to radiation [125]. One of the reasons it was noted is because the background frequency of breast cancers of those Japanese women was extremely low, such that any attributed increase by radiation was noted to be statistically significant. While the main focus of the interpretation of these data has been the radiation exposures, little attention has been given to why the attributed increase was the level seen. In the first place, one interpretation has been that soy products which has been for generations a major component of the Japanese women's diet might have been the reason for (a) small breasts and (b) low breast cancer frequencies. Because soy contains many anti-cancer nutritional components, genistein and Bowen-Birks Inhibitor [126,127], it has been speculated that these dietary components contributed to lowering the breast cancer frequencies of both the control and a bomb survivors. From a mechanistic perspective and our theme that adult stem cells are the target cells for carcinogenic initiation, the next question is: "How do these soy products work on the multi-stage, multi-mechanism process of breast carcinogenesis."

In the first place, human adult breast stem cells have been isolated from normal human breast tissue [83]. These breast stem cells can be neoplastically transformed in vitro.[89] Moreover, while there is no existing evidence that genistein could lower or increase the ionizing radiation genetic damage in human breast stem cells, there is compelling evidence that genistein can induce differentiation of the adult human breast stem cells. [128] Therefore, if either the mother of the daughter, exposed to the a bomb radiation, eat lots of soy products during pregnancy, the female embryo and fetus would have few breast stem cells because the breast stem cell would have been induced to asymmetrically divide rather that symmetrically divide to produce many adult breast stem cells. Further, after birth and during adolescent development, the daughter also consumed lots of soy products. Therefore, from these facts of diet on stem cells during development and adolescent growth, this dietary habit could be a chemo-preventive factor by reducing the breast stem cell pool. This alone would reduce the risk to breast cancer by reducing the number of possible initiated breast stem cells, all other factors being the same. This could be a mechanistic basis of the Barker hypothesis [129]. The hypothesis basically states that whatever might happen in utero to the embryo/fetus could affect the risk or resistance or sensitivity to diseases later in the life of the offspring.

While radiation is assumed to be the initiators of the exposed breast stem cells, could the soy products affect the promotion of cancer? The evidence, on the whole, seems to indicate that these soy components can be chemo-preventive by their ability to interfere with the promotion process, although there is some rodent evidence it could act as a tumor promoter [130]. Again, this points out the need for better understanding of the underlying mechanisms, especially when using either animal bioassays or epidemiological studies. It should now be pointed out that, with the introduction of dairy products into the Japanese diet and the transmigration studies of Japanese, who move to Western countries, soon changed their dietary habits and frequencies of breast cancers to match to of the host country. In addition, it should also be noted that the Japanese women, who contribute to the longest median life span also pay a heavy price for their past dietary practices, namely the high frequency of osteoporosis. Could it be that the soy products which induced differentiation and asymmetrical cell division of the breast stem cell also did the same for the osteoblast precursor stem cells? This then opens up another health aspect of stem cell pool modulation, namely the reduction of stem cells via either diet or environmental agents could affect the aging process itself, as well as the diseases of aging [131,132].

To further analyze how diet can influence breast cancer and getting back to the bovine, milk, cheese, red meat, all factors associated with both breast and colon cancer, were introduced during the domestication of the bovine. Many of the components of these bovine products, aside from the caloric content, is the introduction of dietary components that are known tumor promoters in animal model systems, in vitro model systems, such as those that detect their ability to reversibly inhibit gap junctional intercellular communication [111]. Unsaturated fatty acids, insulin, insulin –like growth factors, among others factors, could cause both the symmetrical cell division in adult breast stem cells (increasing the risk to initiation) and act as tumor promoters of initiated breast stem cells. Note that, prior to the Second World War, few dairy products (cheese, meat, milk) were in the Japanese diet. Today, it is becoming a major component.

Back to the human prostate, when the early humans domesticated the canine, the hunter became more successful. The canine and the human started to share the same diet of red meat that was now grilled. While early humans did not survive long enough to manifest prostate cancers, today with the median life span in developed countries having been significantly increased over the last century, so too has the prostate cancer frequency.

An example of how both an environmental factor and the soy dietary factors play a role in prostate cancer has recently been reported. Ho et al [133] showed that pregnant rodents fed a diet contaminated with bisphenol A gave rise to male offspring that had a high incidence of prostate cancers, even though the male offspring were not exposed to the environmental non-genotoxic chemical after birth. On the other hand, if these pregnant rodents were fed both soy products and the bisphenol-A, the risk to prostate cancer in the male offspring was dramatically reduced. Clearly, if one assumes that the stem cells of the prostate are the target cells for prostate cancers, and that the effects seen occur in utero during fetal development, one can speculate that the bisphenol-A caused the prostate stem cells to symmetrical division, increasing the prostate stem cell pool. This alone, all other factors being the same, would increase the risk to cancer. On the other hand, if during fetal development the components of the soy diet cause the prostate stem cell to divide asymmetrically and to differentiate, then the stem cell pool would decrease, lowering the risk to prostate cancer.

It must be pointed out the bisphenol A is an epigenetic, not genotoxic, toxicant. Dietary chemicals, such as genistein and environmental toxicants, such as bisphenol A, TCDD, PBB, PCB, DDT, can effect, epigenetically gene expression of the offspring when agents are applied in utero. The studies by the Jirtle group showed that the genetic strain of agouti mice could have their coat color modulated by epigenetic agents [134]. The molecular alterations in methylation and histone acetylation suggest that they are associated with the altered phenotypes. However, there is another interpretation. The altered gene expression might be due to altered stem cell pools (recall that the gene patterns of particular adult stem cells will always be different from their differentiated daughter lineage cells that contribute to the agouti phenotype).

In a brief analysis of how dietary nutrients, contaminants and process of preparation, such as frying or grilling, diets, that affect either or both breast and prostate cancer (or any other kind), probably affect the promotion, rather that the initiation process. They could affect initiation, indirectly, by altering the stem cell pool that is exposed to an initiator. Most, if not all, promoters reversibly inhibit cell-cell communication to affect proliferation, differentiation and apoptosis. Promotion is the stage that would most likely be impacted by dietary factors and intervention practices to lower cancer frequencies. Several promoters and anti-promoters come to mind with the advent of cultural evolutionary changes, contributed by the bovine and canine. The animal fats, the excessive calories, the cholesterol, hormones, such as estrogens, insulin, pyrolytic polyaromatic hydrocarbons [68], which both the bovine and canine gave humans (and to the canine by us in return for its hunting and companionship attributes), we can attribute, in part, both the rise in breast cancer and prostate cancers. In the case of breast cancers, the cultural practice, now, of postponing of early marriage and children only raises the breast cancer risk.

It is interesting to note that β-sitosterol, a component of fibers of vegetables and fruits, can lower cholesterol levels [135] and inhibit the ras oncogene effect on cell-cell communication in tumor cells. [62]. It is also, a major component of olive oil [136] and this has been suggested as a possible risk reducer of both cardiovascular and prostate cancer frequencies in the Mediterranean diet. Bovine animals with large mammary glands, unlike the canine with prostate cancers due to its companionship with the humans and their diets, eats lots of plant products containing β-sitosterol (of course, they do not live long enough to develop cancers; however, it they did, it is unlikely they would have a high frequency of mammary cancers).

Conclusion

The implications of understanding the mechanisms of carcinogenesis are immense. Currently, the many known factors that must influence the mechanism of forming a tumor (e.g., genetics, developmental stage, gender, environmental agents, calories, exercise, diet, life-style and cultural behaviours, etc.) appear to prevent the generation of a coherent integrated hypothesis. However, many old ideas, such as the multi-stage, multi-mechanism hypothesis, the stem cell theory, and newer observations in molecular oncology, toxicology of chemical "carcinogens", stem cell biology, oncogene / tumor suppression gene functions, plus the re-discovery of "cancer stem cells", have made it possible to gain a new insight.

While a tumor consists of billions of genotypically- and phenotypically-heterogeneous cells, we do know they all had a single common origin. While still debated, that single normal cell, which was altered during the "initiation" phase of carcinogens, appears to have been a normal, immortal adult stem cell. "Initiation" appears to be a process that blocks that normal stem cell's ability to divide, asymmetrically, under normal conditions of proliferation; in other words, it can not terminally differentiate senesce or apoptose. While the risk to the initiation phase, caused by either mutations or stable epigenetic mechanisms, can be minimized, it can never be reduced to zero. However, the promotion phase, which brings about the clonal expansion of these initiated stem cells or "pre-cancer stem cells", can take decades to generate an invasive and metastatic "cancer stem cell". The promotion of these initiated stem cells can be interrupted or accelerated by environmental-, dietary-, hormone-, inflammatory-, cytokine-, and growth- factors, as well as caloric restriction or gluttony. Cell-cell communication, by either secreted or gap junction-mediated factors, triggers redox-intracellular signalling to alter gene expression, can be either decreased (tumor promotion) or increased (chemo-prevention or anti-tumor promotion). The discovery that the Oct-4 gene can be a marker for both maintaining "stemness" in the normal embryonic and adult stem cells, as well as a marker for the pre-malignant and malignant " cancer stem cells", makes it possible to target these cells with new strategies for chemo-prevention and chemotherapy. Evidence supporting the adult stem cell as the target cell or the cell of origin of the "cancer stem cell" , while supported by experiments with human adult breast stem cells, is also supported by evidence of the existence of adult stem cells in higher plants that can give rise to callas and ultimately a whole plant (137). This gave the authors of that study to state: "...callus resembles the tip of a root meristem, even if it is derived from aerial organs such as petals, which clearly hows that callus formation is not a simple reprogramming process backward to an undifferentiated state as widely believed."

From this new integration of observations and hypotheses, comes another new important implication, namely, one's risk to cancer might be influenced during pregnancy when the mother's dietary or medical treatments could either increase or decrease the adult stem cell pools in various organs. Keeping all other cancer-influencing factors equal, just increasing or decreasing the adult stem cell pool would alter the risk to cancer in adulthood, based on the adult stem cell being the "target" for the initiation phase. On the other hand, what we as inheritors of these adult stem cells from our mothers do to any "initiated" stem cell in our body can either increase or decrease the risk to the promotion phase of carcinogenesis. In other words, *"What our mother's ate or didn't eat (or get exposed to) can influence the number of our adult stem cells; what we eat or do to these initiated stem cells can modulate our risk to cancer."*

REFERENCES

[1] Dobzhansky, T. (1975) Nothing in Biology makes sense except in the light of evolution. *Am. Biol. Teachers, 35*, 125-129.

[2] Hanahan, D. and Weinberg, R.A. (2000). Hallmarks of cancer. *Cell, 100*, 57-70.

[3] Al Hajj, M., Wicha, M.S., Benito-Hernandez, A., Morrison, S.J., and Clarke, M.F. (2003). Prospective identification of tumorigenic breast cancer cells. *Proc. Nat. Acad. Sci. USA, 100*, 3983-3988.

[4] Markert, C.L. (1968). Neoplasia: A disease of differentiation. *Cancer Res., 28*, 1908-1914.

[5] Markert, C. L. (1984). Genetic control of cell interactions in chimeras. *Develop Genet., 4*, 267-279.

[6] Pierce, B. (1974). Neoplasms, differentiation and mutations. *Am. J. Pathol., 77*, 103-118.

[7] Potter, V.R. (1978). Phenotypic diversity in experimental hepatomas: Concept of partially blocked ontogeny. *Br. J. Cancer, 38*, 1-23.

[8] Kerbel, R.S., Frost, P., Liteplo,R., Carlow, D.A., and Elliot, B.E. (1984). Possible epigenetic mechanisms of tumor progression: Induction of high frequency heritable but phenotypically unstable changes in the tumorigenic and metastatic properties of tumor cell populations by 5-azacytidine treatment. *J. Cell Physiol., 3*, 87-97.

[9] Tlsty, T.D., Briot, A., Gualberto, A., Hall, I., Hess, S., Hixon, M., Kuppuswamy, D., Romanov, D., Sage, M., and White, A. (1995). Genomic instability and cancer. *Mutation Res.*, 337, 1-7.

[10] P.W. Laird. (2005). Cancer epigenetics. *Hum. Mol. Genet., 14*, R65-R76.

[11] Boveri, T. (1914). *Zurfrage der Entstehung Maligner Tumoren.* Jena: Gustav Fisher.

[12] Cleaver, J.E. and Trosko, J.E. (1970). Absence of excision of ultraviolet-induced cyclobutane dimers in Xeroderma pigmentosum. *Photochem. Photobiol.*, *11*, 547-550.

[13] Maher, V.M. and McCormick, J.J. (1976). Effect of DNA repair on the cytotoxicity and mutagenicity of UV irradiation and of chemical carcinogens in normal and xeroderma pigmentosum cells. In: J.M. Yuhas, R.W. Tennant and J.D. Regan (Eds.), *Biology of Radiation Carcinogenesis* (pp. 129-145). New York: Raven Press.

[14] Warren, S., R.A. Schultz, C.C. Chang, M.H. Wade and Trosko, J.E. (1981). Elevated spontaneous mutation rate in Bloom syndrome fibroblasts. *Proc. Natl. Acad. Science USA, 78*, 3133-3137.

[15] Brash, D. E., Rudolph, J.A., Simon, X., Lin, A. and McKenna, G.J. (1991). A role for sunlight in skin cancer: UV-induced p53 mutations in squamous cell carcinomas. *Proc. Natl. Acad. Sci. USA*, *88*, 10124-10128.

[16] Ames,B.N., Durston,W. E., Yamasaki, E. and Lee, F. D. (1973). Carcinogens are mutagens a simple test system combining liver homogenates for activation and bacteria for detection. *Proc. Natl. Acad. Sci. USA*, *70*, 2281-2285.

[17] Marsh, D.J. and Zori, R.T. (2002). Genetic insights into famial cancers-update and recent discoveries. *Cancer Letters, 181*, 125-164.

[18] Evans, W.H. and Martin, P.E.M. (2002). Gap junctions: Structure and Function. *Molec. Membr. Biol.*, *19*, 121-136.

[19] Cruciani, V. and Mikalsen, S.-O. (2005). The connexin gene family in mammals. *Biol Chem.*, *386*, 325-332.

[20] Willecke, K., Eiberger, J., Degen, J., Eckhardt, D., Romauldi, A., Guldenagel, M., Duetsch, U. and Sohl, G. (2002). Structural and functional diversity of connexion genes in the mouse and human genome. *Biol. Chem.*, *383*, 725-737.

[21] Eagle, H. (1965). Growth inhibitor effects of cellular interactions. *Isreal J. Med. Sci.*, *1*, 1220-1228.

[22] Revel, J.P. (1988). The oldest multicellular animal and its junctions. In: Hertzberg, E.L. and Johnson, R. (Eds.), *Gap Junction* (pp 135-149). N.Y.: Alan Liss, Inc.

[23] Loewenstein, W.R. (1966). Permeability of membrane junctions. *Ann. N.Y. Acad. Sci.*, *137*, 441-472.

[24] Trosko, J.E. (2007). Stem cells and cell-cell communication in the understanding of the role of diet and nutrients in human diseases. *J. Fd. Hyg. Safety, 22*, 1-14.

[25] Takahashi, K. and Yamanaka, S. (2006). Induction of pluripotent stem cells from mouse embryonic and adult fibroblasts cultures by defined factors. *Cell*, *126*, 663-676.

[26] Shi, Y. (2004). Caspase activation, inhibition, and reactivation: A mechanistic view. *Protein Science, 13*,1979-1987

[27] Wilson, M.R., Close, T.W. and Trosko, J.E. (2000). Cell population dynamics (apoptosis, mitosis and cell-cell communication) during disruption of homeostasis. *Exp. Cell Res.*, *254*, 257-268.

[28] Tumbar, T., Guasch, G., Greco, V., Blanpain, C., Lowry, W.E., Rendl, M. and Fuchs, E. (2004). Defining the epithelial stem cell niche in skin. *Science, 303*, 359-363.

[29] Juckett D. A. (1987). Cellular aging (the Hayflick limit) and species longevity: a unification model based on clonal succession. *Mech Ageing Devel., 38*, 49–71.

[30] Kalimi and Lo blastocyte lack og GJ Lo, C.W. (1996). The role of gap junction membrane channels in development. *J. Bioenerget. Biomembr., 28*, 379-385.

[31] Trosko, J.E., Chang, C.C., Wilson, M.R., Upham, B.L., Hayashi, T. and wade, M. (2000). Gap junctions and the regulation of cellular functions of stem cells during development and differentiation. *Methods, 20*, 245-264.

[32] de Rooij, D. G., Lok, D., Wennk, D. (1985). Feedback regulation of the proliferation of the undifferentiated spermatogonia in the Chinese hamster by differentiating spermatogonia. *Cell Tissue Kinet, 18*, 71–81.

[33] Kimchi, A., Wang, X. F., Weinberg, R. A., Cheifetz, S. and Massague, J. (1988). Absence of TGF-b receptors and growth: Inhibitory responses in retinoblastoma cells. *Science, 290*,196–198.

[34] Borek, C. and Sachs, L. (1966). The difference in contact inhibition of cell replication between normal cells and cells transformed by different carcinogens. *Proc. Natl. Acad. Sci. USA, 56*, 1705-1711.

[35] Yamasaki, H. and Naus, C.C.G. (1996). Role of connexion genes in growth control. *Carcinogenesis, 17*, 1199-1213.

[36] Csete, M. (2005). Oxygen in the cultivation of stem cells. *Ann. N.Y. Acad. Sci., 1049*, 1-8.

[37] Fialkow, P. J. (1979). Clonal origin of human tumors. *Am. Rev. Med., 30*, 135-176.

[38] Nowell, P.C. (1976). The clonal evolution of tumour cell populations. *Science, 194*, 23-28.

[39] Sell, S. (1993). Cellular origin of cancer: De-differentiation or stem cell maturation arrest? *Environ. Health Perspect., 101*, 15-26.

[40] Wernig, M., Meissner, A., Foreman, R., Brambrink, T., Ku, M., Hochedlinger, K., Berstein, B.E., and Jaenisch, R. (2007). In vitro reprogramming of fibroblasats into a pluripotent ES-cell-like state. *Nature, 448*, 318-323.

[41] Macerali N., Sriharan, R., Xie, W., Utikal, J., Eminli, S., Arnold, K., Stadfeld, M., Yachechko, R., Tchieu, J. Jaenisch, R., Plath, K. and Hochedlinger, K. (2007). Directly reprogrammed fibroblast show global epigenetic remodelling and widespread tissue contribution. *Cell Stem Cell, 1*, 55-70.

[42] Okita, K., Ichisak, T. and Yamanaka, S. (2007) Generation of germline-competent induced pluripotent stem cells. *Nature, 488*, 313-319.

[43] Land, H., Parada, I.E. and Weinberg, R.A. (1983). Tumorigenic conversion of primary embryo fibroblasts requires at least two cooperating oncogenes. *Nature, 304*, 596-602.

[44] Hayflick, L. (1965). The limited in vitro lifespan of human diploid cell strains. *Exp. Cell Res., 37*, 614-636.

[45] Berenblum, P.M. (1954). A speculative review: The probable nature of promoting action and its significance in the understanding of the mechanisms of carcinogenesis. *Cancer Res., 14*, 471-477.

[46] Yamagiwa, K. and Ichikawa, K. (1977). Experimental study of the pathogenesis of carcinoma. *CA Cancer J. Clin., 27*, 174-181.

[47] Knudson, A.G. (1971). Mutations and cancer: statistical study of retinoblastoma. *Proc. Natl. Acad. Sci. USA, 68*, 820-823.

[48] Yang, Z., Sui, Y., Xiong, S., Liour, S.S., Phillips, A.C. and Ko, L. (2007). Switched alternative splicing of oncogene CoAA during embryonal carcinoma stem cell differentiation. *Nucleic Acid Res., 35*(6),1919-1932.

[49] Trosko, J.E. (2001). Is the concept of tumor promotion a useful paradigm? *Molec. Carcinogen., 39*, 131-137.

[50] Goodman, J.A. (2001). Operational reversibility is a key aspect of carcinogenesis. *Toxicol. Sci., 64*, 147-148.

[51] Trosko, J.E. and Tai, M.-H. (2006). Adult stem cell theory of the multi-stage, multi-mechanism theory of carcinogenesis: Role of inflammation on the promotion of initiated cells. In Dittmar, T., Zaeker, K.S. and Schmidt, XXX (Eds.), *Infections and Inflammation: Impacts on Oncogenesis* (Contributions to *Microbiology,* Vol. *13*, pp. 45-65). K. Karger AG.

[52] Klaunig, J. and Ruch, R.J. (1987). Strain and species effects on the inhibition of hepatocyte intercellular communication by liver tumor promoters. *Cancer Letters, 36*, 161-168.

[53] Yotti, L.P., Chang, C.C. and Trosko, J.E. (1979). Elimination of metabolic cooperation in Chinese hamster cells by a tumor promoter. *Science, 206*, 1089-1091.

[54] Trosko, J.E. and Chang, C.C. (1988). Nongenotoxic Mechanisms in carcinogenesis: role of inhibited intercellular communication. In: Hart, R.W. and Hoerger, F.D. (Eds), *Banbury Report 31: Carcinogen Risk Assessment: New Directions in the Qualitative and Quantitative Aspects (pp. 139-170).* Cold Spring Harbor, N.Y.: Cold Spring Harbor Laboratory.

[55] Sai, K., Kanno, J., Hasegawa, R., Trosko, J.E., and Inoue, T. (2000). Prevention of the down regulation of gap junctional intercellular communication by green tea in the liver of mice fed pentachlorophenol. *Carcinogenesis, 21*, 1671-1676.

[56] Nielson, M., Ruch, R.J., and Vang, O. (2000). Reservatrol reverses tumor-promoter-induced inhibition of gap junctional intercellular communication. *Biochem. Biophys. Res. Commun., 275*, 804-809.

[57] Upham, B.L. Guˇzvic, M., Scott, J., Carbone, J.M., Blaha, L., Coe, C. Li, L. L., Rummel, A.M., and Trosko, J.E. (2007). Inhibition of Gap Junctional Intercellular Communication and Activation of Mitogen-Activated Protein Kinase by Tumor-Promoting Organic Peroxides and Protection by Resveratrol. *Nutrition and Cancer, 57*(1), 38–47.

[58] Na, H.-K., Wilson, M.R., Kang, K.S., Chang, C.C., Grunberger, D. and Trosko, J.E. (2000). Restoration of gap junctional intercellular communication by caffeic acid phenethyl ester (CAPE) in a ras-transformed rat liver epithelial cell line. *Cancer Letters, 157*, 31-38.

[59] Ruch, R.J., Madhukar, B.V., Trosko, J.E., and Klaunig, J.E. (1993). Reversal of ras-induced inhibition of gap junctional intercellular communication, transformation and tumorigenesis by lovastatin. *Molec. Carcinogen., 7*, 50-59.

[60] Nakamura, Y., Chang, C.C., Mori, T., Sato, K., Ohtsuki, K., Upham, B.L., and Trosko, J.E. (2005). Augmentation of differentiation and gap junction fubction by kaempferol in partially-differentiation colon cancer cells. *Carcinogenesis, 26*, 665-671.

[61] Ogawa, T., Hayashi, T., Tokunou, M., Nakachi, K., Trosko, J.E., Chang, C.C., and Yorioka, N., (2005). Suberoylanilide hydroxamic acid enhances gap junctional

intercellular communication via acetylation of histone containing connexin43 gene locus. *Cancer Res.*, *65*, 9771-9778.

[62] Nakamura, Y., Yoshikawa, N., Hiroki, I., Sato, K., Ohtsuki,K., Chang, C.C., Upham, B.L., and Trosko, J.E. (2005). β- Sitosterol, From Psyllium Seed Husk (Plantago ovata Forsk), Restores Gap Junctional Intercellular Communication in Ha-ras Transfected Rat Liver Cells. *Nutrition Cancer, 5*, 218-225.

[63] Trosko, J.E. and Ruch, R.J. (1998). Cell-cell communication in carcinogenesis. *Front. Biosci.*, *3,* 208-236.

[64] Loewenstein, W.R and Kanno, Y. (1966). Intercellular communication and the control of tissue growth: Lack of communication between cancer cells. *Nature, 209*, 1248-1249.

[65] Cleaver, J.E. (1978). Xeroderma pigmentosum: genetic and environmental influences in skin carcinogenesis. *International Journa of Dermatology, 17*, 435-444.

[66] Warren, S., Schultz, R.A., Chang, C.C., Wade, M.H. and Trosko, J.E. (1981). Elevated spontaneous mutation rate in Bloom syndrome fibroblasts. *Proc. Natl. Acad. Science USA, 78*, 3133-3137.

[67] Ames, B.N., Lois, Swirsky, Gold, L.S., and Shigenaga, M.K. (1996). *Cancer Prevention, Rodent High-Dose Cancer Tests, And Risk AssessmentRisk Analysis, 16*, 613-617.

[68] Trosko, J.E. and Upham, B.L. (2005). The emperor wears no clothes in the field of carcinogen risk assessment: Ignored concepts in cancer risk assessment. *Mutagenesis, 20*, 81-92.

[69] Thilly, W.G. (2003). Have environmental mutagens caused oncomutations in people? *Nat. Genet., 34*, 255- 259.

[70] Upham, B.L., Weis, L.M. and Trosko, J.E. (1998). Modulated gap junctional intercellular communication as a biomarker of PAH epigenetic toxicity: structure--function relationship. *Environ. Health Perspect. 106*(Suppl 4), 975--981.

[71] Weis,L.M., Rummel,A.M., Masten,S.J., Trosko,J.E. and Upham,B.L.(1998). Bay or baylike regions of polycyclic aromatic hydrocarbons were potent inhibitors of gap junctional intercellular communication. *Environ. Health Perspect., 106*, 17--22.

[72] Tai, M.H., Upham, B.L., Olson, L.K., Tsao, M.S., Reed, D.N., and Trosko, J.E. (2007). Cigarette smoke condensate inhibited intercellular communication and differentiation in human pancreatic ductal epithelial cells. *Int. J. Cancer, 120*, 1855-1862.

[73] Minsk, B. and Illensee, K. (1975). Normal genetically mosaic mice produced from malignant teratocarcinoma cells. *Proc. Natl. Acad. Sci. USA, 72*, 3585-3589.

[74] Trosko, J. E. (2006). From adult stem cells to cancer stem cells: Oct-4 gene, cell-cell communication and hormones during tumor promotion. *Ann. N.Y. Acad. Sci., 1089*, 36-58.

[75] Wang X. and Harris, C. (1997). p53 tumor- suppressor gene: clues to molecular carcinogenesis. *J. Cell Physiol., 173*, 247-255.

[76] Barcellos-Hoff, M.H. (2001). Three down and counting: The transformation of human mammary cells from normal to malignant in three steps. *Trends Molec. Med.*, *7*, 142-143.

[77] Bissell, M.J. and Radisky, D. (2001). Putting tumors in context. *Nature Rev. Cancer, 1*, 46-54.

[78] Trosko, J.E., Chang, C.C., Upham, B. and Wilson, M. (1998). Epigenetic toxicology as toxicant-induced changes in intracellular signalling leading to altered gap junctional intercellular communication. *Toxicol. Lett., 102-103*, 71--78.

[79] Potter, V.R. (1973). Biochemistry of cancer. In Holland, J. and Frei, E (Eds.), *Cancer Medicine* (pp. 178-192). Philadelphia: Lea, E. and Febiger.

[80] Al Hajj, M., Wicha, M.S., Benito-Hernandez, A., Morrison, S.I. and Clarke, M.F. (2003). Prospective identification of tumorigenic breast cancer cells. *Proc. Natl. Acad. Sci. USA, 100*, 3983-3988.

[81] Webster, J.D., Yusbasiyan-Gurkan, V., Trosko, J.E., Chang, C.C., and Kiupel, M. (2007). Expression of the embryonic transcription factor Oct4 in Canine neoplasms: A potential marker for stem cell subpopulations in neoplasia. *Vet. Pathol., 44*, in press.

[82] Chang, C.C., Trosko, J.E., El-Fouly, M.H., Gibson, D.R. and D'Ambrosio, S.M. (1987). Contact insensitivity of a subpopulation of normal human fetal kidney epithelial cells and of human carcinoma cell lines. *Cancer Res.*, *47*, 1634-1645.

[83] Kao, C.Y., Nomata, K., Okley, C.S., Welsch, C.W. and Chang, C.C. (1995). Two types of normal human breast epithelial cells derived from reduction mammoplasty: Phenotypic characterization and response to SV40 transfection. *Carcinogenesis, 16*, 531-538.

[84] Linning, K.D., Tai, M.H., Madhukar, B.V., Chang, C.C., Reed, D.N., Ferber, S., Trosko, J.E., and Olson, L.K. (2004). Redox-mediated enrichment of self-renewing adult human pancreatic cells which possess endocrine differentiation potential. *Pancreas, 29*, e64-e76.

[85] Lin, T.-M., Tsai, J.-L., Lin, S.-D., Lai, C.-S., and Chang, C-C. (2005). Accelerated Growth and prolonged lifespan of adipose tissue-derived human mesenchymal stem cells in a medium using reduced calcium and antioxidants. *Stem Cells Devel., 14*, 92–102.

[86] Yang, Y.C., S.W. Wang, H. Y. Hung, C.C. Chang, I.C. Wu, Y.L. Huang, T. M. Lin, J. L. Tsai, A. Chen, F.C. Kuo, W.M. Wang and D.C. Wu. (2007). Isolation and characterization of human gastric cell lines with stem cell phenotypes. *J. Gastroenterology Hepatology,* doi:1111/j.1440-1746.2007.05031.x.

[87] Matic, M., Evans, W.H., Brink, P.R. and Simon, M. (2002). Epidermal cells do not communicate through gap junctions. *J. Invest. Dermat.*, *118*, 110-116.

[88] Matic, M., Petrov, I.N., Chen, S., Wang, C., Dimitrijevich, S.D., and Wolosin, J.M. (1997). Stem cells of the corneal epithelium lack connexins and metabolic transfer capacity. *Different.*, *61*, 251-260.

[89] Kang, K.S., Sun, W., Nomata, K., Morita, I., Cruz, A., Liu, C.J., Trosko, J.E. and Chang, C.C. (1998). Involvement of tyrosine phosphorylation of p185 c-erB2/neu in tumorigenicity by X rays and neu-oncogene in human breast epithelial cells. *Molec. Carcinogen., 21*, 225-233.

[90] Nakano, S., Ueo, H., Bruce, S.A. and Ts'o, P.O.P. (1985). A contact-insensitive subpopulation in Syrian hamster cell cultures with a greater susceptibility to chemically induced neoplastic transformation. *Proc. Natl. Acad. Sci. USA, 82*, 5005-5009.

[91] Ponti, D., Costa, A., Zaffaroni, N., Pratesi, G., Petrangolini, G., Coradini, D., Pilotti, S., Pierotti, M.A. and Daidone, M.A. (2005). Isolation and In vitro propagation of tumorigenic breast cancer cells with stem/progenitor cell properties. *Cancer Res., 65*, 5506-5511.

[92] Chang, C.C., Sun, W., Cruz, A., Saitoh, M., Tai, M.H. and Trosko, J.E. (2001). A human breast epithelial cell type with stem cell characteristics as targets for carcinogenesis. *Radiat. Res., 155*, 201-207.

[93] Takahashi, K. and Yamanaka, S. (2006). Induction of pluripotent stem cells from mouse embryonic and adult fibroblast cultures by defined factors. *Cell, 126*, 663-676.

[94] Okamoto, K., Okazawa, H., Okuda, A., Sakai, M., Muramatsu, M. and Hamada, H. (1990). A novel octamer binding transcription factor is differentially expressed in mouse embryonic cells. *Cell, 60*, 461-472.

[95] Niwa, H., Miyazaki, J. and Smith, A.G. (2000). Quantitative expression of 0ct3/4 defines differentiation, de-differentiation or self-renewal of ES cells. *Nat. Genet. 24*, 372-376.

[96] Rosner, M.H., Vigano, M.A., Ozato, K., Timmons, P.M., Poirier, F., Rigby, P.W. and Staudt, L.M. (1990). A POU-domain transcription factor in early stem cells and germ cells of the mammalian embryo. *Nature, 345*, 686-692.

[97] Monk, M and Holding, C. (2001). Human embryonic genes re-expressed in cancer cells. *Oncogene, 20*(20), 8085-8091.

[98] Tai, M.H., Chang, C.C., Kiupel, M., Webster, J.D. and Trosko, J.E. (2005). Oct-4 expression in adult stem cells: Evidence in support of the stem cell theory of carcinogenesis. *Carcinogenesis, 26*, 495-502.

[99] Momiyama, M., Omori, Y., Isizaki, Y., Nishikawa, Y., Tokairin, T., Ogawa, J. and Enomoto, E. (2003). Connexin 26 mediated gap junctional communication reverses the malignant phenotype of MCF-7 breast cancer cells. *Cancer Sci., 94*: 501-507.

[100] Barcellos-Hoff, M.H. (2001). It takes a tissue to make a tumor: epigenetics, cancer and the microenvironment. *J. Mammary Gland Neoplasm, 6*, 213-221.

[101] Atlasi, Y., Mowla, S.T., Ziaee, S.A. and Bahrami, A.R. (2007). Oct-4, an embryonic stem cell maker is highly expressed in bladder cancer. *Internatl. J. Cancer, 120*, 1598-1602.

[102] Kelly, P.N., Dakic, A., Adams, J.M., Nutt, S.L. and Strasser, A. (2007). Tumor growth need not be driven by rare cancer stem cells. *Science, 317*, 337.

[103] Umemoto, T. Yamato, M., Nishida, K., Yang, J., Tano, Y. and Okano, T. (2005). Limbal epithelial side-population cells have stem cell-like properties, including quiescent state. *Stem Cells, 24*, 86-94.

[104] Kim; M., Turnquist, H., Jackson, J., Sgaglas, M., Yan, Y., Gong, M., Dean, M., Sharp, J.G., and Cowan, K. (2002). The multidrug resistance transporter ABCG2 (Breast cancer resistance protein 1) effluxes Hoechst 33342 and is overexpressed in hematopoietic stem cells. *Clinical Cancer Res., 8*, 22-28.

[105] Trosko, J.E. (2007). Stem cells and cell-cell communication in the understanding of the role of diet and nutrients in human diseases. *J. Fd. Hyg. Safety,* 1-14.

[106] Milton, K. (2000). Back to basics: Why foods of wild primates have relevance for modern human health. *Nutrition, 16*, 480-483.

[107] Kiple, K.F. (Ed). (2000). *The Cambridge World History of Food*. Cambridge University Press.

[108] Teaford, M.F. and Ungar, P.S. (2000). Diet and the evolution of the earliest human ancestors. *Proc. Natl. Acad. Sci. USA, 97*, 13506-13511.

[109] Mariani-Constantini, A. (2000). Natural and cultural influences on the evolution of the human diet: Background of the multifactorial processes that shaped the eating habits of Western societies. *Nutrition, 16*, 483-486.

[110] Popkin, B.M. (2007). The world is fat. *Sci. Amer., 297*, 88-95

[111] Trosko, J.E. and Ruch, R. J. (2002). Gap junctions as therapeutic targets. *Curr. Drug Targets, 3*, 465-482.

[112] Franco,E.L., Correa,P., Santella,R.M., Wu,X., Goodman,S.N. and Petersen,G.M. (2004). Role and limitations of epidemiology in establishing a casual association. *Semin. Cancer Biol., 14*, 413--426.

[113] Goodman G.E., Thornquist, M.D., Balmes, J., Cullen, R.M., Meysken, F.L., Omenn, G.S., Valanis, G.S. and Williams, J.H. (2004). The beta-carotene and retinol efficacy trial: Incidence of lung cancer and cardiovascular disease mortality during 6 year follow-up after stopping beta-carotene and retinol supplements. *J. Natl. Cancer Instit., 96*, 1743-1750.

[114] Shuin, T., Nishimura, R., Noda, K., Umeda, M., and Ono, T. (1983) Concentration-dependent differential effect of retinoid acid on intercellular metabolic cooperation. *Gann, 74*, 100-105.

[115] He,K., Nukada, H., Urakami, T. and Murphy, M.P. (2003). Antioxidant and pro-oxidant properties of pyrroloquinoline quinine (PQQ): Implications for its function in biological systems. *Biochem. Pharmocol., 65*, 67-74.

[116] Henning, H., Wenk, M.L., Dohahoe, R. (1982). Retinoic acid promotion of papilloma formation in mouse skin. *Cancer Letters, 16*, 1-5.

[117] Cohen, G.M., Bracken, W.H., Iyer, R.P., Berry, D.L., Selkirk, J.K., and Slaga, T. J. Anticarcinogenic effects of 2,3,7,8-tetrachlorodibenzo –p-dioxin on benzo(a) pyrene and 7,12-dimethylbenz (a) anthrcene tumor initiation and its relationship to DNA binding. *Cancer Res., 39*, 4027-4033.

[118] Kushida, M., Sukata, T., Uwagawa, S., Ozaki, K., Kinoshita, A., Wanibusbuchi, H., Morimura, K., Okuno, Y. and Fukushima, S. (2005). Low dose DDT inhibition of hepatocarcinogenesis by diethylnitrosamine in male rats: Possible mechanisms. *Toxicol. Appl. Pharmacol., 208*, 285-294.

[119] Lee, G.H. (2000). Paradoxical effects of Phenobarbital on mouse hepatocarcinogenesis. *Toxicol. Pathol., 28*, 215-225.

[120] Kelloff,G.J., Lippman,S.M., Dannenberg, A.J., Sigman, C.C.H.L., Reid, B.J., Szabo, E., Jordan, V.C., Spitz, M.R., Mills,G.B., Papadimitrakopoulou, V.A., Lotan,R., Aggarwal,B.B., Bresalier, R.S., Banu Arun, J.K., Lu,K.H., Thomas, M.E., Rhodes, H.E., Brewer, M.A., Follen, M., Shin,D.M., Parnes, H.L., Siegfried, J.M., Evans, A.A., Blot, W.J., Chow, W.-H., Blount, P.L., Maley, C.C., Wang, K.K., Lam, S., Lee, J.J., Dubinett, S.M., Engstrom, P.F., Meyskens, Jr. F.L., O'Shaughnessy, J., Hawk, E.T., Levin, B., Nelson, W.G., Hong, W. K. (2006). Progress in Chemoprevention Drug Development: The Promise of Molecular Biomarkers for Prevention of Intraepithelial Neoplasia and Cancer—A Plan to Move Forward. *Clin. Cancer Res., 12*, 3661-3697.

[121] Upham, B.L., K.-S. Kang, H.-Y Cho, J.E. Trosko (1997). Hydrogen peroxide inhibits gap junction intercellular communication in glutathione sufficient but not glutathione deficient cells. *Carcinogenesis., 18*, 37-42.

[122] Coffey, D.S. (2001). Similarities of prostate and breast cancer: Evolution, diet and estrogens. *Urology, 57*, 31-38.

[123] Grover, P.L. and Martin, F.L. (2002). The initiation of breast and prostate cancer. *Carcinogenesis, 23*, 1095-1102.

[124] Trosko, J.E. (1984). Scientific views of human nature: Implications for the ethics of technological intervention. In D. H. Brock (Ed). *The Culture of Biomedicine (*Vol. *1.*, pp. 70-97) Newark: University of Delaware Press.

[125] Thompson, D.E., Mabuchi, K., Ron, E., Soda, M., Tokunaga, M., Ochikubo, S., Sugimoto, S., Ikeda, T., Terasaki, M., Preston, D.L. (1994). Cancer incidence in atom bomb survivors. Part II: Solid tumors 1958-1987. *Radiat. Res., 137*, S17-S67.

[126] Murrill, W. B., Brown, N., Zhang, J.X., Manzolillo, A., Barnes, S. and Lamartiniere, C.A. (1996). Prepubertal genistein exposure suppresses mammary cancer and enhances gland differentiation in rats. *Carcinogenesis*, *17*, 1451-1457.

[127] Kennedy, A.R. (1998). The Bowman-Birk inhibitor from soy beans as an anticarcinogenic agent. Am. *J. Clin. Nutr.*, *68*,1406s-1412s.

[128] Hsieh C.Y. and Chang, C.C. (1999) Stem cell differentiation and reduction as a potential mechanism for chemoprevention of breast cancer. *Chinese Pharm. J., 51*, 15-30.

[129] Barker, D.J. P., Mothers, Babies, And Health Later In Life. (2nd ed.). Churchill Livingstone. New York.

[130] Ju, Y. H., Allred, C.D., Allred, K.F., Karko, K.L., Doerge, D.R. and Helferich, W.G. (2001). Physiological concentrations of dietary genistein dose-dependently stimulate growth of estrogen-dependent human breast cancer (MCF-7) tumors implanted in athymic mice. *J. Nutr., 131*, 2957-2962.

[131] Trosko, J.E. (2003) Human stem cells as targets for the aging and diseases of aging processes. *Medical Hypo.*, *60*, 439-447.

[132] Trosko, J.E. (2007). Aging as the 'System's' Breakdown of Communication between the Quality and Quantity of Stem Cells. In *The "Manifesto" For a Long Life*. In Press.

[133] Ho, S.M., Tang, W.Y., de Frauto, J.B., and Prins, G.S. (2006). Developmental exposures to estradiol and bisphenol A increases susceptibility to prostate carcinogenesis and epigenetically regulates phosphodiesterase Type 4 Variant 4. *Cancer Res., 66*, 5624-5632.

[134] Dolinoy, D.C., Weidman, J.R., Waterland, R.A. and Jirtle, R. I. (2006). Maternal genistein alters coat color and protects AVY mouse offspring from obesity by modifying the fetal epigenome. *Environ. Health Perspect. 114*, 567-572.

[135] Moghadasian, M.H. and Frohlich, J.J. (1999). Effects of dietary phytoterols on cholesterol metabolism and atherosclerosis: Clinical and experimental evidence. *American J. Med., 107*, 588-94.

[136] De la Puerta, R., Martinez-Dominguez, E., and Riuz-Gutierrez, V. (2000). Effect of minor componbents of virgin olive oil on topical antiinflammatory sassays. *Z. Naturforsch. C.*, *55*, 814-819.

[137] Sugimoto, K., Jiao, Y., Meyerowitz, E.M. (2010). Arabidopsis regeneration from multiple tissues occurs via a root development pathway. *Devel. Cell* 18, 463-471.

INDEX

A

D

F

H

I

J

K

L

M

N

O

P

Q

R

S

T

U

V

W

X

Y

Z